No Game for Boys to Play

STUDIES IN SOCIAL MEDICINE

Allan M. Brandt, Larry R. Churchill, and Jonathan Oberlander, *editors*

This series publishes books at the intersection of medicine, health, and society that further our understanding of how medicine and society shape one another historically, politically, and ethically. The series is grounded in the convictions that medicine is a social science, that medicine is humanistic and cultural as well as biological, and that it should be studied as a social, political, ethical, and economic force.

KATHLEEN BACHYNSKI

No Game for Boys to Play

The History of Youth Football and the
Origins of a Public Health Crisis

The University of North Carolina Press *Chapel Hill*

This book was published with the assistance of the Lilian R. Furst Fund of the University of North Carolina Press.

Set in Arno Pro by Westchester Publishing Services
Manufactured in the United States of America

The University of North Carolina Press has been a member of the Green Press Initiative since 2003.

Library of Congress Cataloging-in-Publication Data
Names: Bachynski, Kathleen, author.
Title: No game for boys to play : the history of youth football and the origins
    of a public health crisis / Kathleen Bachynski.
Other titles: Studies in social medicine.
Description: Chapel Hill : University of North Carolina Press, [2019] |
    Series: Studies in social medicine | Includes bibliographical references
    and index.
Identifiers: LCCN 2019008153| ISBN 9781469653693 (cloth : alk. paper) |
    ISBN 9781469653709 (pbk : alk. paper) | ISBN 9781469653716 (ebook)
Subjects: LCSH: Youth league football—United States—History—
    20th century. | Youth league football—Health aspects—United States. |
    Football for children—Health aspects—United States. | Tackling
    (Football)—Health aspects. | Football injuries—Public opinion—
    History—20th century. | Masculinity in sports—United States.
Classification: LCC RC1220.F6 B33 2019 | DDC 617.1/027633262—dc23 LC record
    available at https://lccn.loc.gov/2019008153

Cover illustration: *Football Player Sitting on Field*. iStock.com/jpbcpa.

James Wright, "Autumn Begins in Martins Ferry, Ohio," in *The Branch Will Not Break* (Middletown, CT: Wesleyan University Press, 1963), is used by permission.

Portions of chapters 2 and 4 previously appeared in "The Duty of Their Elders—Doctors, Coaches, and the Framing of Youth Football's Health Risks, 1950s–1960s," *Journal of the History of Medicine and Allied Sciences*.

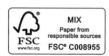

MIX
Paper from
responsible sources
FSC
www.fsc.org   FSC® C008955

To my grandparents and my uncle Finbar

Autumn Begins in Martins Ferry, Ohio

By James Wright

In the Shreve High football stadium,
I think of Polacks nursing long beers in Tiltonsville,
And gray faces of Negroes in the blast furnace at Benwood,
And the ruptured night watchman of Wheeling Steel,
Dreaming of heroes.

All the proud fathers are ashamed to go home.
Their women cluck like starved pullets,
Dying for love.

Therefore,
Their sons grow suicidally beautiful
At the beginning of October,
And gallop terribly against each other's bodies.

Contents

Figures, Graph, and Tables

TABLES

Acknowledgments

This book exists thanks to multiple football teams' worth of friends, family, and colleagues. I am deeply indebted to more people than I can name for their wisdom, expertise, and generosity.

I began this research as a doctoral dissertation while studying at Columbia University's Center for the History and Ethics of Public Health. The project never would have gotten off the ground without my committee of David Rosner, James Colgrove, Betsy Blackmar, Ron Bayer, and Jennifer Hirsch, who provided invaluable intellectual guidance and unfailing encouragement. The faculty, staff, and students at the Mailman School of Public Health modeled so many rigorous and creative forms of interdisciplinary public health scholarship that shaped this project.

At the American Academy of Arts and Sciences, Larry Buell, Paul Erickson, Minou Arjomand, Daniel Couch, Houman Harouni, Daniel Morales, Jessie Wilkerson, and Kristi Willsey all offered thoughtful feedback on multiple chapters of this project. Julian Kronick provided wonderful administrative support. Stephen Hardy not only traveled from New Hampshire to serve as a commentator for a chapter but also generously provided feedback on the entire project. Down the street from the Academy, Harvard's History of Medicine working group warmly welcomed me, and Allan Brandt generously helped steer me along the path from dissertation to book.

At NYU School of Medicine, I was fortunate to receive extraordinary support as a Rudin postdoctoral fellow, with wonderful colleagues and mentors at the Division of Medical Humanities and Division of Medical Ethics. I am particularly grateful to Art Caplan, David Oshinsky, Katie Grogan, Sasha Kruger, Alison Bateman-House, Carolyn Chapman, Kelly Folkers, Lisa Kearns, and Brendan Parent for their many words of advice and encouragement. Members of the History of Science workshop at NYU's Gallatin School of Individualized Study also provided insightful comments on a chapter draft.

Friends and colleagues Stephen Casper, Merlin Chowkwanyun, Daniel Goldberg, Emily Harrison, Masako Hattori, Nick Juravich, Nicole Longpré, Benjamin Mason Meier, Robin Wolfe Scheffler, Brett Siegel, Ian Shin, and Megan Wolff variously read drafts, talked shop, shared feedback, put together conference panels, and provided wise counsel. Niall Bachynski, Meredith

Barnes, Jack Borrebach, Peter Cashwell, Megan Farkas, Emily Hauser, Alex Hindin, Charles Lee, Ravi Mehta, and Laura Sockol also read sections of this book, checked in with me when I needed to meet writing deadlines, and helped me format illustrations. Elizabeth Bachynski and Matt Gagne read and helped copy edit the entire manuscript. I am fortunate to have such wonderful friends and family who went so far beyond the call of duty and indulged so many conversations about youth football.

One of the greatest pleasures of this project has been the generosity of librarians, archivists, local historical societies, and interested individuals who provided immeasurable assistance. I'm so grateful to Cindy Slater of the Stark Center at the University of Texas at Austin for her assistance. My thanks to the librarians at Columbia, Harvard, NYU and the New York Public Library who answered questions about citations, retrieved requests, and scanned pages. I do not know the names of all the librarians and staff across the country who diligently fulfilled countless interlibrary loan requests, but you made my research possible.

Marianne Hooper of the King of Prussia Historical Society was extraordinarily generous in sharing materials from the society, opening her home to me, and introducing me to community members with an interest in the local youth football league. I am also grateful to Ross Deachman of Plymouth, New Hampshire, who answered my questions and mailed me copies of photos depicting how sporting goods equipment used to be manufactured. Representatives of the Maynard Historical Society, Ypsilanti Historical Society, Holt-Delhi Historical Society, University of Georgia Libraries, Houghton Library, Joyner Library, Louis Round Wilson Special Collections Library, and the Snell Memorial Foundation kindly responded to my inquiries and granted me permission to use photographs from their collections in this book. Virginia Pelton graciously granted permission to include Ernie Pelton's yearbook photo.

I also thank Russ Crawford for sharing suggestions and insight from his research on American sports during the Cold War, and Michael Oriard for his wonderful encouragement to a junior scholar embarking on a book about football.

I am so grateful to my editor Lucas Church for his expert guidance and many patient reassurances offered to a first-time author, and to all the staff at the University of North Carolina Press who brought this book into being. Thanks also to the staff at Westchester Publishing Services for their thorough copy editing of this manuscript.

Most importantly, thank you Mom, Dad, Erin, and Niall for your unfailing love and support.

Abbreviations in the Text

AAHPER	American Association for Health, Physical Education, and Recreation
AAN	American Academy of Neurology
AAP	American Academy of Pediatrics
ACSM	American College of Sports Medicine
AFCA	American Football Coaches Association
AMA	American Medical Association
ASA	American Standards Association
ASTM	American Society for Testing and Materials
CDC	Centers for Disease Control and Prevention
CPSC	Consumer Product Safety Commission
CTE	Chronic Traumatic Encephalopathy
JAMA	Journal of the American Medical Association
KPHS	King of Prussia Historical Society
NCAA	National Collegiate Athletic Association
NEA	National Education Association
NFHS	National Federation of State High School Associations
NFL	National Football League
NOCSAE	National Operating Committee on Standards for Athletic Equipment
NYSPHSAA	New York State Public High School Athletic Association
SGMA	Sporting Goods Manufacturers Association
WPA	Works Progress Administration

No Game for Boys to Play

Introduction

In 1905, Shailer Matthews, a professor and future dean of the University of Chicago's Divinity School, urged the abolition of "a social obsession—a boy-killing, education prostituting, gladiatorial sport. It teaches virility and courage, but so does war. I do not know what should take its place, but the new game should not require the services of a physician, the maintenance of a hospital, and the celebration of funerals."[1]

Matthews was referring to tackle football, and he was far from the sport's only critic at the turn of the twentieth century. In fact, Matthews wrote at a time of roiling debates over football safety. In 1902, the *Journal of the American Medical Association* (*JAMA*) had reported twelve fatalities ("enough to supply a respectable Spanish-American war"), eighty serious injuries, and innumerable "smaller items" such as sprains, lost teeth, and torn ears from that year's football season.[2] One commenter observed that future generations would be surprised "that there should be a medical history of a 'sport,' but the figures fully justify the term."[3] College administrators urged reform.[4] In 1906, the Intercollegiate Athletic Association of the United States, later renamed the National Collegiate Athletic Association (NCAA), was established to oversee the sport at the college level.[5]

Several decades later, doctors and coaches continued to confront public uncertainty about football safety. In 1931, Joseph H. Burnett, a team physician, published a survey of football injuries in Massachusetts high schools. He began by describing the prevailing parental concerns that had prompted the study. "'If I had a son I'd never let him play football—it's too dangerous.' How many times have those associated with football heard that or similar remarks?" Burnett hoped that his injury survey would alleviate these concerns.[6]

At midcentury, the introduction of plastic helmets rekindled debates. In 1961, sportswriter Jim Murray worried that this new equipment was making football more dangerous. Reform was essential, he warned, to prevent the goal line from becoming "the ghoul line." Murray emphasized the risk of head and neck injuries. "Any further progression in the direction of brutality instead of ballet and they may have to stop counting touchdowns and start counting concussions."[7]

In 2013, U.S. President Barack Obama echoed Burnett's 1931 characterization of parental fears when he told the *New Republic*: "If I had a son, I'd have to think long and hard before I let him play football."[8] The president's remarks came amid widespread media coverage of the dangers of concussions in football, as well as lawsuits filed against the National Football League (NFL) and NCAA by former players who alleged that the leagues had failed to adequately protect them or inform them of the risks. Four years later, U.S. President Donald Trump complained that NFL rule changes intended to address concussion concerns were "ruining the game."[9] Another prominent round of anxiety was under way. Yet again, educators, doctors, journalists, and American presidents raised the questions: Should football be reformed? Would changes improve or destroy the game? Was the sport too dangerous for boys to play?

By the time that Presidents Obama and Trump weighed in, debates over youth football had become focused primarily on the sport's consequences for players' brains. In response to scientific evidence about the risks of tackling for long-term neurological health, San Francisco 49ers linebacker Chris Borland made headlines by walking away from the sport at age twenty-four, after just one season in the NFL. Borland emphasized that the issue was not limited to NFL players: "With the science that's available right now, the fact that we are knowingly subjecting five-year-olds to a brain disease, to me, will baffle anthropologists for centuries to come."[10] An essayist expressed similar astonishment in 2014 over the long-standing and extraordinary prominence of football in the lives of American boys: "What does it mean that our society has transmuted the intuitive physical joys of childhood—run, leap, throw, tackle—into a corporatized form of simulated combat? That a collision sport has become the leading signifier of our institutions of higher learning, and the undisputed champ of our colossal Athletic Industrial Complex?"[11]

Such questions about the safety of youth football, its intimate association with American educational institutions, and its existence as a form of entertainment for adults have persisted to a remarkable extent throughout the twentieth and into the twenty-first century. What exactly are the health consequences of football? Does the sport build strong bodies and turn boys into men or harm the health of vulnerable children?

Arguments over the answers to these questions are as old as the game itself. This book examines the history of debates over the safety of youth football—not only changing medical understandings of the sport's health effects but also the social and cultural attitudes that shaped those understandings. With its focus on safety debates, *No Game for Boys to Play* provides a bridge between sports history and public health history, examines the values and beliefs animating the development of one of America's most popular activities for boys, and considers how football's effects on children's bodies came to be framed as a matter of public health and well-being.

College and high school football developed widespread popularity in the first half of the twentieth century, but the sport expanded even more remarkably after World War II, overtaking baseball in many ways as America's national pastime. Leagues for elementary and middle school aged boys took off, while television helped make the NFL the most popular professional sports league in the United States.

Over the decades, the full-body collisions involved in tackling remained key to football's wide appeal, even as those repeated impacts presented more frequent and serious injury risks than other popular American sports. The physical dangers ranged from brain trauma to spinal cord injuries and dislocated joints. Ever since the sport's earliest days, numerous doctors and educators repeatedly expressed the view that football was not an appropriate sport for boys to play. Yet, largely overshadowing more than a century of medical and educational concerns, a counter narrative celebrating football's risks and its heavy hitting not only thrived but profoundly shaped the youth game.

This book focuses on youth football, defined as players of high school age and younger, because the vast majority of football athletes have been children. Comparatively few athletes continue to play tackle football in college, let alone professionally or as older adults. By contrast, every year millions of American boys participate in football. Because children are not fully able to weigh the sport's long-term risks and benefits, their participation raises different ethical questions than adult athletes. In addition, children's still-developing bodies are differently susceptible to injuries than those of fully grown adults. Consequently, examining the youth level of play has significant implications from a public health perspective.

For over a century, debates over the safety of youth football have raged among doctors, lawyers, coaches, equipment engineers, and sporting goods manufacturers, as well as the general public, including journalists, parents, and the players themselves. One goal of this book is to examine when and how public health and medical professionals became involved in efforts to improve football safety. When did health professionals begin to study systematically the epidemiology of football injuries and to evaluate the effectiveness of equipment and other protective interventions? How did medical and popular understandings of sports safety change over time? Further, in what ways did medical opinions not only highlight risks but also downplay them? What were the centers of controversy, and which influential individuals and groups were involved in critical moments of change in youth football safety debates?

A related goal of this book is to examine how broader social and cultural changes shaped conversations about young athletes' physical safety. For example, how did changing demographics among youth football players influence debates? How did professional and college football influence youth football and vice versa? How did football for prepubescent boys develop differently from football for older teenagers? What cultural norms and attitudes—such as notions of manhood, boyhood, race, and national identity—were involved, and how did these change? By addressing these questions, this book places football and other sports injury prevention efforts in critical social, cultural, and historical contexts.

No Game for Boys to Play also examines the role of sporting goods manufacturers in these debates. Many histories of public health have described public health threats posed by a range of consumer products, from tobacco to lead. In contrast, manufacturers of sports equipment offered products explicitly advertised to protect consumers' health. They thus often formed alliances with public health and medical professionals, rather than opposing their interventions. In promoting their business interests, sporting goods dealers and manufacturers influenced ideas about football's health effects and the role that their products might play in mitigating risks.

Book Overview

No Game for Boys to Play is divided into four thematically organized sections. The first examines the emergence of high school and college football in the United States, the sport's connections with American ideas about race and national identity, and football's ensuing expansion to include prepubescent boys. I find that popular beliefs about the social value of tackle football for boys partly masked the sport's physical risks but in other ways framed those risks as positive: football was associated with a particular vision of masculinity that included the ability to withstand significant physical danger. Amid fears of the "feminization" of men, youth football represented an arena where women could be largely excluded and where men were charged with overseeing young boys' development.

The second section focuses on midcentury efforts to study football as a medical issue, including the development of sports medicine and debates over what constituted an injury attributable to playing football. Football injury research was largely shaped by men associated in some way with the sport, such as coaches, former athletes, or team physicians. As a consequence, many researchers appear to have underestimated the risks associated with youth football because they believed a priori in the sport's value.

Third, I explore how doctors, coaches, sports administrators, and sporting goods manufacturers managed the physical and financial hazards of football, and to whom they attributed responsibility for the injuries that occurred. By focusing primarily on improving protective equipment and insurance coverage, doctors and researchers sought to "save football" in the face of accumulating evidence of the sport's risks. Meanwhile, shifting ideas about legal responsibility for injuries contributed to an increase in the number of lawsuits, particularly against helmet manufacturers. In response, manufacturers treated the prevention of football injuries as the responsibility of individual players, parents, and coaches.

Finally, I examine the changing demographics of youth football and the increasing corporate power of the NFL. The sport's racial and ethnic composition, as well as the geographic and economic conditions of communities in which school football rose to greatest prominence, were key in shaping debates. These factors influenced whose bodies were at risk, and for which athletes and communities the perceived social benefits of football carried the greatest significance.

There are several important limitations of this project to consider. The first is the paucity of archival material specifically oriented to youth football programs. College and professional associations such as the NCAA and the NFL have the resources to maintain extensive documentation of materials, such as meeting minutes, conference agendas, and letters. Amateur and youth organizations operating on shoestring budgets, however, largely lack the means to develop and maintain archives. Notably, the largest youth football league in the United States, Pop Warner Little Scholars, did not have archival material available for research use at the time of writing.[12] This introduces significant bias into the kinds of source material available. The primary source of youth football archival material used in this book, the Dave and Mary Vannicelli Collection of the King of Prussia Historical Society (KPHS), was made available due to the generous donation of archival materials provided by the founders of a local youth football league. While these documents provide an illustrative example of how one youth league operated, systematic comparisons of safety debates across different geographic regions of the United States or different types of league structures were not possible.

Additionally, this book largely examines the arguments put forward by the range of adults who supervised, supported, protested, or profited from youth football. These adults were disproportionately white men. Women and nonwhite perspectives are relatively underrepresented among both the professional and lay commentators whose views are documented in written records. Furthermore, while several stories and quotes provide some indication of how young players themselves viewed the risks and benefits of the game, this project provides relatively limited insights into the perspectives of child athletes on the risks they were taking.

Despite these important limitations, studying debates over the safety of a popular collision sport for boys is a powerful way to understand major themes in the history of American sport, health, culture, and politics. This history continues to shape ongoing debates over football's risks. Since the nineteenth century, numerous rule, equipment and demographic changes have transformed the sport. Yet over a century since Shailer Matthews decried youth football, many elements of his critique remain pertinent to the contemporary game. Football remains an American obsession tied to educational institutions and a spectator sport that some consider gladiatorial. Coaches continue to emphasize the values of courage and toughness they believe the sport teaches. Advocates and critics alike have drawn comparisons between football and war. Moreover, youth football continues to require "the services of a physician, the maintenance of a hospital, and the celebration of funerals."

While a number of physicians and other observers have long been aware of head injuries in football, only recently have these injuries been framed as a public health crisis. As historian Emily Harrison noted in 2014, "what gained attention a century ago as a medical problem among young men playing football in elite colleges is now a serious problem of public health."[13] This history indicates that a wide range of cultural priorities other than child health have shaped youth football safety debates. Indeed, in many ways, youth football injuries and deaths represent an inscription of adult values onto boys' bodies. Controversies over football safety repeatedly flared up when those values seemed threatened. The history of debates over the safety of youth football is, in part, a history of beliefs about how to raise boys to meet particular ideals of manhood.

Part I

The Rise of Youth Football

CHAPTER ONE

The Modern Knight Errant

Nation, Race, and the Origins of American Football

For good or for bad the progress of [football] has been as steady and irresistible
as the progress of the spirit of colonization.
— John Corbin, "The Puritan and the Football Player," 1897

On a beautiful October day in 1897, Richard Vonalbade "Von" Gammon took
his position in the University of Georgia's football lineup. He was considered
one of the team's best athletes. Von Gammon hailed from Rome, Georgia,
where his father was a leading merchant and councilman, and his mother pre-
sided over the local chapter of the Daughters of the American Confederacy.
His prominent father was "never so happy as when the young man emerged
from some contest covered in glory," and his son rarely disappointed.[1] As a
quarterback, Von Gammon had led Georgia to an undefeated record the previous fall. This season, he had been moved to fullback to take advantage of his
many talents on the field.[2]

During a play in the game's second half, Gammon was covering a defensive back position. As the Georgia defense smashed into their University of
Virginia opponents, Gammon was thrown into the air. Amid the scuffle, he
fell hard on his head and lost consciousness. The young athlete was taken to a
nearby hospital, where doctors determined that the hit had "produced in all
probability concussion of the brain." Von Gammon died shortly after his
father arrived. He was a few months shy of his eighteenth birthday.[3]

The fatality was just one in a string of football tragedies that 1897 season.
Also in October, nineteen-year-old Andrew Hasche died after suffering a broken neck "at the bottom of a heap of players" in a game at Casino Beach, Long
Island.[4] In November, Eddie Buckman of Stoneham, Massachusetts, "one of
the brightest boys in the town," died of injuries he suffered playing in an open
lot with eight or nine other boys. Most of the Stoneham youngsters who
had gathered to play ranged in age from ten to fifteen years. The doctor
who had attended Buckman told newspapers, "There should be a law passed
to prevent boys who have not attained somewhere near the mature age from
engaging in football contests. . . . There should be a law against football."[5]

But the 1897 football debates reached a crescendo with the death of Von
Gammon (see figure 1). He was not a boy playing in an open lot or on the

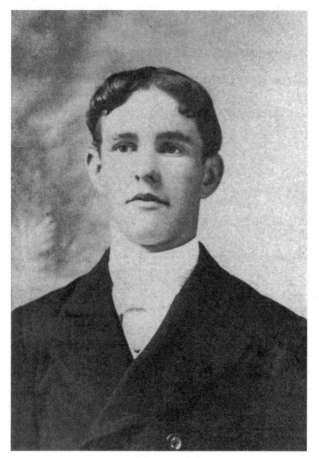

FIGURE 1 This 1897 yearbook photo depicts Richard
Vonalbade "Von" Gammon the year he died from a football
injury. Courtesy of the Hargrett Rare Book and Manuscript
Library/University of Georgia Libraries.

beach but a popular college student competing for a public university
team. Moreover, while football had already assumed a prominent place
among many Ivy League schools in the north, the sport was not quite as
entrenched in southern university culture in the 1890s. Many Georgians
regarded organized sports with the disapproval they accorded other dis-
reputable pastimes, such as horse racing and gambling. Southern newspapers decried football as a "source of evil," a "demoralizing, money-making
scheme," and a "first-class display of savagery." Several weeks after Gammon's death, the Georgia House of Representatives voted 91–3 to ban the
game.[6]

In response, supporters of football rallied to its defense. One Virginia school headmaster insisted that "gentlemanly boys" could play football for months without injury. He complained that condemnations of the sport were an unjust fad. All youthful activities carried risks, and "parents must take their chances on bringing up a boy sound and unmaimed."[7] The *New York Times* similarly asserted that the "noble game" of football was not so dangerous as to require prohibition.[8] Ultimately, in December 1897, Georgia governor William Yates Atkinson vetoed the antifootball bill. In his message to the House of Representatives justifying his veto, Atkinson explained that "the sports of every great people, ancient and modern, have been hard and severe."[9]

The legislative contest over the fate of football in Georgia had turned not simply on athletes' physical safety but also on whether it was proper for "gentlemanly boys" to play football. Should "great people" engage in rough sports? This question was intertwined with shifting understandings of civilization, race, and masculinity. Did football and its physical risks foster American ideals of manliness? Or did the violent sport represent "savagery" and stand in opposition to standards of "civilized" manhood? The answer would determine the fate of football in the United States.[10]

Development of American Tackle Football and Mechanics of the Game

By the time of the 1897 debates, football was still a relatively new sport. American tackle football had originated from rugby and soccer, sports that also involved two teams of players competing for control of a ball. In each, the ball could be kicked through a goal or run across a line in order to score points. Football shared these qualities, but the quintessentially American game developed its own particular set of rules in the late nineteenth century.

Modern football primarily took shape at elite colleges in the northeastern United States, then spread to players of high school age and even younger. But the sport may have its earliest origins among high school boys in the 1860s. A number of leading football luminaries would accept the Oneida Football Club of Boston, composed of boys from several area high schools, as the first organized football club. Its first match likely occurred on November 7, 1863, on Boston Common, according to a newspaper account of this "interesting game of Football" published two days later. In the 1920s, surviving club members proudly highlighted that as schoolboys they had played a new version of football several years before any college students at Princeton, Rutgers, Harvard, or Yale attempted the game. In 1925, these Oneida Club alumni established a stone monument at the entrance to Boston Common in honor of the club's athletic achievements, emphasizing their victorious record. The seven surviving teammates inscribed on their plaque that in all their matches "the Oneida Goal was never crossed."[11]

The origins of modern college football, however, are usually traced to a November 6, 1869, game in New Brunswick, New Jersey, between Princeton and Rutgers. Princeton modified rules of the London Football Association, a rugby club, to allow for twenty-five players to a side, kicking or butting the ball with the head, scoring six goals to win a game, and placing goalposts twenty-five feet apart. In the ensuing years, other Ivy League schools, including Columbia, Cornell, Harvard, and Yale, began to join in with their own various sets of rules. To attempt to standardize the game, several of these schools formed the Intercollegiate Football Association (IFA) in 1876.[12]

In a series of meetings over the following years, football took form, with the previously used round rubber ball discarded in favor of an egg-shaped leather ball and the number of players on a team reduced to eleven. In 1880, IFA officials implemented a new method of putting the ball into play: an athlete would place the ball on the ground in front of him and either kick the ball or snap it back with his foot. This introduced the modern American football scrimmage. The scrimmage established the principle of possession of the ball, distinct from a more haphazard rugby scrum where neither team had the right to possess the ball or put it into play. In 1882, the IFA adopted a system of "downs" that had been proposed by Walter Camp, a player and coach who became known as "the father of American football." Camp's system prescribed the number of consecutive tries a team had to attempt to advance a particular number of yards down the field before they would be required to surrender the ball to their opponents. To gauge the distance players covered, Camp further proposed a system of marking off yards on the field, known as a gridiron. Camp was responsible for another profound rule change in 1888, when tackling players below the waist was legalized. Football thus developed into a sport where repeated series of full-body collisions were involved in attempting to gain control of the ball and move it down the field.[13]

Equipment was introduced gradually. Football star John Heisman would recall that in the earliest days players wore no padding or protection of any sort. In the 1890s and 1900s, however, players began to wear "shin guards, rubber nose guards, and homemade soft pads for elbows." Much of this padding was made of leather and wool and soon covered vulnerable parts of the players' bodies. As an 1897 *Chicago Daily Tribune* article delicately observed, "Especial precaution has been made this year for the hips, and a protuberance greater there than anywhere else shows extra padding." After the introduction of these relatively soft protective pads, Heisman recounted, next "came leather helmets and sole leather shoulder pads—sometimes reinforced with metallic plates—and thigh and knee pads of more or less murderous composition. Inflexible and unyielding pads often did damage to the opponent." From its earliest introduction into the sport, then, football equipment could serve to protect its wearer or to cause harm to other players.[14]

Although leather head protection would become so ubiquitous that football players could be described as "leatherheads," the headgear was initially viewed with skepticism. According to one author, around the turn of the twentieth century, "An enterprising manufacturer put the first pneumatic head harness on the market made of soft black rubber with an inflated crown. The old timers thought such head guards 'sissy,' contending that no 'real football player' would wear one." Whether the tough-looking gear enhanced a player's masculinity or symbolized safety fears and thus rendered him a coward was another persistent source of controversy.[15]

Tellingly, newspapers described football players as appearing "in full armor," likening the equipment to the protection soldiers might wear heading off to war.[16] Football quickly became immensely popular in American military academies. An 1892 *Harper's Weekly* article explained, "If there is any game fitted to the training of the soldier, it is this one." As "a mimic battle-field," football emphasized "a spirit of self-sacrifice." Such descriptions suggested that football players, like soldiers, must be prepared to expose themselves to great physical risk for the greater good.[17]

Accounts of football matches often celebrated athletes' blasé attitudes toward injuries. Visible wounds were treated as battle scars indicative of an athlete's manliness. "Such trifles as blackened eyes, wrenched knees and broken noses are rather welcomed than otherwise, for the bruises of battle received on the gridiron field are badges of honor in college circles."[18] Harvard team doctors described the football athletes they treated as having a uniquely high disregard for pain and a culture of laughing off injuries. "Concussion was treated by the players in general as a trivial injury and rather regarded as a joke." Football had emerged as a uniquely American collision sport linked with a military ethos of self-sacrifice and glorification of physical pain.[19]

Football and American Identity

By 1893, an editor of the *New York Herald* observed that Thanksgiving Day was no longer a solemn American festival of thanksgiving, but "a holiday granted by the State and the nation to see a game of football." The sport's growing popularity reached a pinnacle at college matches scheduled after Thanksgiving church services. The 1893 Thanksgiving Day championship game at New York City's polo grounds attracted 40,000 football fans. Each had paid five dollars to see Princeton challenge Yale.[20] The match was "a major event on the social calendar of the city's elite, equivalent to a fashionable tennis tournament, the opening of the racing season at Jerome Park, the annual horse show, or the opening of the opera season."[21]

It was no coincidence that football became closely associated with Thanksgiving, a national holiday that had also emerged as an important facet of American cultural life only several decades prior. As historian S. W. Pope has argued, "The popular notion of American myth and destiny expressed through football commentary was entirely consistent with the myth of Thanksgiving." Football celebrated physical prowess, team unity, organized effort, and the acquisition of territory. The rituals of football and Thanksgiving each fostered notions of shared national origins and American identity.[22] Football players represented these ideals and were likened to military heroes of a romanticized past. In 1894, the *Washington Post* dubbed the football player "the modern knight errant."[23]

Football's knights errant were usually to be found at exclusive institutions such as Harvard and Yale. At the turn of the twentieth century, American football became linked with white, Anglo-Saxon, protestant students at elite colleges and universities. Proponents of football insisted that the sport was not only appropriate for civilized American gentlemen but enhanced and reinforced these students' status. Ivy League coaches explicitly characterized football as an exemplar of white masculinity. In 1900, Harvard's football coach stated, "Football is the expression of the strength of the Anglo-Saxon. It is the dominant spirit of a dominant race, and to this it owes its popularity and its hopes of permanence."[24]

Americans were not alone in seeking to express national and racial identity through athletics at the turn of the twentieth century. As a range of risky competitive sports took new forms, the globalization of modern athletics in many ways served to make "the expression of national identity . . . through sport a global phenomenon."[25] Promoters of judo in Japan, rugby in New Zealand, and ice hockey in Canada all shaped these sports in ways intended to represent these countries' histories and cultures.[26]

The expansion of football in the United States was part of this global phenomenon, while also connected to particular ideas about American identity. In this period of expanding imperialistic aspirations, U.S. leaders linked aggressive sports and their physical dangers to business and military success. As Senator Henry Cabot Lodge explained in an 1896 address to Harvard alumni, "The time given to athletic contests and the injuries incurred on the playing field are part of the price which the English-speaking race has paid for being world-conquerors." The physical risks of competitive school sports were thus justified by racialized ideas of colonization and conquest. Politicians and university administrators characterized athletic success as the ideal preparation for the English-speaking American men who were expected to build and expand the nation.[27]

Although football was touted as reinforcing the superiority of Anglo-Saxon men, participation by minority American racial and ethnic groups dated to the earliest days of the sport. In the 1890s, several predominantly white college football teams in the northern United States included black players. Because football was promoted as an arena of white superiority, participation in football by a minority group was at odds with a variety of prevailing racist stereotypes. In this context, the achievements of minority athletes on the football field had the potential to demonstrate that young boys and men typically considered inferior were in fact equal to their white peers.[28]

Nowhere was this aspiration more evident than in the development of the youth football program at the Carlisle Indian Industrial School. Located in central Pennsylvania, Carlisle was founded in 1879 as an off-reservation boarding school intended to assimilate Native American students into white, Christian American culture. Captain Richard Henry Pratt, the school's founder and superintendent, characterized Carlisle's educational philosophy as "Kill the Indian in him, and save the man." With the increasing popularity of football at Ivy League colleges, Carlisle's leaders realized that the sport offered an avenue for showcasing the school's educational program. As sportswriter Sally Jenkins observed, school administrators and staff regarded football as "a stage on which Carlisle could exhibit a different kind of 'show Indian' to the public, one who was every bit as intelligent and civilized as the elite college boys." In 1906, Carlos Montezuma, a Yavapai doctor who served as resident physician at Carlisle for several years, promoted this view to white Christian reformers who sought to acculturate Native Americans. "Let us get into civilization," he urged. "If there is no other way but by kicking the pigskin, then let us get in that way."[29]

On this view, football represented a powerful avenue for imparting Anglo-Saxon culture and values to Native students. This strategy of relatively marginalized communities adopting a sport associated with elite members of society was not unique to the United States. Cricket in India provides an interesting point of comparison; the British sport was seen as a way of "implanting English ideals of manliness, stamina, and vigor into Indian groups seen as lazy, enervated, and effete."[30] Football at Carlisle, however, was also touted as a public relations effort to garner support for the school's specific educational program that claimed to "civilize" its students. Widely viewed contests in which Native American teenagers challenged Harvard and Yale athletes on the gridiron appeared to be the most effective means to reach the public.

Much of the attention the Carlisle Indians attracted did not result in the hoped-for recognition of Native students as intelligent and civilized but rather reinforced prevailing biases. An 1894 *Washington Post* article began, "It is an unusual thing to see an Indian bestir himself sufficiently to take part in any sort of amusement which is liable to disturb his peaceful serenity, but in the Carlisle Indian School they have a set of young bucks who have taken up the American game of football." Widespread media coverage of the students' "performance of civilization" on the football field constantly reminded the Native American players of their second-class status.[31]

In 1899, Carlisle hired accomplished white coach Glenn Scobey "Pop" Warner to coach the school's football team. In the following decade, major American newspapers avidly covered the team's remarkable exploits. No Carlisle football player—and indeed, perhaps no Native American athlete—received more attention than renowned athlete Jim Thorpe. "In elevating Thorpe to superstar status, the newspapers painted a 'human face' on the fledgling sport of college football."[32]

Racist stereotypes were just as central to the creation of Thorpe's superstar status as they were to the origins of American football. In 1911, the *Philadelphia Inquirer* reported that when he arrived at Carlisle "three short years ago, Jim Thorpe was just a simple and unsophisticated Indian, that was all," yet "there was a latent ability that was destined to make this careless child of Nature the athletic marvel of the age." According to this narrative, it took Pop Warner, a white coach, to discover Thorpe's "slumbering" athletic skills. Newspapers claimed that the training and exposure to organized sports Thorpe received from white coaches and administrators transformed "this simple-minded Indian" into "the best half-back the football game has ever developed." As historian Philip Deloria has observed, the performance of Native athletes such as Thorpe "offered white audiences spectacles of a lost time of natural physicality and strength."[33] As one of the first American football heroes, Thorpe represented the "civilizing" influence of an Anglo, Christian education as well as embodying the "natural" Indian athlete.

Physical Risks and "Civilized" Values

Richard Henry Pratt, the founder and superintendent of the Carlisle Indian Industrial School, was initially concerned about football injuries. But he reportedly rationalized introducing the sport into the school by noting that students could just as easily suffer injuries while doing farm work. Pratt emphasized that no other activity in Carlisle's history had "attracted the attention and comment" of the school's football season. The decision to allow Carlisle students to play represents an early exemplar of how health concerns were eclipsed by football's perceived social benefits. In this racialized context, the sport's spectacle nature was crucial. If football matches could not only impart "civilized" values to Native students but also display the efficacy of a Carlisle education to a broader public, the risks would be justified.[34]

At stake in the Carlisle Indians' matches against predominantly Anglo-Saxon teams was the question of who could be considered civilized gentlemen. As historian Michael Oriard has observed, the issue of what it meant to be a man has underlain "virtually every narrative of football."[35] This question intersected with the racial meanings of school-sponsored football. Dominant social hierarchies constrained efforts to challenge prevailing racist stereotypes and limited recognition of the contributions of nonwhite athletes to the development of modern football. For years, the accomplishments of the Carlisle Indian athletes were largely overshadowed by celebrations of the achievements of their white coach, Pop Warner. Warner would be credited with introducing many major innovations to football, including such tactics as the huddle, the idea of numbering plays, the body block, the double-wing formation, the spiral pass, and the spiral punt.[36] Nevertheless, Carlisle administrators promoted football as a way to "demonstrate what education means to the Indians."[37]

On the other hand, those who opposed the rough sport of football as entertainment commonly objected to upper-crust men participating in such an unseemly spectacle. As an 1897 *New York Times* editorial argued, "A young gentleman engaged in getting an education ought not to exhibit himself for money, and he and his fellows ought not to raise a mere sport to the dignity of an occupation." Tellingly, this editorial incorporated football into a discussion of lynching, a form of social violence associated with masculinity and race. The *Times* argued that both evils could be cured by altering financial incentives. The families of lynching victims should be entitled to the right to recover damages against the sheriff of the county where the lynching took place. Meanwhile, in the case of football, "the process must be reversed. Take away the gate money and the game will revert to its proper status of innocuous pastime."[38]

But neither of these "curable evils" would be resolved by the *Times*'s proposal. If anything, the reality of college football increasingly deviated from the ideal of an amateur game for gentlemen where no money changed hands. Furthermore, the sport's physical toll was attracting significant media attention. Newspapers highlighted dramatic injuries and deaths that took place on the gridiron. As early as 1892, a *Chicago Daily Tribune* commentary warned that should football become a national pastime, it "must be reformed or it will cripple and physically ruin thousands of young men."[39] Two years later, the *Tribune* published an opinion piece elaborating on the risks of football as it expanded to "the schoolboys who are preparing for college." The author contended that the dangerous game was an uncivilized way to train American youth. Football stood apart as the only sport "which brings the whole bodies of players into violent collision . . . the violent personal concussion of twenty-two vigorous, highly trained young men is not only permissible, but is a large part of the game." Such a competition "which may be won by disabling your adversary, or wearing out his strength, or killing him, ought to be prohibited, at all events, among [civilized people's] youth."[40]

Throughout the 1890s, an accumulation of fatalities such as Von Gammon's lent weight to arguments that football had crossed the murky line from gentlemanly daring to savagery. By the turn of the century, college football had attracted significant unfavorable attention. Several prominent university leaders argued that, while such risk taking might be justified in occupations such as fire protection and seafaring, "no mere sport" should imperil life.[41] Other observers confidently predicted that football would soon fall into disfavor.[42] In a 1906 report for the *Boston Medical and Surgical Journal*, team doctors for Harvard's football squad concluded that the football injuries they had seen were "inherent in the game itself," and that "the percentage of injury is much too great for any sport."[43]

To save football, university leaders called for reform. They garnered high-powered support for their efforts, including from none other than President Theodore Roosevelt. Roosevelt had a tough, military image, particularly due to his service during the Spanish-American War leading a regiment nicknamed the Rough Riders. As a politician, Roosevelt embraced this image and promoted "the doctrine of the strenuous life." He encouraged boys and men to embrace physical danger, notably by playing "rough games," as a means to success. Tackle football fit squarely within this vision. Roosevelt had been among the first to analogize the sport's risky collisions to life itself, famously writing, "In life, as in a football game, the principle to follow is: Hit the line hard; don't foul and don't shirk, but hit the line hard!" He helped popularize the view that the collisions involved in football were not only a source of entertainment for spectators but also a source of character building and life lessons for the young athletes engaged in those collisions.[44] An abundance of early twentieth-century literature for young boys reinforced these ideas with tales of schoolboys achieving success both on the football field and in life.[45]

Roosevelt endorsed football as a means of training college students and supported reforms to preserve the sport. He ultimately contributed to establishing the NCAA to oversee football and other sports in response to numerous American colleges considering abolishing football in 1905–1906. This famous "football crisis" led to rule changes intended to cut down on injuries but perhaps more importantly was portrayed as eliminating the uncivilized elements of the sport. One 1905 cartoon depicted President Roosevelt and a college president advancing a football against their bestial opponents who represented "brutality in football" (see figure 2). By removing the "brutish" elements of football, Roosevelt was hailed as having preserved the sport as an option for civilized gentlemen.[46]

Nonetheless, an ongoing, racialized tension between the sport's civilized and brutish components remained. In fact, this tension was no doubt part of football's popular appeal. The sport was promoted as both a training ground for elite American men and as a dangerous spectacle associated with savagery. In likening football's progress to the spirit of colonization, American writer John Corbin contended that these coexisting attitudes toward dangerous sports were "as old as the Anglo-Saxon nation." But football's strength, he suggested, lay in its ability to impart moral, even puritanical, virtues of discipline and "a dauntless soul," while simultaneously allowing young men the thrill of "the quickening forces of nature within them." On this account, while the sport's value depended on its "chivalrous" ethics, giving free rein to "the wonderful flow of physical strength within [men's] veins" was all the more necessary "in a new country, when the struggle is still waging with the gigantic forces of nature."[47]

As is evident in the narratives surrounding Native American athlete Jim Thorpe, an athlete's racial identity influenced the perceived balance of these competing factors. Native students were considered to have a greater need for football's civilizing effects, while Anglo students required an outlet where

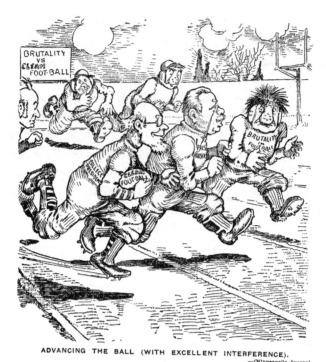

ADVANCING THE BALL (WITH EXCELLENT INTERFERENCE).
—(Minneapolis Journal

FIGURE 2 This November 26, 1905, cartoon depicts a
contest between "clean football" and brutality in the sport.
Theodore Roosevelt political cartoon collection, 1884–1940
(MS Am 3056). Courtesy of the Houghton Library,
Harvard University.

they could develop their physical strength to wrestle with and conquer
"forces of nature." Football matches between the Carlisle Indians team and
Ivy League colleges were particularly revealing of how these competing ideals
were inscribed within the sport and projected onto players of different ethnic
backgrounds. Football had come to represent particular American conceptions of civilization and savagery in ways that drew crowds, recruited enthusiastic students, and appealed to school administrators.

Secondary Education and "the Rules of Life"

With the intervention of the U.S. president and other leaders to preserve
the sport, football continued to thrive and expand onto the field of high
school campuses. The sport was not new to American high school students;
they had played informal football matches in parks and fields since the

second half of the nineteenth century. By the 1880s, some students in north-eastern and midwestern cities were organizing their own leagues absent faculty supervision. Their games often attracted spectators, encouragement from alumni, and interest from local communities. In Brooklyn, high school students from four schools organized a series of games to compete for the 1893 title of the "boss kickers of Brooklyn." That year, the *New York Times* asserted that the rivalry between the high school teams was "as keen as that shown between the regular college elevens, and locally the interest is nearly as great."[48]

But the early twentieth century heralded an even greater expansion and organization of football among teenagers. Interregional matches began taking place, although the development of high school football remained uneven. Regional disparities were in dramatic evidence when Brooklyn Polytechnic students, champions of greater New York, traveled to Chicago in 1902 to compete against Hyde Park High School. In what historian Robert Pruter has deemed "perhaps the most one-sided high school intersectional contest of all time," Hyde Park defeated Brooklyn Polytechnic 105 to 0. Because "a more even contest had been expected," the *New York Times* drily observed, "the rapid scoring grew somewhat monotonous."[49] While acknowledging that the younger boys had been "a little slow in picking up the game," an enthusiastic 1905 *Washington Post* article claimed that there was "barely a high school which does not possess its college eleven." As this phrase suggests, football was still primarily associated with "college elevens" at the turn of the century, although more high school players were taking up the game.[50]

Similar to the debates about football and civilization at the college level, some high school officials tried to prohibit the game. The 1905 football death of Vernon Wise, a seventeen-year-old Oak Park high school student, prompted a local campaign against the sport. "Stop football, stop it," Wise's father reportedly begged the school principal, who agreed.[51] In 1909, the New York Board of Education banned football from city high schools. One board member explained that the game fostered "a desire to maim," while Commissioner Frederic R. Coudert characterized football as "homicidal, barbaric and brutal."[52] The board of education's decision elicited protests from football's defenders, who contended that "there is no special hazard in the game if it is properly planned and properly controlled."[53] In 1910, New York reinstated football in public high schools under new rules that would purportedly reduce the most serious safety threats. Some of these rule changes, which were adopted by the American Intercollegiate Football Rules Committee in May 1910, prohibited pushing, pulling, and interlocking interference and reduced the length of games to four fifteen-minute quarters.[54]

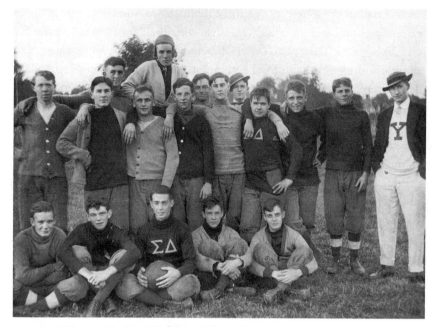

FIGURE 3   The 1908 Ypsilanti High School football team poses for a team photo. Ypsilanti Historical Society Fletcher-White Archives, University of Michigan Library Digital Collections. Courtesy of the Ypsilanti Historical Society.

As efforts to ban football failed, high school officials instead sought to supervise the sport. Students sometimes welcomed and sometimes resisted increasing faculty control of their teams.[55] A photo of Ypsilanti High School's 1908 football team suggests this transitional period (figure 3). The sigma delta appearing on several students' jerseys represents a high school fraternity. Yet only three years later, as part of a broader trend of increasing administrative control over athletics, the Michigan state legislature would abolish high school fraternities in 1911.[56]

Informal games in parks and fields gave way to interscholastic matches that were organized and officiated by adults. Ensuring that only eligible students participated in competitions, providing adult and institutional supervision for matches, and implementing rule changes (such as adding a third official) helped make football "more palatable" to school officials and parents concerned about the safety and suitability of the game for young players.[57] By the 1923–1924 school year, only three states lacked statewide oversight of interscholastic contests.[58] High school football players increasingly had access to adult coaching, protective equipment, and administrative support

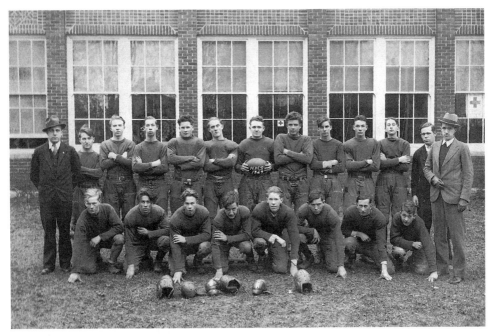

FIGURE 4 Examples of the leather headgear players wore are displayed in front of the kneeling players on the 1929 Holt High School football team of Holt, Michigan. Many players are also visibly wearing shoulder pads. Courtesy of the Holt-Delhi Historical Society.

(figure 4). In fact, the first coaches of Holt, Michigan's high school football team were the school's principals.[59]

Increasing adult oversight of high school football was part of a larger trend of incorporating competitive athletics into American schools.[60] At the college level, a 1929 survey found that out of 177 directors of physical education programs, only four directors held master's degrees in physical education or education, but 85 percent had qualified for the position through their success as a football coach. Sports, particularly football, became profoundly intertwined if not synonymous with physical education programs for men and boys during the early twentieth century.[61]

Interscholastic sports were also increasingly seen as part of the educational mission of secondary schools. Historian S. W. Pope has observed that the movement away from gymnastics and toward team sports reflected "the new educational psychology of John Dewey (and others), who believed that children should learn from experience." Many educators interpreted competitive team athletics as a source of practical opportunity to experience the "rules of life," namely victory and defeat, in a way that other physical activities could not offer. As historian Brad Austin characterized this reasoning, "Where better could students experience the thrills of success and the agony of failure than on the athletic fields and courts?"[62]

In addition, progressive and religious leaders promoted football as a means to instill moral values in boys. The belief that athletic competition fostered moral self-improvement, often known as "muscular Christianity," had roots in Victorian conceptions of health and became popular among a number of American Christians.[63] In 1904, the Reverend A. E. Colton of the American Bible Society wrote that his son left his high school football season "in prime condition for the hardest kind of tackling and protracted endeavor with languages, physics and mathematics. Thus we gladly pay tribute to the great game which is doing so much for developing our young men physically and morally, preparing them for the hard grinding battles of coming days."[64] If football improved academic performance and even prepared boys to engage in future battles to defend civilization, then its physical aggression could be coded as civilized and moral, rather than brutish and savage.

Interscholastic sports received further justification during World War I as a means to meet national defense needs and foster physical fitness among citizens, particularly in response to reports that one-third of American men called for military service were physically unfit.[65] In January 1917, President Woodrow Wilson told a delegation from the Maryland and Massachusetts Leagues for National Defense that "unquestionably, physical training is needed. . . . but it can be had without compulsory military service."[66] Adopting the president's statement as their slogan, a newly formed Committee for Promoting Physical Education in the Public Schools of the United States sought to introduce physical education without military features into public schools.[67] Chaired by John Dewey and composed of a number of other leading educators, this committee placed a model bill before the general assemblies of California, Indiana, and Connecticut in 1917. By 1923, thirty-two states had passed legislation requiring physical education as part of the high school curriculum.[68]

Dewey's committee explicitly characterized physical education as essential to American citizenship. Organized athletic competitions were portrayed as a means to instill teamwork and responsibility in boys, contributing to "the building up of the character of the manhood of America."[69] Daniel Chase, the first president of the New York State Public High School Athletic Association (NYSPHSAA), recalled drafting fourteen points of "good sportsmanship" in 1920, to be printed in all of the association's earliest handbooks. These included the admonition that a good sport should play for the joy of playing, be a good team worker, accept adverse decisions gracefully, back his team in every honest way, and play hard until the end.[70]

In 1926, Chase left the state Department of Education to serve as the executive director of the recently formed International Sportsmanship Brotherhood. A *New York Times* profile of this organization asserted that sportsmanship had educational value that would translate to the business world, and "were this not true the games and sports of a nation would make but little contribution to character."[71] Such notions of sportsmanship and fair play were considered essential in justifying the educational value of athletic competition.[72]

Competitive sports such as football were thus billed as preparing future leaders and offering a form of physical training as an alternative to military service. This framing of sports owed much to an influential essay by philosopher William James on the need for a "moral equivalent of war" to advance civilization.[73] In 1922, R. Tait McKenzie, a physician and professor of physical education, proclaimed, "Athletic activity is the best substitute for war, and every virile people must have either one or the other." A *New York Times* report on McKenzie's lecture noted that the professor clearly had James's essay in mind, and inquired whether educators had given "any thought of providing a moral equivalent of football."[74]

This quip indicated the extraordinary rise of football, as well as concerns that rather than providing an alternative to war, school-based competitive sports instead posed new moral problems. Some administrators argued that athletics had taken on an unhealthy level of importance. They occupied "the time and attention of the pupils in the schools and of the community in general in a manner most unwholesome for the contestants and for the spectators as well."[75]

How did football become so strongly associated with school and community identity in many American locales? In his examination of the importance of high school sports in northeastern Pennsylvania, historian Paul Zbiek suggests several factors that may have contributed to football's particular prominence. As a fall sport played in a large open field, in a setting that could accommodate crowds of thousands (unlike an indoor gym), football was well suited to mass spectatorship. The sport's hard-hitting, rough play appealed to both coal miners and upper class families who associated the sport with their alma maters, combining "a working class attitude with the trappings of academia." Zbiek further argues that the geography of regions such as the Wyoming Valley fostered athletic rivalries and excitement. The proximity of small towns, their links with particular ethnic and socioeconomic identities, and the ability of boys to play team sports together from grade school through high school, all contributed to a broader sense of community investment in the outcome of a match.[76]

The heavy involvement of adults in both managing and watching youth sports worried some educators. Frederick Rand Rogers, the New York State director of health education, feared that the educational value of athletics was being warped. In a 1929 book, he decried the transformation of school athletics into an adult-oriented activity. The nature of youth sports as a public spectacle for adult community members, and even a means to raise funds for schools, was harming children. Rogers explained, "when adults insist upon spending their leisure time watching children at play, and not through any interest in the children themselves except as actors on a stage, the wisdom of a culture which provides the leisure is open to serious indictment. Probably the remedy lies in more education. But any education which accustoms *adolescents* to spectacles of *adults excited over adolescent athletics* is an unhealthy form of training for the children. The school must solve its problems more effectively if it is to save itself."[77]

Rogers's reference to the problems of schools pointed to a deeper institutional self-interest underlying spectator sports. The rhetoric of football's proponents emphasized its educational value to students. But critics such as Rogers perceived school administrators using football as a means to address financial and other institutional shortcomings. Such a strategy, he contended, was fundamentally flawed: education and sports as professional entertainment were "incompatible by nature."[78]

Modern Schools Where Football Is Taught

Concerns about the spectacle nature of contact sports, particularly football, would persist throughout the twentieth century. Such anxieties also underscored how the remarkable popularity of high school and college athletic contests in communities had influenced attitudes toward collision sports, civilization, and education. School administrators and other leaders promoted football as a spectator sport that conferred moral benefits to students. Their efforts overwhelmed opposing attitudes that it was inappropriate for boys and young men to "exhibit" themselves in front of crowds for money. The growth of competitive school sports proved consistent with the ideas of a broad range of progressive leaders and thinkers, from Theodore Roosevelt to John Dewey.

The framing of football as training for future leaders and "civilizing" Indian athletes also obscured objections based on the sport's physical dangers.

Americans were well aware of the physical risks of football since its inception. Commentators in newspapers and medical journals had pointed out the dangers of repeated full-body collisions, including relatively rare but tragic deaths of young boys and men, often from head injuries. In addition to listing the names of players who had died playing football in 1903, *JAMA* editors informed readers "we believe that in this particular game the human wreckage far outweighs the good." But such objections were largely sidelined by the promotion of a vision of American masculinity that included the ability to withstand significant physical injury.[79]

In 1906, American satirist Ambrose Bierce quipped that *academe* could be defined as "an ancient school where morality and philosophy were taught," but an *academy* was "a modern school where football is taught."[80] Bierce's satirical definition exposed how school football was associated with a new set of educational ideals related to masculinity, race, civilization, and American identity. By the first decade of the twentieth century, the sport was firmly established in American colleges and expanding at the high school level. Concerns about football's risks did not disappear. But future debates over the safety of youth football would take place in a new context. The full-body collision sport had been integrated into academic programs for boys expected to become the future business and military leaders of the United States. As a consequence, questioning the social benefits of football would prove even more difficult.

CHAPTER TWO

We Are Not a Nation of Softies

Youth Football from the Great Depression to the Cold War

This boy's fear of being called a sissy . . . is the ruling spirit of high school football.
— William Brady, 1952

Forty-four years after Von Gammon's death in Georgia, about 75,000 fans crowded the Yale Bowl. It was October 24, 1931, and the spectators were closely following the tightly contested Army-Yale football game. In the fourth quarter, returning a kickoff, cadet Richard Brinsley Sheridan Jr. made a flying tackle head-on. Considered "one of football's most spectacular sights," this method of tackling was also highly dangerous. Sheridan broke his neck and never regained consciousness. The young cadet died after two days on an artificial respirator with his family, football coach, an Army delegation, and West Point chaplain at his side.[1]

Sheridan's death prompted "the most violent excoriation football has been subjected to since 1905."[2] Like Von Gammon's death, the fatality of an Army cadet threatened beliefs that football prepared boys and young men to be business and military leaders. The *New York Herald Tribune* reported on calls "to the very heavens for revision and emasculation [of football] to a point where young men, who are expected to amount to something in the world of business and affairs in time to come, can be permitted to participate."[3]

The process of "emasculating" football in order to retain its educational value would also include addressing the spectacle nature of the sport in schools. The *New Haven Register* editorialized that a complete survey of football injuries and deaths among students should "silence the most rabid fanatic, who today shouts: 'Play the game! Take what's coming to you and smile!'" The number of young players who were injured, "many in a manner which may later develop weaknesses that will have to be carried throughout life, actually cries aloud for action."[4]

In response to the outcry, the Intercollegiate Football Rules Committee introduced "the most far-reaching modifications adopted in the playing rules of the game in a quarter of a century." The changes included making the flying block and tackle illegal, allowing more frequent substitutions, and forbidding players from striking opponents on the head, neck, or face. In fall 1932, the first season after the new rules were adopted, the *New York Times* reported on ten football-related deaths. All but one had occurred among boys, and the toll "came mainly through head injuries." While the new safety code appeared to have reduced deaths at the college level, the rule changes had "failed to eliminate the hazards to prep school, high school and sandlot combatants."[5] Sportswriter Allison Danzig observed that the supportive response of coaches, officials, and athletic executives to the new rules "reflected the belief that something constructive had been done to reduce the risks of the game without working any radical change in the character of the play."[6] By this period, even the outrage sparked by a player's death was insufficient to inspire substantial change to how the sport was played at all levels. Football was deeply entrenched in American culture and institutions of higher education. Administrators prioritized preserving the game while tweaking rules in response to safety concerns.

During the Great Depression and World War II, the construction of new athletic facilities, in conjunction with arguments connecting athletics and national defense, laid the groundwork for a remarkable expansion of youth football in the 1950s. Players younger than high school age, including boys of more diverse ethnic backgrounds, increasingly took up the game. Meanwhile, although safety debates continued, the particular masculine ideals associated with football acquired ever greater influence amid concerns of "soft" boys in need of male supervision.

Big-Time Football

Limited finances during the Great Depression circumscribed the growth of high school extracurricular activities, including athletics. Historian Robert Pruter has argued that "high school sports were essentially put on hold" during the 1930s and early 1940s.[7] This was not entirely the case; spectators continued to flock to big games. In 1937, Chicago's annual Prep Bowl match drew an estimated 120,000 fans, "making it one of the largest crowds for any sporting event in the United States, at any time, on any level."[8] Many schools continued to benefit financially from cash receipts from football games.[9]

While high school football remained popular, however, limited funds generally did hamper the expansion of existing athletic programs. In some regions, attendance diminished. Several Pennsylvania high schools reduced the price of admission to football games from a dollar to fifty cents, yet crowds declined nonetheless as many fans still could not afford the reduced prices.[10] Tight budgets were even blamed for serious football injuries and deaths attributed to inadequate supervision, facilities, and equipment.[11]

Conjoined with prominent player deaths such as Sheridan's, the funding challenges left football more vulnerable to criticisms. A number of administrators and coaches characterized the Depression as an opportunity to refocus school athletics on student well-being. Among them was renowned football coach Pop Warner, then especially known for his success coaching star athlete Jim Thorpe at the Carlisle Indian school. Echoing President Franklin Roosevelt's call for "a new deal for the American people," in a 1933 *Saturday Evening Post* article Warner proposed a "new-deal code to restore normal, sane conditions to college and school athletics, and to football in particular."[12]

According to Warner, the transformation of football into a big business designed to generate money for academic institutions had warped the purpose of amateur athletics. To rectify the situation, he argued that "we should revalue athletics in terms of the good they can do for the athletes themselves."[13] This would involve "deflating" high school and college football. Provided it could be kept a sport and not a business, Warner expressed his expectation that football would "thrive more than ever as the great American sport, with every able-bodied youngster playing it, even in his grammar-school days."[14] Even this prominent critic of the overcommercialization of athletics, then, envisioned football as appropriate for younger children as well as high school and college students.

Meanwhile, the American appetite for football remained strong. Aided by New Deal programs, the 1930s saw the construction of infrastructure that would contribute to making football a ubiquitous sport in high schools across the United States. Throughout the duration of the Works Progress Administration (WPA), workers built or improved about 5,600 athletic fields and nearly 3,300 stadiums, grandstands, and bleachers (see figure 5). In fact, in 1946 the WPA acknowledged in its final report that there was "an early tendency to overbuild" parks and recreational buildings, given that such facilities "furnished a ready use for WPA labor."[15] Many of these stadiums were designed for high school football, frequently using a popular football-track combination design which included a quarter-mile running track surrounding the football field.[16]

Stadium construction projects provided much-needed work in local communities and were consistent with popular ideals of masculinity and civic autonomy. For example, in 1938, the WPA financed the construction of Oakley High School Stadium in Oakley, Kansas. The stadium was used to host football games and track meets since its 1939 completion by a team of unskilled laborers, primarily local farmers who were struggling financially.[17] As Holly Allen observed in her examination of gendered New Deal narratives, "highly

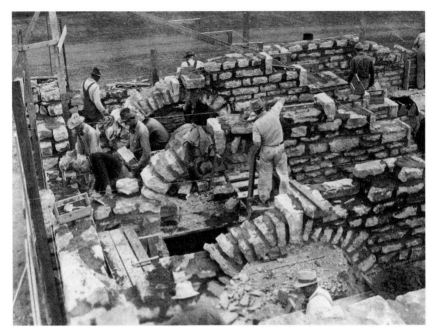

FIGURE 5 WPA construction of Cleburne High School Stadium, Johnson County, Texas, 1940. Records of the Works Progress Administration, Record Group 69, National Archives and Records Administration.

visible, tangibly productive, and affirming of project workers' masculinity, construction projects dominated the rhetoric and iconography of federal work relief."[18] The construction of football stadiums in local communities, intended for the use of men and boys to engage in athletic competitions, affirmed male workers' masculinity and self-reliance in the face of unemployment and an expanding federal government. Such construction projects also legitimized competitive sports as "wholesome" leisure activities.[19]

After the United States entered World War II, gas rationing, difficulty retaining coaches, and other constraints further threatened school sports. Many schools curtailed team schedules or temporarily suspended their football programs.[20] By the end of 1942, the National Federation of State High School Associations (NFHS) estimated that about 5 percent of the nation's schools had dropped their football programs, 25 percent reduced their coaching staffs, and 35 percent limited football team travel.[21] At one public high school on New York City's Lower East Side, more than 800 students went on strike to protest the loss of their team, indicating the importance many students attached to the football program. However, the school's principal defended the decision as a wartime necessity, explaining to students "that the suspension was inevitable and a war sacrifice that they would have to make."[22]

Yet high school football by no means ceased during this period. Neither did concerns over the sport's safety. In 1942, Logan Clendening, a nationally known physician and medical historian with a syndicated health column published in 383 daily newspapers, questioned the safety of high school football in his column. Without citing sources for his statistics, he asserted that boys who played high school football had a one in four chance of getting injured and a one in five chance of receiving a permanent injury that would last a lifetime, such as loss of teeth, a dislocated knee, or a fractured pelvis. They had a one in 1,000 chance of dying and a one in 10,000 chance of having a leg amputated, he continued. Clendening claimed that college players were at lower risk of injury due to having more mature bones and access to better protective equipment. Consequently, he argued that football should be prohibited for high school students until at least their senior year. To any coaches who disliked his views, Clendening impudently warned that football coaching was in itself a hazardous occupation, with coaches at risk for heart failure.[23]

Despite ongoing medical critiques, with the end of World War II and the easing of wartime restrictions, high school football surged. In addition to suggesting pent-up demand for football, the sport's expansion occurred in the context of increasing prosperity, high school attendance, and suburbanization.[24] In postwar southwestern Pennsylvania, for example, as area coal mines closed, schools in nearby towns lost enrollment, and nearly all became involved in school district mergers.[25] This consolidation of smaller school districts into larger, often more suburban districts—a trend that had begun before World War II and continued after the war ended—influenced the game.[26] A larger student body might facilitate the formation of a football program or make an existing program more competitive. For instance, James F. Byrnes High School was created as the result of the reorganization and consolidation of multiple schools in Spartanburg County, South Carolina, in 1950. The new high school opened in 1955 and kicked off its first football season that same year.[27] In expanding, wealthier districts, additional funding supported increasingly sophisticated football programs with such amenities as weight rooms, football stadiums, and summer training camps.[28]

Historian Michael Oriard argues that, in the 1940s and 1950s, magazine profiles of "football towns" produced a generic image of small-town high school football, implicitly symbolizing "idyllic small-town America everywhere."[29] Yet even such depictions acknowledged the big business aspect of football in these communities. For instance, a 1946 profile of the White Plains, New York, football team opened by observing the enormous economic influence of the sport: "Elevation of football at the White Plains High School to virtually a college level, with adults thronging the $2,500,000 stadium, has given to the sport such fiscal status that it is the chief support of all extra-curricular activities."[30] A few years later, the *New York Times* reported that White Plains would institute new policies, such as limiting students to six semesters of athletics, so that a boy could not deliberately postpone graduation in order to continue playing football.[31]

Critics of the commercialization of football continued to worry about the impact on children's health as well as their education. In a 1952 commentary for the *Saturday Evening Post*, former high school football coach Don Group charged schools with neglecting student athletes' physical welfare, stating that "some schools don't even go through the motions of safeguarding the boys."[32] He decried the failure of schools to implement basic precautionary measures, such as having a team physician under contract to treat injured players. Asserting that schools were "exposing boys, through negligence, to crippling injuries," Group argued that "big-time football" was harming high school students.

Despite such critiques, by the 1950s, the business of high school football was booming, sometimes even to the perceived detriment of other sports. The general manager of the Cleveland Indians baseball team reportedly felt that the appeal of playing college football among high school boys was "robbing baseball of promising material."[33] As Bob Harrell, who coached Texas high school and college football teams from 1938 to 1963, recalled, "After the war football just took off, and there weren't enough coaches to go around."[34] The NFHS secretary estimated that in 1950–1951, approximately 9,000 high schools offered football, with about 600,000 high school boys playing the sport.[35] According to the National Center for Education Statistics, 3,568,000 American boys aged fourteen to seventeen were enrolled in high schools in 1950.[36] These figures suggest that roughly one in six American boys enrolled in high school at midcentury played football.

Citizens Fit for a Dangerous World

The remarkable expansion of youth football after World War II had roots in the promotion of competitive sports as a way to prepare young American men to meet military threats. A 1940 address to the American Football Coaches Association (AFCA) provides a particularly clear example of the relationship coaches and school administrators endorsed between athletics and national defense. William Lewis Mather, president of Lafayette College in Pennsylvania, urged "the development of a generation of young men who have the red blood, who have the stamina, who have the loyalty, to protect the American way of life." No more effective group existed to meet this challenge than the coaches and administrators of college football and other sports, Mather contended. Observing that France had fallen to Germany that year because of "weakness within," he argued that athletic departments had a responsibility to build up "clean manhood" in order to preserve civilization. Whether or not the United States would ultimately enter World War II, "there isn't a chance in the world that the boys in your gymnasiums, in your locker rooms, will not be called upon, when they graduate, to participate in a tremendous economic and social and political conflict forced upon us by the totalitarian powers."[37]

Advocates for physical education and athletic competitions pointed to world events and geopolitical strife as evidence for the importance of their programs. In 1954, the president of the American Association for Health, Physical Education and Recreation (AAHPER) told the association, "In the high schools are the young men and young women who will become the workers and defenders of the nation tomorrow."[38] The threat of communism further inspired calls for improved physical education as an urgent matter of national interest and national defense. A 1954 study found that American schoolchildren fared poorly on a measure of muscular fitness as compared to European children, heightening anxieties over the fitness of American youth.[39] A 1955 *Sports Illustrated* article dubbed the research study "The Report that Shocked the President."[40] President Eisenhower invited coauthors of the study Hans Kraus and Bonnie Prudden to a White House luncheon to discuss their report.[41] Prudden, director of the Institute for Physical Fitness at White Plains, New York, told the president, celebrity athletes, sports officials, and other attendees: "American mothers are afraid of their children hurting themselves. This is a Band-Aid society. If a child breaks an arm, the arm may be in a plaster cast six weeks. That is not a catastrophe. The catastrophe is that so few opportunities for adventure remain to children—and the few that do remain are often curtailed by overanxious parents."[42]

At the President's Conference on Fitness of American Youth, convened in June 1956, Vice President Nixon warned that "we are not a nation of softies" but could become one "if proper attention is not given to the trend of our time, which is toward the invention of all sorts of gadgetry to make life easy and, in so doing, to reduce the opportunity for normal health-giving exercise."[43] In response to the concerns raised at these meetings, on July 16, 1956, President Eisenhower issued an executive order to establish a President's Council on Youth Fitness.[44]

Nixon spoke of football from personal experience. He had been an avid, though not especially gifted, player. A childhood friend recalled that Nixon "used to be the dummy for everybody to tackle. He wasn't coordinated enough for a football player. He had two left feet, I think."[45] Nixon served as "scrimmage cannon fodder" in high school and was never more than a third-string substitute on Whittier College's football team.[46] Nonetheless, he attached great meaning to his participation, invoking the experience in crafting his public persona. Nixon wrote in his memoirs that his happiest college memories involved sports, recalling, "Ever since I first played in high school, football has been my favorite sport. . . . I think that I admired [Coach Wallace "Chief" Newman] more and learned more from him than from any man I have ever known aside from my father."[47]

Eisenhower, who had played football at West Point, similarly pointed to his own athletic experience as evidence of football's importance in training men to become leaders: "I believe that football, almost more than any other sport, tends to instill into men the feeling that victory comes through hard—almost slavish—work, team play, self-confidence, and an enthusiasm that amounts to dedication."[48] His successor, John F. Kennedy, published several articles in *Sports Illustrated* lamenting the unfit, "soft American," and promoting sports to instill in youth "the vigor we need." Kennedy reorganized the President's Council on Youth Fitness and placed it under the leadership of a college football coach, Charles "Bud" Wilkinson of the University of Oklahoma (see figure 6).[49]

American presidents, coaches, and sports administrators thus framed organized football in terms of training leaders, promoting the "American way of life," and protecting the United States from foreign threats. Football could meet this need not only in schools but also in external leagues then emerging for young boys, notably the Pop Warner Conference. National Pop Warner registration certificates stated that coaches would agree to comply with the conference's standards "along lines of Scholarship, Sportsmanship and Safety First Football as a medium of inspiring the nation's youth in the American Way of Life."[50] A 1959 *Los Angeles Times* story claimed that "today, as an acceptance to the challenge to our American way of life, we have the National Pop Warner Conference teaching physical condition, religious tolerance and economic freedom principles to more than half a million youths in the country annually."[51]

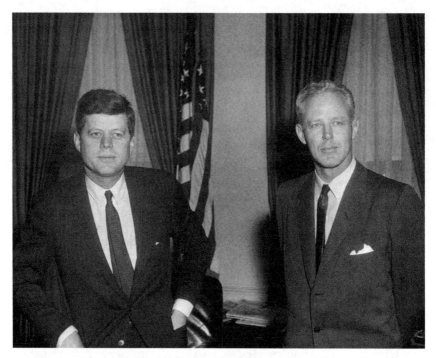

FIGURE 6 President John F. Kennedy meets with football coach Charles "Bud" Wilkinson, the new director of the Youth Fitness Program, on March 23, 1961, in the Oval Office. Courtesy of the John F. Kennedy Presidential Library and Museum.

How could the sport of football instruct young athletes in "economic freedom principles"? Football's competitive nature was portrayed as preparing boys to succeed in competitive, free market economic systems, while its nature as a team sport would prepare boys to cooperate with colleagues in their professional futures. A 1960 report on school athletics, published by a commission of the National Education Association (NEA) and the American Association of School Administrators, asserted: "We believe that cooperation and competition are both important components of American life."[52] Vice President Nixon emphasized the importance of experiencing competition and failure as preparation for adult life: "Young Americans need the fighting spirit, the determination, the teamwork and the discipline which competitive athletics inevitably instill. . . . Our young men are going to enter a competitive world where they experience failure as well as success. Let's not kid ourselves, they won't be properly prepared for life if they have been shielded from the disappointment of a failure."[53]

Football, then, would prepare boys to succeed as adults working in the American free market system. As historian David Wallace Adams put it, football was "an ideal forum for creating the new American man—half Boone, half Rockefeller."[54] Opposition to competitive sports was even conflated with support for the USSR, and football was highlighted as a particularly wholesome way to lessen the threat of communism. For example, in 1958, radio commentator Bill Stern asserted that boys "like to hoot and holler and wave pennants and if they can't do it at the football stadium you may well be sure that they will do it in the party cell."[55]

In addition to mitigating external threats, football was promoted as addressing internal problems by helping boys from marginalized groups assimilate into the prevailing American culture. Notably, at mid-twentieth century, it was believed that football could help "Americanize" children of diverse ethnic backgrounds, as historian Russ Crawford has described in his study of the use of sports to promote an "American way of life" during the Cold War. In 1946, the *Saturday Evening Post* ran a cartoon depicting a football coach telling his players, "Zablotskiwizc, play left half, Karenoftski, right half, Polkontowicz, quarterback, and you, Smith, Smythe, Smitt, however you pronounce it, fullback." This image humorously illustrated the perception that children of a variety of ethnic backgrounds were increasingly playing football.[56] Furthermore, the implied Eastern European background of players' names suggested that football could help bring children into the American mainstream who might otherwise be associated with the Communist threat. At the college level of play, sociologist Jeffrey Montez de Oca has argued that "college football in the early Cold War was most effective in opening an institutional path to men of ethnic European descent, whether as players or as fans."[57]

Prior to the integration of black and white schools following the Supreme Court's 1954 *Brown v. Board of Education* decision, many African American boys played football but in segregated "Negro" leagues that did not attract the media attention that their white counterparts received. They also received less financial support and were often less formally organized. For example, Pat Paterson, a high school coach whose career spanned from 1939 through 1967 and who founded the Negro Interscholastic League, recalled that early in his career, "players were recruited off the sandlots by both players and coaches. It was a common practice back then." After taking over as head coach, Paterson sought to make the program more rigorous and to ensure that only boys who attended school could play. In his study of African American high school football teams in Texas, Michael Hurd notes that "even the midweek scheduling of games for black teams carried a 'less than' feel." High school football competitions were traditionally scheduled on Friday nights at white schools, while black football players typically competed on Wednesdays or Thursdays.[58]

Among other nonwhite groups, high school sports sometimes represented an institutional path to racially integrated activities where other academic offerings remained segregated. For example, an examination of the racial dynamics of high school football programs in south Texas notes a policy of tracking Anglo and Mexican students into different academic curricula (with Mexican Americans placed in remedial and vocational courses) at midtwentieth century. Consequently, entertainment and extracurricular activities such as football often proved one of the limited venues where racial and ethnic mixing occurred in high schools.[59]

Even in integrated athletic programs, however, students of diverse backgrounds often "stood together but apart." For example, although yearbook photos and rosters depicted racially mixed sports teams, a 1952 photo of spectators at a high school game shows the Anglo students occupying the front rows together, with the Mexican students immediately behind them. The different groups of students observed the game together while keeping their distance. Furthermore, the time involved in attending games and practices, as well as the expenses associated with participation, deterred many of the poorest students, including predominantly Mexican migrant workers, from playing football. One man who attended Edinburg High School in Edinburg, Texas, in the late 1960s told researcher Joel Huerta that the cost of student health insurance had prevented him and some of his friends from participating in school athletics. "I just couldn't come up with the twelve bucks or whatever it was. Coach said, 'I'm really sorry, but I just can't let you go on.'"[60] Football was clearly limited in its ability to overcome major social problems. The sport was nonetheless promoted at mid-twentieth century as a way to strengthen social ties, address a perceived fitness crisis, and prepare boys to defend their country from external threats.

Anxious Mothers and Sissy Boys

From the remarks of physical education researchers to the vice president of the United States, the 1950s fitness crisis was framed in gendered terms. Overanxious mothers were portrayed as hovering over their children with Band-Aids, rendering their sons' childhoods overly secure and feminized. The view that boys needed to be toughened up by experiencing a certain amount of risk was promulgated at the highest levels in presidential fitness programs of the 1950s. As one columnist observed, boys anxious to convince their skeptical mothers to allow them to play football would likely "make full persuasive use of the fact that the President has come out strongly in favor of more competitive sports among youth."[61] Politicians and sports administrators argued that football offered growing boys the opportunity for physical contact in a modern world where gadgetry otherwise made life too easy. "I believe that competitive body contact sports are good for America's young men," Vice President Nixon told the AFCA at a 1958 luncheon.[62]

Such comments were part of a wider discourse about overprotective mothers that was influenced in particular by American author Philip Wylie. A novelist who had first achieved fame with works of science fiction, Wylie subsequently turned his pen to nonfiction. He critiqued social mores in several polemical works which "straddle[ed] a number of different genres." Wylie's best-selling 1942 book *Generation of Vipers* popularized the term "momism," defined as "excessive attachment to, or domination by, the mother."[63] Doctors, scientists and other commentators referenced and expanded on this notion in the popular press, warning of the dangers of domineering mothers stifling their children's growth. As one psychiatrist wrote in the *Saturday Evening Post,* "One can have little patience with these moms who worry constantly and needlessly about the health of healthy children. . . . Undue solicitude on mom's part is harmful."[64]

Thus, mothers were blamed not only for the illnesses and injuries their children suffered but also for being unduly protective.[65] By preventing their children from taking risks, these mothers supposedly placed American youth, particularly boys, at risk of becoming unfit. As historians Steven Mintz and Susan Kellogg have observed, "It seems clear that the underlying source of anxiety pervading child-rearing manuals during the postwar era lay in the fact that mothers were raising their children with an exclusivity and in an isolation without parallel in American history."[66]

Fathers, on the other hand, were expected to encourage their sons to take risks and to limit mothers' influence if necessary.[67] Fathers were typically assigned responsibility for preventing their boys from becoming a "sissy," which the coordinator of the New York State Health Commission defined as a child "who gets too much satisfaction from what his mother does for him and not enough from what he does for himself."[68] Tackle football would protect boys from becoming sissies by fostering male supervision and excluding feminine influence. The term *sissy* was homophobic; football was not just about making boys into men but making them into straight men. Indeed, in the 1960s satirist Russell Baker would dub young men uninterested in sports "asportual," writing that the great majority of such men "live in shame of their peculiar tastes and seek to conceal them by pretending to enjoy sports as much as the normal man."[69]

The function of American football in promoting a particular vision of masculinity was so obvious that, across the Atlantic, British correspondent Don Iddon found in football the perfect target to mock American athletes' pretensions to toughness. Whenever "American football players in their out-landish padded costumes and helmets appear on an English screen, the audience hoots with laughter," he wrote. To the British, he claimed, such protective equipment represented not toughness but cowardice and weakness. He placed the blame for such "pampering and effeminacy," of course, squarely on American mothers. "The colossal cult of the American 'Mom' and her mawk-ish devotion to her 'boys' are sapping the fiber of the American athlete."[70]

Yet the risks boys took to avoid the stigma of being a sissy alarmed some medical practitioners. Physician William Brady, who wrote a health column for the *Los Angeles Times,* warned that the fear of being perceived as a sissy was causing players to obey coaches' orders to the point of harming their own well-being. He recounted a story of a boy who had sustained a concussion while playing football and hid his constant headache for fear that he would be considered weak. The child's parents only learned of his symptoms when his vision began getting blurry, and he ultimately had to spend a month in the hospital. Brady concluded, "In my judgment no high school boy should play football—especially not interscholastic or varsity football, and certainly not under the guidance, training or influence of an outside coach."[71]

Similarly, in a 1958 article examining the dangers of high-pressure sports, journalist John Lagemann warned that "the greatest danger of permanent de-formity comes from the sports injury which is concealed because the child is afraid of being called a sissy by his coach and his fellow players." He recounted the tale of twelve-year-old Billy, who bumped heads with another player dur-ing tryouts for a junior high school football team. Billy told nobody of the resulting pain in his neck, continued to play for weeks, suffered another colli-sion, and had to spend six weeks in traction after an x-ray revealed that he had a dislocation of the first cervical vertebra.[72]

Despite these voices of caution, football was presented as offering a unique opportunity to impart masculine virtues that would ultimately pro-tect boys from greater hazards than a knock or two on the field. In a 1954 newspaper column, Columbia University football coach Lou Little asserted, "I think it's dangerous for boys *not* to play football. Nowadays, particularly, when so much courage, moral and physical, is demanded of our sons."[73] Ac-cording to this view, exposing boys to a certain amount of risk would benefit their mental and physical health and enable them to face the challenges of the modern world. In fact, competitive sports would benefit boys by teaching them to endure a certain amount of pain and that "it does not hurt to get hurt."[74]

Football for Little Tykes in the 1950s

The belief in the merits of high school football had overwhelmed concerns that the sport might adversely affect older adolescents' health or that large crowds of spectators cheering on student athletes might be troublesome in an educational venue. In fact, football had grown so immensely popular that some observers could not foresee it expanding any further. The authors of a 1951 study on the cultural diffusion of the sport speculated, "It may be that football has reached the apex of its audience appeal."[75] Yet this conjecture was quickly disproved. The numbers of spectators and participants continued to increase, and a significant portion of this expansion consisted of boys younger than high school age.

While high school football was enormously popular, younger players were much less likely to play in junior high or elementary schools. Educators were reluctant to host competitive athletics for prepubescent children. Administrators were concerned not only about safety but also about the expense of administering a football program relative to the number of students who could participate. As one school principal remarked, "Boys of this age are not ready physically or emotionally for intense competition, and a program for a few cannot be justified in terms of the amount of time and money required."[76] During the 1950s and 1960s, many professional medical and education groups expressed their disapproval of any highly organized sport, including football, for young children.[77] A notable 1952 report published by an AAHPER joint committee recommended against any "interschool competition of a varsity pattern" for children below the ninth grade.[78]

In his comments to journalists on the report, however, the committee's chair was nonetheless concerned that the committee might be perceived as overly cautious or as spoilsports. He told an Associated Press reporter, "I'd like to have the idea emphasized that we're for sports and we're for competition. I don't want people thinking we're a bunch of fuddy-duddies."[79] In their report, the committee encouraged alternative and less competitive forms of physical activity, including sports days and informal games.[80] Consistent with broader concerns about the dangers of an overemphasis on winning, a 1950 survey found that most elementary schools offered no competitive athletics for their students, and none of the schools surveyed offered any competitive sports below the fourth grade.[81]

Educators were more open to offering competitive sports at the junior high level. A survey to which 2,329 junior high schools responded found that more than 85 percent offered interscholastic athletics in the 1957–1958 school year.[82] Yet junior high school administrators were only slightly less reluctant than their elementary school counterparts to permit tackle football. A 1962 survey of junior high school administrators in California found that most believed that tackle football was not desirable for junior high school students, although three-quarters of respondents favored interscholastic athletics at this level.[83]

In fact, respondents to this survey singled out tackle football as a uniquely worrisome game. "All things considered, the consensus of opinion of the coaches at the junior high level seems to be that, except in the case of tackle football, interscholastic athletic competition is a beneficial part of the physical education program."[84] Respondents considered that football required greater supervision, protective equipment, and coaching than other sports, and that junior high schools were not able to supply the necessary support. Only 15 percent disagreed with the statement that many schools could not afford the equipment and facilities needed "to make participation in this type of competition relatively safe for their players." One respondent wrote that the sport necessitated "a great deal of specialized coaching as no one should play football unless the fundamentals have been taught rather completely."[85] Such comments suggested that administrators considered football too expensive, complicated, and unsafe to offer at the junior high school level. Consistent with these attitudes, the survey found that only 20 percent of junior high schools in the state of California competed in tackle football.

School-based tackle football programs for children before high school remained relatively limited. Yet voluntary sports organizations outside schools grew at a remarkable pace. In 1952, a joint Committee on Highly Organized Competitive Sports and Athletics for Boys Twelve and Under noted that the increase in organized sports that had prompted their work had largely occurred outside the school system.[86] In emphasizing the complexity of the subject, the committee identified some of the most notable organizations on the youth sports scene. "Clearly, no one study or research project will produce noncontroversial evidence that Little League, Pop Warner, Biddy Basketball or any of their home-grown counterparts are overwhelmingly 'good' or 'bad.'"[87]

When it came to organized youth football, the Pop Warner league was an extraordinary force. Founded in Philadelphia in 1929 by Joseph Tomlin, a former high school football player, the league was named in 1934 after the famous and influential football coach.[88] Initially Pop Warner athletes were predominantly older teenagers and adults, but during World War II the league lost most of its older players to the military. As many of its teams folded or merged, the league's finances suffered as well. After the war, Pop Warner rebounded, fielding eighty-eight teams in 1946, of which thirty-six had players aged fifteen or younger.[89] Its membership shifted toward younger players, as many returning adult service members abandoned playing football.[90]

In 1947, Joseph Tomlin opened a national office in order to establish Pop Warner football programs in Washington, Baltimore, and New York.[91] In 1956, the Pop Warner Conference decided to become an exclusively youth football association, allowing only boys aged sixteen and under to participate, and with a particular emphasis on children aged thirteen and under.[92] League organizers hoped to expand beyond the Philadelphia community and build a national football league for youth players, modeled in many ways on the success of Little League Baseball for youth baseball players.[93] In the 1950s, teams were established in Northern and Southern California.[94] By 1957, the *New York Times* reported that approximately 266 cities had engaged in Pop Warner football that year.[95]

In 1959, the conference was reorganized and legally incorporated as Pop Warner Little Scholars, a new name that reflected its focus on young players and projected an emphasis on the educational benefits of participation.[96] The league's organizers intended to promote both athletic and academic accomplishments among their "little scholars."[97] The duty of determining whether players met the minimal academic standards to participate was often assigned to one player's mother on each team. This "grade mother" was charged with "regularly reporting players' grades to the coach; those who slip below a C average are usually banished to the bench."[98]

The league's growing popularity sometimes helped to overcome long-standing rules limiting tackle football among younger children. For instance, in Los Angeles, Venice High School hosted 1958's first annual Pop Warner Football Bowl championship match. This event broke a thirty-five-year board of education rule that had prohibited tackle football by pre–high school players on school property.[99] This example suggests that even if schools were reluctant to permit elementary and junior high school tackle football under their jurisdiction, officials might allow children to play the sport on school grounds under the aegis of an external league.

Although Pop Warner emerged as one of the largest and most famous football leagues in the country, it was by no means unique. Smaller youth leagues were organized in communities across the United States by groups such as local boys clubs or the Catholic Youth League.[100] In 1956, the *New York Times* estimated that over 90,000 children were playing on 2,000 organized "midget" football teams across the United States, for children ranging from 60-pound seven-year-olds to 160-pound teenagers. This glowing article on Long Island football attributed the sport's expansion to parental realizations that it was "useless" to forbid their boys from playing. "They realize the next best thing to do is to organize the activity, provide competent supervision and buy adequate equipment."[101]

A Sport for the American Nuclear Family

News stories describing the growth of youth football in flattering terms nonetheless acknowledged parental concerns, even if only to dismiss them or to suggest they were dissipating. For instance, a 1957 profile observed that football for young children was "on the boom" in Orange County, California, "and apprehension over whether a boy in his tender years is able to absorb the bumps that go with the game as it is played in high schools and colleges has just about disappeared."[102] A favorable 1958 *Wall Street Journal* article about the increase in spending on sporting goods equipment despite an economic recession sounded one note of caution—sales of youth football equipment. "A lurking dread of football still exists in many mothers' hearts and sports manufacturers admit that the major growth in this activity for little tykes is still 'about three or four years away.'"[103]

As this comment about mothers' hearts suggests, equipment manufacturers and promoters of youth football tended to cast parental concerns about safety in gendered terms. These attitudes extended to perceptions of mothers' involvement in youth football. According to this framing, children eager to play football, coaches, and league administrators all needed to persuade anxious mothers that their boys would not be subject to great dangers while tackling. To illustrate his contention that parents were unreasonably keeping their children "aloof" from the game, a coach recounted the story of a boy who might have played football, but "the boy's mother said she would give him a Thunderbird if he didn't play."[104] This was an extreme example of the supposedly unfair and perhaps futile lengths to which mothers might go to prevent their sons from participating. One commentator observed that "well-informed youngsters" would plead to be permitted to participate in competitive sports despite "whatever mother may envision in terms of split lips or broken collarbones."[105]

Mothers not only needed to be reassured but also prevented from overly influencing the masculine game. In 1955, team coaches and managers drew up a code of ethics for the Pop Warner Conference that explicitly addressed maternal interference with the sport. A list of behaviors that "intelligent parents" would never engage in included creating "a 'Momma's boy' stigma by a mother cuddling her son in front of other players and public with words and gestures."[106] While mothers were expected to keep their distance from the field, their presence on the sidelines was welcomed as an indication of the sport's safety and support among women. "Mothers who used to be worried when their sons participated in the rough game of football now jam the sidelines and cheer their offspring onto greater effort."[107] Mothers were also encouraged to be involved in supporting the team off the field by providing financial and secretarial assistance. For example, at Niles-McKinley High School in Niles, Ohio, the "Mothers' Club" assisted in preparing the team banquet and providing money for the football program.[108]

In 1959, the *Christian Science Monitor* published an article by a reader describing her experiences as the mother of a seventh-grade football player. She cleaned uniforms, repaired damaged equipment, and drove young players and cheerleaders to the football field, concluding, "I can spend my weekends with scrub brush and detergent, working on football pants. And we feel that it is all a real family experience."[109] Similarly, the *Los Angeles Times* profiled a "Pop Warner mom," Hazel Besserer, who exemplified this ideal mother who supported Pop Warner football without threatening the masculine culture on the field. The article described the types of roles considered appropriate for mothers: preparing food and snacks, patching uniforms, listening to recitations of plays, doing clerical work, and putting together the league newspaper. Besserer recounted how the different roles of each family member could make Pop Warner football an "all-family deal": "Little sisters act as cheerleaders. Fathers act as head coaches or team fathers. And in addition to dishing out hot dogs (and advice) we gals perform as team mothers."[110] By offering roles for each member of the family, football represented a means by which Americans aspiring to cultural ideals of the suburban, middle-class, heterosexual nuclear family could strive to conform.[111]

Girls who cheered for their brothers could also have the opportunity to be judged on their poise, personality, and character. The King of Prussia Indians football team's competition for the Queen of the First Annual Indian Bowl was held in 1963. "Here are the young beauties. . . . See how good you are at judging" offered one newspaper account. The girls, aged nine to thirteen, were all either a sister of a player on one of the King of Prussia football teams, or a daughter of one of the coaches. Deborah Ann Fillman, whose mother coached cheerleaders on the eighty pound football team, won the first crown. Fillman posed for a photo "between her two comely attendants," both sisters of youth football players.[112]

While mothers scrubbed muddy football pants and sisters cheered on the sidelines, fathers were responsible for coaching boys on the field. It was not merely adult supervision that was required to ensure player safety, but a particular *male* form of supervision. Male coaches and fathers were responsible for overseeing their sons' safety but also for making them men. Male authority figures needed to "toughen up" their young charges by exposing them to a certain amount of risk, while also managing that risk so that children were not harmed. On this view, male-supervised roughness was beneficial for boys. As a reporter summarized the remarks of one university football coach, "Football is a game designed to make men out of boys. It is healthy for young men to bump heads on Saturday afternoon."[113]

Football or Fallout Shelters

Beliefs in football as a uniquely effective means to turn boys into men gained ever greater currency in the years from the Great Depression through the Cold War era. Concerns about the big business aspects of the sport remained, and tackle football's proliferation at even younger ages after World War II fostered a new set of health and educational concerns. Yet calls for limits on tackle football were ultimately obscured by the political and social culture of the Cold War. Parental anxieties were repudiated as infantilizing and emasculating boys who needed to be exposed to rough, physical contact. Locking boys in nuclear fallout shelters was even presented as the ridiculous and objectionable alternative to allowing them to tackle one another. "If your boy is or soon intends to be playing high school football, your conscience likely has acid indigestion," one article told parents. "So what shall we do? Build a fallout shelter and confine him to a playpen?"[114]

From coaches to American presidents, tackle football was widely celebrated as a physically and morally beneficial activity for boys. It was promoted as a uniquely American sport to prepare boys of diverse ethnic backgrounds to defend the nation against threats, compete as business leaders, and develop desired qualities of toughness and risk taking. Safety concerns were discounted as the anxieties of overly protective women. To reassure worried mothers, football's proponents highlighted that the organized sport was carefully supervised by adult men, who provided oversight and protective equipment. Despite decades of medical concerns, football had emerged as perhaps the preeminent embodiment of American masculinity. Football fields had become a proving ground where American boys of all ages could demonstrate that the United States was not a nation of softies.

CHAPTER THREE

Your Men Can Smash Through
Designing and Marketing Football Equipment

Nothing does as much for the status or the ego of a boy as a football helmet, one just like the college teams wear . . . Suddenly he is inches taller. Visibly tougher. Obviously a man among pros and All-Americans.
—Joan Beck, 1961

In 1905, the *Washington Post* asserted that whereas football was once a "diluted" English game with "little real meat to it," the sport had rapidly transformed into an American pastime. As evidence, the newspaper claimed that one factory was churning out twenty times more football supplies than it had five years prior. Now American cities might have two uniformed football teams on average, the *Post* estimated. Undoubtedly, manufacturers had "clothed more ambitious youngsters with canvas jackets this year than they ever have before." Football's remarkable popularity was a "common truth" that every sporting goods dealer in the United States "cheerfully granted."[1]

It was no coincidence that the *Post* framed the rapid development of football in terms of uniformed teams, factory output, and the cheers of sporting goods dealers. The proliferation of equipment certainly signaled football's popularity. But in many ways it also defined the American sport emerging at the turn of the twentieth century. The production of standardized sporting goods, in conjunction with a "network of expert coaches, journalists, administrators, manufacturers, and dealers," was increasingly demarcating the boundaries of organized athletics.[2]

In addition to defining the nature of organized football, protective equipment and its makers shaped perceptions of the sport's health effects. In conveying messages about football safety, equipment manufacturers had to carefully thread a needle. They needed to portray football as sufficiently risky to require extensive protective gear but not so dangerous that the purchase of pads and helmets could not minimize the harms. In addition, advertisements associated equipment with desirable social values for boys, such as personal fulfillment, athletic achievement, confidence, and the ability to aspire to future football careers at higher levels of play.

By mid-twentieth century, the unusually large amount of gear involved in football had been inextricably tied to the nature of the game. The equipment also proved crucial to the expansion of organized football to elementary and middle school boys. Pads and helmets symbolized the sport's dangers and, it was believed, conferred the protection necessary to render such a risky game feasible for young children. Doctors and coaches expressed concerns that innovations in equipment design presented new risks, but they were reluctant to eliminate any gear. Instead, their focus on improving equipment only reinforced its centrality to youth football. Helmets would make boys tough, and helmets would keep them safe.

Manufacturing Football Gear

The expanding production of football equipment took place in the context of a burgeoning sporting goods market. In the United States, the Sports & Fitness Industry Association, originally established as the Sporting Goods Manufacturers Association (SGMA), has long stood as the leading trade association of manufacturers and retailers of sports equipment. SGMA was founded by manufacturers of baseball supplies in New York City in 1906. Jason Fletcher Draper of the Draper-Maynard Sporting Goods Company in Plymouth, New Hampshire, was elected the association's first president.

Draper's company exemplified the late nineteenth century transition from handmade goods to industrially produced sports equipment. In 1840, Draper's father and uncle had started the business as a home workshop for tanning and glove making. By 1906, the Draper-Maynard Sporting Goods Company employed more than 100 men and women and was engaged in factory production of sporting goods for national markets. By the time SGMA was established, the mass factory production of sports equipment was already well under way, including football-specific items (see figures 7 and 8). The 1900 U.S. Census listed 144 sporting goods manufacturers (excluding bicycles and billiards), including big names such as Spalding and Rawlings, as well as many smaller firms competing for business.[3]

In its account of its own history, SGMA emphasizes its long-standing association with football safety. SGMA was founded shortly after the creation of the NCAA in response to outcry over college football injuries and deaths. Acknowledging that the gathering of athletic manufacturers was not assembled directly in response to the football injury crisis, "it is significant that the SGMA and NCAA began working together to make football, as well as other sports, as injury-free as possible."[4]

One of the most important football equipment manufacturers, however, was not established until several decades later. In 1922, John Tate Riddell, a

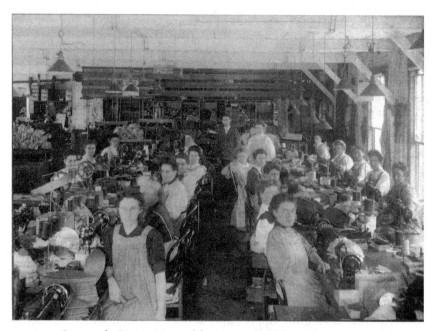

FIGURE 7 In 1904, the Draper-Maynard factory was divided into three separate divisions: baseballs, leather goods, and uniforms, with leather goods remaining the mainstay of the newly organized factory. After the leather was cut by men, it was taken to the sewing room where stitchers, predominantly women, sewed items such as boxing gloves, baseball mitts, and footballs. The stitchers shown in this image (c. 1900–1910) are in the leather sewing room for stitching footballs. Rodney Freeman, Katherine C. Donahue, Eric Baxter et al., "The Draper-Maynard Sporting Goods Company of Plymouth, New Hampshire, 1840–1937," *The Journal of the Society of Industrial Archaeology* 20 (1994): 139–51. Photo courtesy of the Ross Deachman collection.

football coach at Evanston High School in Illinois, tried to solve a problem his players were experiencing with their shoes: the wood or leather cleats nailed to the bottom of the shoes did not work in wet weather. Furthermore, the nails sometimes caused injuries. In response to these difficulties, Riddell designed the first removable screw-on cleat. He equipped his entire football team with these interchangeable, hard rubber cleats. By 1923, Northwestern University's football team was wearing them too. In 1927, Riddell decided to quit teaching and coaching, and opened his own company to manufacture the equipment.[5]

Based in Chicago, Riddell's company began by producing these new football cleats and also manufacturing the first soft-spike baseball shoe. Ultimately, Riddell's most influential innovation was not in athletic footwear but in football helmet design. In 1939, Riddell introduced the first plastic helmet,

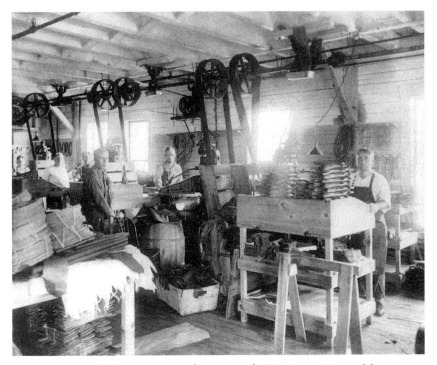

FIGURE 8 In this leather cutting room (c. 1900–1910) of the Draper-Maynard factory, football patterns are seen on the wall. These patterns were placed on leather, then pressed to cut out the shapes of the footballs. Rodney Freeman, Katherine C. Donahue, Eric Baxter et al., "The Draper-Maynard Sporting Goods Company of Plymouth, New Hampshire, 1840–1937," *The Journal of the Society of Industrial Archaeology* 20 (1994): 139–51. Photo courtesy of the Ross Deachman collection.

"the granddaddy of helmet innovations," using tenite, a tough cellulosic plastic. He further developed the sling suspension, a design that provided a pocket of air between the player's head and the hard outer shell of the football helmet. Improving the design and plastic materials required several years of additional experimentation. Gerry Morgan, who joined Riddell in 1945 and later became the company's chairman, recalled that it took until 1950 to finally obtain the right thermoplastic that could absorb impacts and withstand temperature changes. He highlighted the challenges the company faced in designing effective and comfortable helmets, observing that "the human head is the damnedest thing to fit."[6]

In addition to the technical difficulties that required time and new materials to resolve, the onset of World War II led to a relative hiatus in football helmet making. During the war, Riddell instead devoted many of its resources to military helmet production. The U.S. Army provided the company with business by adopting a modified version of their plastic helmets for paratroopers to use. After seeing a Riddell football helmet displayed in a Georgia sporting goods store, an army parachute troop officer liked the greater ventilation and safety afforded by the "off the head" style of Riddell's sling suspension design. In collaboration with the army, Riddell and his company of 150 employees made some modifications to the helmet, such as a shortening of the ear guards to facilitate the ability of parachute troopers to fire their rifles from their shoulders. Gerry Morgan recalled, "Every GI who went through training wore one and we gave [the patent] to the government for what I regret was a ridiculously low fee."[7]

After World War II, Riddell returned to its focus on football helmets. Its product line received a major boost when the company began selling helmets to NFL teams. The Chicago Rockets were Riddell's first professional customers, followed by the Cleveland Browns. In traveling with teams to adjust designs, Gerry Morgan developed a bar attached to the helmet to protect the face of Cleveland Browns quarterback Otto Graham. This development eventually led to the double bar and the face mask, which would prove to be a central point of debate over helmet safety in the 1960s. By 1949, Riddell had the largest share of the professional football market.[8]

Riddell's connections with professional football and the military helped propel the company to the forefront of football helmet manufacturing. By the mid-1970s, all NFL teams but one had their players wear Riddell helmets. Riddell's success contributed not only to the proliferation of its brand but also to establishing plastic football helmets as essential to both safety and to the style of the game. The majority of NFL athletes were modeling both the equipment and playing strategies for younger players. As the *Chicago Tribune* noted, "The Riddell name is clearly emblazoned on the front of the helmets millions of American see slamming and banging into each other on television every weekend from September through January."[9]

Riddell was unique in its prominence and specialization in football equipment but far from alone in its growth and success in the sporting goods market. Both football participation and equipment sales grew dramatically in the decades after World War II. Total U.S. consumer purchases of sporting goods equipment skyrocketed, climbing even during the recession of 1958.[10] Indeed, the *Wall Street Journal* contended that the sporting goods industry seemed to be "one of the most sturdily recession-resistant industries in the United States." Reporting that the three big producers of sports equipment—A. G. Spalding & Co., Wilson, and MacGregor—all saw sales in 1958 greater or equal

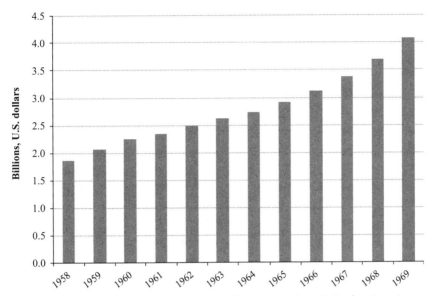

GRAPH 1   Total sporting goods sales, 1958–1969 (in billions of U.S. dollars). Adapted from Richard Snyder, "The Sporting Goods Market at the Threshold of the Seventies," National Sporting Goods Association, 1969.

to those of the previous year, the *Wall Street Journal's* staff reporters speculated that the industry might be aided by the country's youthful demographics. There were 5 million more American teenagers than even just five years prior, the leading edge of what would become known as the "baby boomer" genera-tion of children born after World War II. School athletic programs were ex-panding as a result. The sporting goods boom continued through the 1960s; economist Richard Synder found that total sporting goods sales in the United States more than doubled from 1958 to 1969. He dubbed the sales of sporting goods to be "a vast, record-breaking human endeavor."[11]

The popularity of tackle football and the amount of equipment the sport required presented a particularly promising business opportunity. Manufac-turers noted that in the fall 1958 season, more than 11,000 high schools would be fielding football teams, an increase of 1,000 schools from the previous year. Meanwhile, 100,000 younger boys were playing with the Pop Warner and National Boys Football leagues. Even at the Pop Warner level of play, the range of required equipment included helmets, pads, uniforms, and face and teeth protectors, at an estimated cost of $30 per player in 1961.[12]

Although the data do not show how many boys used this equipment to play organized tackle football as opposed to flag or sandlot games, the sales of footballs provide one way to estimate football participation. According to this measure, too, the sport's popularity continued to climb past the 1950s and through the 1960s. In 1966, according to SGMA, retail sales of footballs increased to a larger extent than any other common sporting goods item from 1960 to 1965. Furthermore, sporting goods retailers' percent of total retail trade in the United States rose from 2.4 in 1954 to 3.4 in 1968, highlighting the growth and importance of the industry to American business as a whole.[13]

Advertising Equipment

One key way that sporting goods manufacturers influenced public understanding of football safety was through advertising their equipment. In the late nineteenth century, emerging sporting goods powerhouses such as Spalding not only promoted their own brands but emphasized the need for their new industry's very existence. As early as 1893, Spalding advertisements depicted equipment produced by independent craftsmen as undermining players' performance. One such ad portrayed a baseball player struggling to round the bases in shoes produced by "some inexperienced cobbler." These advertisements argued that handcrafted gear no longer sufficed; only manufacturing firms could provide the higher quality, standardized equipment necessary for athletes to participate in organized sports.[14]

But sports ads, like ads for other products, would soon make more abstract promises related to personal values and aspirations. Sports marketing and management researchers have argued that in the 1920s sporting goods advertisements shifted from promoting product quality to more intangible appeals. This is consistent with analyses of marketing appeals in other industries. For example, Kodak did not stress the superior luminescence of its photographic film but rather highlighted the promise and satisfaction of memories preserved. Similarly, sports advertisements increasingly emphasized how equipment could enhance personal style, identity, and fulfillment.[15]

Advertisements for protective gear, however, inherently signaled to consumers that sports carried a certain element of risk. The importance of communicating that equipment could effectively minimize those risks thus interacted with the emphasis on personal fulfillment and achievements. For decades, sporting goods manufacturers consistently promoted their equipment to athletes and coaches as both protecting players against injuries and improving athletic performance.

For example, in 1935, Rawlings published a football equipment advertisement entitled "Banish fear of injuries" in *Athletic Journal*, a trade journal aimed at coaches. The subsequent text emphasized that without fear of injuries, athletes could play tougher. "Your men can smash through and play their hardest when outfitted with Rawlings equipment. . . . They'll buck, tackle and block with that air of confidence born only through banishment of injury fears." The Wilson Sporting Goods Company told coaches that "the ability of your team to win" depended on the action, protection, and comfort afforded by their lines of football equipment. Their gear included saddle-seat football pants, cantilever shoulder pads, corset-back helmets, thigh guards, and kidney pads that were built to cover players' hip bones, kidneys, pelvic bones, and lower ribs. The J. A. Dubow Manufacturing Company observed that while good football equipment alone couldn't win championships, by preventing injuries and giving players assurance, quality equipment was a key part of the "victory complex."[16]

These advertisements communicated that football equipment could minimize risks and that eliminating fear was crucial to athletic achievements. In so doing, they promoted ideals associated with particular forms of twentieth-century American masculinity. Banishing fears and inspiring confidence and toughness would enable boys to "smash through" their opponents. Protective gear facilitated such aggression while purportedly shielding players from its harmful physical consequences.

Advertisements aimed at coaches and prospective athletes promulgated remarkably similar claims through the decades. Sales pitches to younger players included an additional appeal that child athletes could emulate their older role models. Such ads became more common in the 1950s, when prepubescent boys increasingly began playing organized football. For example, in 1959, Rawlings published an advertisement in *Boys' Life*, the official youth magazine of the Boy Scouts of America. The ad featured NFL coach Buddy Parker and evidently targeted young prospective football players. Pictured next to a boy wearing a football helmet, Parker recommended Rawlings equipment, explaining that the manufacturer's helmets and shoulder pads not only protected against injury, "but they give the confidence and freedom of action needed for good blocking and tackling." Parker and the players named in the advertisement were members of the Rawlings advisory staff, and the ad promoted a "Tobin Rote helmet" and a "Bobby Layne official youth football," both named for professional football stars of the day.[17]

Even when they did not include the explicit sponsorship of professional coaches or football players, advertisements targeted at younger children emphasized that the equipment would afford youth athletes the same protection as their older football heroes. In the September 1960 issue of *Boys' Life*, for

example, MacGregor depicted a boy wearing a football helmet and a reproduction of a Baltimore Colts uniform, "just like the pros wear!" In September 1961, Wilson asked young readers if they were ready for big-time football,
stating that "Wilson gives you the same type of protective equipment worn
by leading high school, college and professional teams. You get the same helmet and pads worn by top gridiron stars, scaled to your size to give you maximum protection." Football equipment was a means by which children in
youth leagues could aspire to future high school, college, and even professional football stardom. Pads and helmets were thus imbued with many
meanings, from eliminating fear of injuries to enabling boys to identify with
football heroes.[18]

In addition to linking their equipment with athletic role models, sporting
goods manufacturers studied how to make the best use of boys' relationships
with their family. In 1958, the Institute for Motivational Research particularly
focused on fathers in its examination of sales, advertising, and merchandising
challenges confronted by the Rawlings Sporting Goods Company. The institute was an advertising consultancy firm whose founder would later be
dubbed "the patron saint of motivational research." The institute's study devoted much space to developing a "typology of paternal participants" and
how the company could craft its appeals accordingly. The study was primarily
focused on baseball gloves, but the report suggested that its findings could be
applied to Rawlings's other product lines, and even that the company should
emphasize "the continuity of sports in all seasons" by offering packages
including a baseball glove, a basketball, and a football.[19]

The report identified three types of fathers, each of whom provided a particular target for advertising appeals. The first was the "vicarious athlete," who
sought to recapture his own athletic past and participated in athletics through
his son. The vicarious athlete perceived the best equipment as enabling his
son to perform well. Secondly, the "genuine athlete" believed in the value of
sports participation as an integral part of a healthy life. Finally, the "indifferent
athlete" was a father whose primary interest was in developing a strong relationship with his child. He was thus drawn to sports not as a good in itself but
as an instrument to strengthening a father-child relationship. Identifying these
relationships as key to sporting goods purchases, the report recommended
that Rawlings craft appeals to each of these types of fathers. For example, to
appeal to the indifferent athlete father, Rawlings could produce advertisements that depicted fathers and sons in action, enjoying sports together.[20]

The October 1955 cover of *Boys' Life* depicted an idealized relationship between fathers and sons playing football, with an added twist: the two sons

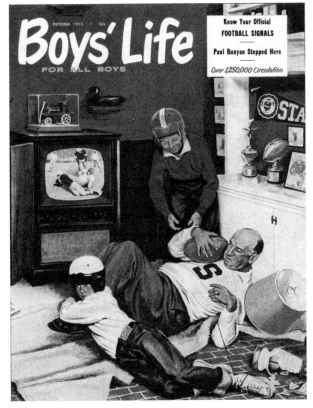

FIGURE 9 The October 1955 cover of *Boys' Life* magazine
depicted boys in protective equipment playing football with
their father in front of a televised football match. Image by
cover artist Carol Johnson. © *Boys' Life* magazine/Boy Scouts
of America.

and father on the cover were mirroring the positions of the professional football players seen on the television in their living room (figure 9). Interest-
ingly, the two sons wore football headgear but not their father. This likely
indicates that youth football was already associated with the organized version of the game that required protective equipment. Fathers, on the other
hand, were perceived as informally "roughhousing" with their sons. The *Boys'
Life* scene reinforced the importance of protective gear for youth. Helmets
protected vulnerable boys from injuries and enabled them to aspire to future
athletic success. Tellingly, the father's college football trophies and photos appear on a nearby shelf. This imagery, both in equipment advertisements and
boys' magazines, illustrated how male role models, from professional players
to fathers, could promote the desirability of youth football participation.

Yet mothers were not wholly absent from the youth sports advertising picture. They also could be vicarious athletes. The pilot study of Rawlings's marketing techniques quoted one mother as saying, "Because I was so non-athletic I'd like them [my children] to do it. I realize that I missed so much."[21] To acknowledge the interest of women in sports, and especially their role in purchasing equipment for sons or nephews as gifts, the report suggested that Rawlings stress the "whole family" appeal of youth sports. Such advertising techniques reinforced popular beliefs about women's involvement in sports, particularly tackle football, as being relegated to supplying their sons with equipment, rides to games, snacks, and other types of assistance from the sidelines. As discussed in chapter 2, tackle football was portrayed as providing a role for each member of a heterosexual nuclear family that conformed to prevailing gender norms.

Advertisements also featured numerous claims about protective equipment being scientifically designed. Although no standards for football helmets or other equipment existed before the 1970s, such claims were widely promulgated for decades. For example, in 1932, the Witchell Sheill Company advertised its "scientific football shoes" featuring "eleven points of superiority." In 1946, the Brooks Shoe Manufacturing Company promoted its "scientifically constructed shoes" which would "positively" prevent football injuries.[22] In 1947, MacGregor Goldsmith described its new plastic football helmet as "the product of many years' painstaking research and experimentation." In 1950, Spalding advertised its "scientifically padded" helmet to provide the "utmost protection." In 1954, Rawlings asserted that its helmet could dissipate "over 75% of sharp and sudden impact," providing "the Safest, Surest Head Protection ever developed for football."[23]

The basis of the claim that a Rawlings helmet could dissipate the impact of more than 75 percent of blows to players' heads is unclear. Yet many unsourced but scientific-sounding statements persisted in decades of football equipment advertising. Such techniques were certainly not limited to sports equipment. Claims promoting "scientific design," undocumented statistics about product effectiveness, and endorsements from experts were common features of many forms of American advertising in the twentieth century. Perhaps most notoriously, the tobacco industry used images and endorsements from physicians to claim that cigarettes would improve consumer health. Many football advertisements similarly drew on American confidence in scientific research and laboratory design to promote their products. In making such claims, manufacturers invoked the prestige of scientific research and medicine to sell products that addressed a broad range of health and safety concerns outside the control of organized medicine.[24]

But unlike tobacco manufacturers, whose advertisements masked the risks of an unhealthy product associated with chronic disease, sporting goods manufacturers were promoting products intended to prevent injuries. Their advertisements implicitly, and often explicitly, acknowledged that football could be a dangerous activity. Advertisers of protective gear thus had to portray a nuanced portrait of the hazards associated with collision sports: they needed to depict youth football as sufficiently risky to require the purchase of extensive equipment but not so risky as to be inappropriate for young children. Equipment ads communicated that technology and engineering were effective in mitigating risks, and often specifically emphasized manufacturers' alliances with coaches and doctors in working to protect children. For instance, a 1951 Rawlings ad for rubber-plastic football helmets highlighted that the headgear "complies fully with the safety recommendations of the American Football Coaches Association, doctors and trainers, *AND* is built with Rawlings' half-century of 'know-how.'" Such claims indicated that a combination of medical, coaching, engineering, and manufacturing expertise informing the design of protective gear afforded the greatest possible protection.[25]

Administrators, Educators, and Protective Gear

As football leagues for younger children expanded in the 1950s, organizers often emphasized the equipment that they offered—and the money they spent on it. For instance, a 1958 article on the Mar Vista Giants, a team sponsored by the Mar Vista Optimist Club and entered in the Pop Warner Midget Football League, noted that "the Optimists have spent $1250 on the club. They have helmets, face masks, shoulder pads, football pants, tennis shoes with soft rubber cleats, and purple and gold jerseys."[26] Sports administrators claimed that the "bump-absorbent material" of football uniforms worked to prevent injuries.[27] The equipment itself was a major selling point for organized play as compared to sandlot games. A 1956 *New York Times* article on organized youth football set up the story by first describing children who played unsupervised in vacant lots: "Their equipment is meager at best. Few wear helmets or shoulder pads. Most of them don't know what a pair of hip guards look like—nor do they care." By contrast, youths playing on organized teams were outfitted with "the best football equipment available."[28]

Yet the favorable press and confident advertising appeals did not convince all youth sports decision makers. Educators and administrators remained divided on the efficacy of protective equipment and the overall influence of manufacturers on football safety. A 1954 *Athletic Journal* review of debates over the value of athletic competition for children noted that Delbert Oberteuffer, who chaired the men's department of physical education at The Ohio State University for twenty-five years, was highly critical of youth football. In particular, he was cynical about the role that sporting goods manufacturers had played in promoting equipment for youth, thereby contributing to the extension of football programs for younger players. Oberteuffer argued that "the American public should know there are really only two reasons why football has been pushed down into the lower grades where it does not belong! One, so that lower grade teams can be used as a farm system for high school and college varsities; and second, so that more expensive football gear can be sold by the commercial sport goods houses."[29]

Clifford Fagan, the executive secretary of NFHS, disputed such complaints. Fagan argued that no group had made greater contributions toward the goal of eliminating sports-related injuries than manufacturers. "They maintain and staff laboratories which devote their entire efforts to the development and construction of better equipment. Today's helmets, shoes, pants and pads are so much better in every respect that they cannot be compared with those used even a decade ago." Fagan pointed to the scientific design and technological advancements underlying equipment development as fundamental to increasing safety. He contested the belief that low-cost equipment could provide an adequate level of protection, emphasizing that this misconception caused the most damage in youth sports. "You pay for what you get in athletic equipment, the same as you do for any other commodity."[30]

Fagan promulgated the same view that sporting goods advertisements disseminated: safety could be bought, and protective equipment was fundamental to safety in tackle football. While acknowledging that the added cost of colors, stripes, or other decorations did not "add one iota" to the protection afforded by a piece of equipment, Fagan nonetheless contended that apart from such unnecessary frills, "the price determines the quality. Price determines the protection." Fagan further warned against schools handing down gear from one squad to another, typically from a varsity level team to a lower-level team. He decried the practice of relying on gate receipt sales to fund equipment purchases. All players were entitled to the best equipment, regardless of their skill level or monies obtained through ticket admissions. If funds were insufficient, schools needed to use tax revenues to obtain equipment for their athletes. If such a policy was unacceptable, schools ought to drop athletic programs that they could not adequately support.[31]

Fagan's view was shared by many youth football administrators in both school settings and private leagues. When injuries did occur, better equipment was often put forth as the necessary solution. For instance, parents, industries, and service clubs donated $13,500 to get the Pop Warner Tackle Football League under way in Westchester and Playa del Rey, California. In 1957, the league's first year of existence, one boy suffered a broken collarbone. The league's vice president attributed this injury to subpar gear and told the *Los Angeles Times* that in response, "We decided to buy the best equipment. This will eliminate the possibility of any boy getting hurt because of inferior equipment."[32]

The sharp differences between Fagan and Oberteuffer's attitudes toward the influence of sporting goods manufacturers highlight fundamental tensions in safety debates related to protective equipment. Fagan praised manufacturers for developing and improving quality equipment that was essential to protecting players. He argued that schools were responsible for ensuring that all students had access to this equipment. In this view, the protective function of equipment was democratic and visible: all athletes deserved access to the same protection, and investment in top-quality gear clearly signified a program's commitment to safety. On the other hand, Oberteuffer portrayed protective equipment as a moneymaking scheme for sporting goods manufacturers. To him, investment in equipment did not represent safety but instead conflicted with the best interests of children. The proliferation of gear was a means by which business could promote and profit from the inappropriate extension of tackle football into younger age groups.

Both perspectives on the role of sporting goods manufacturers would persist in debates over the safety of youth football. Yet the embrace of manufacturers' contributions to enhancing equipment was far more widespread than cynicism about the influence of financial motives. By the mid-twentieth century, it was widely assumed that extensive equipment was an essential safety feature to which football owed its very existence. As a columnist for the *Chicago Tribune* asserted in 1950, "If such protective measures had not been adopted it is questionable whether football would have survived as one of our national sports."[33]

Improving Equipment

Along with advertisements, substantial technological developments also shaped public perceptions of equipment as essential to youth football safety.

Even with the multitude of pads and headgear already ubiquitous in tackle football, the 1950s saw calls for new and improved protective gear.

Evaluating the effectiveness of helmets in protecting brains would prove challenging, but the risk of exposed teeth to injury was more visible and more straightforward to address. With the expansion of organized football, concern about the frequency of tooth injuries led to the study, improvement, and mandate of the mouth guard. A survey of the 1950 college football season drew particular attention to the problem. This study found an 18 percent incidence of teeth chipped or knocked out among football athletes. The issue affected players at all levels, from "kids in sand lots to 'pros,'" wrote the author in *Dental Survey*. But available mouthpieces were too clumsy and uncomfortable for widespread use, making "breathing difficult and talking virtually impossible."[34]

As a result, dentists increasingly promoted the use of better mouth protection in tackle football and offered techniques for fabricating improved mouth guards. In 1954, pointing to several sources of data, including statistics he had collected at a Kansas high school, dentist Howard Dukes wrote that mouthpieces should become standard football equipment. He highlighted a 1952 *Life* magazine article on college football that had featured photographs of toothless Notre Dame football players. Dukes claimed that the images of toothless athletes had made parents "much more reluctant to allow their boys to play football."[35] Such noticeable damage to players' faces might threaten the respectability of football as an athletic option. Coaches also supported the addition of mouth protectors, with one report in *Scholastic Coach* noting that they would reduce both injuries and the costs associated with treatment.[36]

In response to these studies and concerns, the National Alliance Football Rules Committee—composed of the NFHS, the National Junior College Athletic Association, and the National Association of Intercollegiate Athletics—mandated the use of mouth guards for high school and junior college football beginning in the 1962 season. In 1964, the American Dental Association claimed that since the face guard had become mandatory, injuries in and around the mouth had declined about 50 percent. Furthermore, 99 percent of 238 high school football players surveyed agreed that wearing mouth protectors was a good way to protect the teeth. Coaches, dentists, and players thus all expressed enthusiasm about this new piece of protective equipment.[37]

Refining an older piece of football equipment—the helmet—proved much more challenging. No testing or design standards constrained what helmets could be sold to consumers at midcentury. Stephen Reid, a researcher and team physician at Northwestern University, pointed out that football helmets could be purchased anywhere from toy departments to sporting goods stores. Furthermore, "the head gear varies in quality from mere toys to the Cadillac class."[38] Through the 1960s, the American Medical Association (AMA) warned parents that helmets sold as toys could not withstand low impacts, were sharp enough to cause lacerations, and had internal padding that provided no protection on impact. The safety of children who wore such helmets was "in serious jeopardy."[39]

Many schools, particularly those that served poor or marginalized communities, could not—or chose not—to invest the money in providing their students with "Cadillac class" helmets. A 1955 study of expensive football equipment used in Texas high schools necessarily included schools willing to spend "a tremendous amount of money" on football equipment. Yet smaller schools had smaller budgets and higher rates of shoulder injuries. The study's conclusion speculated that this might be due to schools "economizing on items of equipment that were covered and unseen by the viewing public."[40] Oglala Lakota author Charles Trimble recalled of his school days at the Pine Ridge Indian Reservation in South Dakota in the late 1940s, "Our original uniforms were straight out of the Jim Thorpe era—mothball smelly, lightly padded and outright dangerous to play in. We were ridiculed by the BIA [Bureau of Indian Affairs] boarding school jocks that we were the only team around that could fold up our helmets after the game and keep them in our back pockets."[41]

In addition to warning the public about inadequate helmets, physicians called for more research in prominent medical journals. They asserted that changes in helmet construction could cut down on football injuries. In particular, the AMA's Committee on Sports Injuries, established in 1953, focused on football head injuries as one of the first problems to come before the committee. The committee encouraged "the production of a newer, safer type of football helmet." In 1957, Allan Ryan, the committee's chairman, asked Edward Dye, a safety engineer with Cornell's Aeronautical Laboratory, to prepare a set of recommended minimum performance standards for protective headgear.[42] A 1955 *Sports Illustrated* article described the available football equipment of the day as "an unscientific patchwork of steel-hard fibers and plastic which not only fails to protect the wearer but has converted him into a human battering ram."[43]

School sports administrators, too, had been calling for improved equipment for years at both the high school and college level. The September 1948 issue of the *Kentucky High School Athlete* told its readers that all school groups were interested in better, more affordable equipment, given the publicity that football injuries received and the high costs of athletic equipment. As a result, major sporting goods manufacturers were working "at top speed" to produce helmets and shoulder pads that offered greater protection, even as they cautioned against the overly optimistic belief "that certain pieces of equipment constitute a panacea which will eliminate all fatalities and serious injuries. In a contact game, it is doubtful whether all hazards will ever be eliminated."[44]

The American Football Coaches Association (AFCA), representing football coaches across the United States, also continually insisted on the importance of better protective gear, with a particular focus on helmets. Indeed, nearly two decades before, coach Pop Warner had warned attendees at the AFCA's 1931 conference that the hard material used in football headgear was contributing to injuries and that a softer material ought to be used to protect players. The strongest recommendation from the AFCA's 1946 report, in capital letters in the original, stated: "Appoint at once a qualified committee to scientifically study the construction and material used in the present headgear. This study committee, it is hoped, can recommend a headgear that will materially reduce the large number of present fatalities caused by skull fractures and cerebral hemorrhage."[45]

There is no evidence that this recommendation resulted in any action taken. Indeed, the authors of the AFCA's 1951 report would acerbically note that "there seems to be little reason for making new recommendations," because those previously submitted "were only infrequently, if ever, put into practice."[46] Nonetheless, nearly every year during the decade 1951 to 1960, the AFCA report included recommendations to initiate helmet research to improve football safety. As of 1960, however, the recommended research had not yet been published.[47] Despite all the calls for research from doctors, coaches, and sports administrators, there were few laboratories devoted to assessing athletic equipment. Neither were there significant sources of funding to conduct such research. Furthermore, evaluating the variety of available equipment posed a significant challenge. In his studies of football helmet impacts, with the hopes of ultimately identifying minimum requirements for a safe helmet, Reid reported that conditions that prevailed on the football field could not be simulated in the laboratory.[48]

A Helmet Crisis, 1961

The increasing adoption of plastic helmets among organized youth football teams in the 1950s and 1960s prompted debates over whether this new material was an improvement over preexisting leather headgear. Discussions emphasized not only which helmet provided greater protection but also which design inspired greater confidence in players, and even which might provide greater reassurance to concerned mothers.

A 1957 survey of football head injuries and protective helmets in use among Colorado high schools, for example, included an examination of arguments for plastic versus leather helmets. Coaches who responded in favor of plastic helmets felt they offered better head and neck protection but also that they were longer lasting, more attractive, liked by boys, and gave players confidence. Those in favor of leather helmets thought these were sturdier, offered better protective cushioning, and could be more economically repaired. A final argument in favor of using leather helmets, "and it is felt that this reason was offered in all seriousness, was that there was less noise when contact was made." While this reason might seem "rather amusing from the coaching standpoint, however, if women are close to the playing field it might very well be a talking point in favor of leather helmets."[49]

That a football coach would mention in such a survey the noise that plastic helmets made when young athletes collided with one another illustrates yet another way football equipment represented both danger and safety. The sound of plastic against plastic amplified the excitement of hits for spectators but also had the potential to upset those mothers perceived as needing reassurance that their boys could safely tackle one another. In the 1950s, a coach who prioritized assuaging maternal fears might still favor leather head protection. Ultimately, however, plastic helmets would be widely adopted (see figure 10), with implications for athlete safety as well as the spectacle nature of football.

In 1961, an influential medical report sparked widespread public debate about whether plastic helmets were protecting athletes. Richard Schneider, a neuroscientist at the University of Michigan, and his colleagues examined serious and fatal football injuries in *JAMA*. Reviewing the mechanisms involved in several severe football-related injuries and deaths, these researchers observed that the recently introduced rigid plastic face guards could act as a lever causing injury. One detailed case report, for instance, recounted how an eighteen-year-old football player attempting to make a tackle had his face guard struck by the knee of an opposing player. This forced his cervical spine into hyperextension, causing immediate and complete quadriplegia. Based on such cases, Schneider and his colleagues recommended several changes to the design of football helmets, including using a less rigid, more resilient material, and shortening the length of the face guard so that it would not protrude several inches from the face. The authors nonetheless concluded that

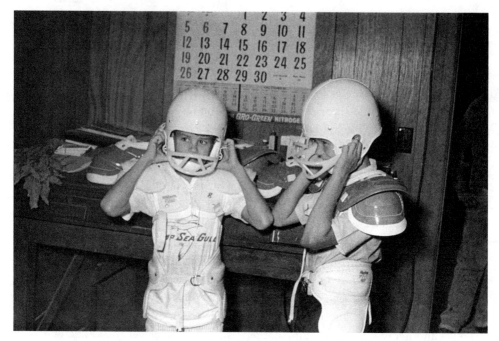

FIGURE 10 Two young boys try on football helmets and pads. The *Daily Reflector* Image Collection, September 3–4, 1965 (dates from negative sleeve). Courtesy of the Joyner Library, East Carolina University.

among the estimated 2.5 million individuals who played football in the United States each year, "there are only an infinitesimal number of fatal injuries."[50]

Despite this seemingly reassuring conclusion, the article prompted media coverage warning parents, particularly mothers, of the disturbing finding that helmets might not always enhance safety. The *Chicago Daily Tribune* presented the scenario of a young boy deriving a sense of pride and toughness from his helmet, while his concerned mother felt relief at the protection it provided. As the mother watches her son playing in "organized games that start as young as the sixth grade in some communities, she thinks: At least the helmet will protect him from hurting his face or head." Not so, the article frighteningly continued. Instead, the football helmet could represent an added danger and even serve as a vicious weapon on the field.[51] Meanwhile, Jim Murray, a sportswriter with the *Los Angeles Times*, observed that "something depressing has happened to Football, 1961. . . . the sudden boom in head and neck injuries may speed a day when a team won't need a head coach so much as a head neurosurgeon nor a bench so much as an operating table." He went so far as to warn his readers that "football is creeping up on reckless driving as an important cause of death in this country," an ominous observation based on a common comparison, as described in chapter 5.[52]

Much of the debate centered on whether the recently introduced plastic helmets with face guards increased or decreased the risks as compared to their older leather counterparts. Sportswriter Bob Addie suggested that the new plastic helmets, when used as weapons by players, "may be more harmful than all the broken noses and facial injuries" that the face cages were intended to prevent. "It's a 15-yard penalty to grab a runner by the cage but the penalty may be small, indeed, when compared with the damage which could be caused by a head snapping back."[53]

Some coaches of youth and college teams argued that the transition from leather to plastic helmets had actually increased the risks. The athletic director of the University of Tennessee told the *New York Times* that the NCAA was concerned that an uptick in head and neck injuries might be due to modern equipment.[54] A football coach at the University of Denver agreed: "There is a real question whether plastic head guards are the cause of an increased number of accidents."[55] Coaches observed that the hard, unyielding plastic magnified the impact of the equipment when a player's head collided with part of another player's body. Another college coach characterized the plastic helmets as "devastating weapons" and recommended a return to their leather predecessors.[56] In 1962, Mal Stevens, orthopedic surgeon and former football player and coach, told the *Boston Globe* he thought plastic helmets ought to be outlawed.[57]

But in an article for the *Journal of School Health*, Clifford Fagan, the executive secretary of the NFHS, disagreed with claims that returning to the use of leather helmets might reduce injury rates. "As a matter of fact, the consensus of experts is that the return to the use of the leather helmet would be taking a step backward. The plastic helmet is, at the present time, providing the best protection available."[58] Ultimately, some observers argued, protective equipment was not the primary culprit for the game's risks. Instead, coaches themselves needed to take more responsibility for limiting the brutality of football. Writing for the *Los Angeles Times* and referring to a major sporting goods company, sportswriter Jim Murray argued that "the character of the game itself is up to the coaches, not A. G. Spalding."[59]

Sporting goods manufacturers, too, assigned responsibility to coaches for upholding the "character of the game." In the following years, they would join doctors, trainers, and sports administrators in decrying the dangerous technique of using the helmet as a weapon, also known as "spearing," that was associated with the introduction of plastic helmets. Manufacturers emphasized that their product should not be considered responsible for such risks. In a

1976 interview with the *Chicago Tribune*, Gerry Morgan continued to blame high school coaches who taught such dangerous strategies. He lamented that the more manufacturers had improved equipment, the more "it seems it's been to the detriment of the game."[60]

Coaches, in turn, emphasized the importance of their profession in addressing equipment concerns. "We've certainly got to find out whether any weakness in equipment or in training can be overcome so we can better protect these youngsters," insisted Jack Curtice, president of the American Football Coaches Association. Curtice further speculated that the problem might be attributable to a lack of proper adult supervision. "We've been pushing sports competition for our youth so much maybe we haven't enough trained people to supervise it in our growing population."[61]

In the wake of the 1961 media outcry over injuries, in May 1962, the AMA sponsored a national conference on head protection for athletes in Chicago. All the presentations addressed issues related to head protection in football. Despite the focus on helmets, an introduction describing the problems posed by the conference topic sounded a skeptical note about the ultimate safety benefits such equipment might offer. An examination of the mechanics of head impacts and protective helmets, observed the authors, "discloses that we are severely limited in the protection which can be afforded even with ideal materials and design."[62] Doctors and engineers questioned how much protection even an optimal helmet might afford the players who "smashed through" one another on the gridiron.

Although not everybody agreed that plastic helmets were providing the best protection available, by mid-twentieth century nearly all adults involved in football seemed to agree on the centrality of equipment to injury prevention. The nature of particular debates was influenced by the equipment in question. The prevention of dental injuries was both particularly urgent and relatively easy to assess given the visibility of tooth damage and loss. Data on mouth guards clearly indicated their effectiveness, and their introduction to the sport proved largely uncontroversial. On the other hand, changes to helmet design proved far more contentious, particularly given the lack of clear data both on head injuries and on helmet effectiveness. But even amid fears that plastic helmets might in fact be dangerous to their users and other players who came into contact with them, eliminating helmets was not offered as a solution. Instead, helmets needed to be improved upon with different materials or a different design.

Protective equipment had proven central to the early development of football and its mid-twentieth century expansion to elementary and middle school players. The gear was associated with the increasing organization of youth leagues and the emphasis on adult supervision to protect youth. Pads and helmets also enabled the very aggression that both raised those safety concerns and appealed to ideals of a tough form of masculinity. Successful marketing efforts frequently celebrated the potential for hard hits on the field made possible by sturdy pads and helmets. These collisions conveyed the kind of manhood to which a young boy might aspire by playing football. In many ways, football equipment fostered a vicious cycle: equipment innovations enabled greater force and aggression, which created a perceived need for even more equipment. In so doing, protective gear represented coexisting American attitudes toward football. Adults wanted to protect young players, while also wanting to see boys deliver ever harder and more dramatic hits.

Part II

Understanding and Preventing
Football Injuries

CHAPTER FOUR

The Duty of Their Elders

Doctors, Coaches, and Safety Expertise, 1950s–1960s

Whenever young men gather regularly on green Autumn fields, or Winter ice,
or polished floors to dispute the physical possession and position of various
leather and rubber objects according to certain rules, sooner or later somebody
is going to get hurt.
—Thomas B. Quigley, 1959

In 1959, Carl Willgoose, a professor of health and physical education, was
alarmed by a growing trend of football teams with younger players. Boys were
no longer waiting until high school to don pads and helmets. Writing for the
Journal of School Health, Willgoose noted that in Nassau County, New York,
a single village football league would attract hundreds of boys to a call for
players. "There is a pee wee division for 10 year olds, a junior varsity division
for 11 year olds, and a midget division for 12 year olds. . . . Football for younger
boys may already be here to stay."[1] "Pee wee" football raised a different set of
health and safety questions than other popular organized youth sports, such
as Little League Baseball.

Willgoose was uncertain whether football was a medically sound option
for children. He was concerned about physical injuries as well as emotional
health. Small boys were playing "under the kind of pressure conditions which
involve newspaper displays, athletic editorials, large adult crowds in attendance, and a game tension comparable to high school or college athletics."
Willgoose concluded with a call for research to examine whether the health
benefits of highly competitive contact sports for young children outweighed
the risks.[2]

Indeed, the growing number of boys younger than high school age playing
football in private leagues was of increasing public and medical concern. "He is
somewhere between 8 and 14, and he wants to play football. In fact, he is playing football. Is it good for him?" asked the *Chicago Daily Tribune* in 1955.[3] Parents looking for an answer to this question solicited medical advice and also
looked to educators, football coaches, and sports administrators for guidance.

With more elementary and middle school aged boys playing organized
football in the 1950s and 1960s, adults supervising the game needed to address

its risks and defend its benefits for young children. Examining how doctors and football coaches established their professional authority on youth football reveals how their justifications for this collision sport were connected to broader cultural trends. The framing of football's risks was influenced by beliefs about the moral value of youth sports, and expertise on the subject was gendered. Doctors and coaches, who were virtually all men, emphasized their firsthand knowledge of an all-male sport that was widely promoted as a means of teaching boys to become men.

Furthermore, there was significant overlap between these groups of adult male authorities: many doctors who conducted research into football injuries were also involved in supervising the sport, as either coaches, team physicians, or parents. The tension between promoting football and studying its risks influenced how many doctors and coaches conceived of the dangers and constrained the solutions they proposed.

Largely lacking epidemiological data on risk factors for injuries, doctors and coaches instead based their views on youth football safety on other sources. These included available tabulations of injuries and deaths, extrapolation of this data to younger populations, clinical experience, and personal experience of the sport. On these bases, doctors and coaches each sought to establish their authority on matters of youth football safety. They conveyed health information to parents and described strategies for making the game safer.

In so doing, doctors and coaches promoted the perspective that football could be made sufficiently safe for young children to play. Protective equipment featured prominently as a safety strategy. Medical advice to prevent injuries frequently focused on making athletic trainers or physicians available to youth teams, requiring physical exams for athletic participation, and increasing the involvement of football coaches and parents to supervise youth. This emphasis on adult supervision, or "supervisory imperative," necessarily contained an element of self-interest: doctors and coaches argued for expanding the role of doctors and coaches.[4] This supervisory imperative was also informed by the promotion of competitive athletics as a means for adult men to transmit particular cultural values to young boys.

Counting Injuries

Since the emergence of tackle football, doctors had commented on the sport's health effects, often emphasizing the particular vulnerability of youth. For example, a 1907 *JAMA* editorial highlighted that out of the fourteen football players killed that fall, none had been over twenty years in age. The editorial concluded that there need be no hesitation "in deciding that football is no game for boys to play."[5]

Through the early decades of the twentieth century, several doctors published reports in leading American medical journals on the football injuries they had observed in their practices. Physicians who were most likely to observe football injuries included orthopedists, surgeons, pediatricians, and school physicians. Doctors affiliated with schools that had football teams tended to serve predominantly white, wealthy communities. Colleges were most likely to have a school or team physician to look after their athletes, although some elite prep schools did as well. But public secondary schools often did not have such medical staff able to treat and track injuries. Consequently, youth football injuries were probably greatly underreported, and published injury counts generally did not include high school players at less affluent schools. Nonetheless, these counts represent important early efforts at documenting football injuries as a medical concern.

For example, in the 1930s, Thomas N. Horan served as a resident physician at Cranbrook School. At this private boys' preparatory school in Bloomfield Hills, Michigan, 80 percent of the boys played football. In 1934, Horan reported on the number and types of injuries he had seen among Cranbrook students playing in the previous four football seasons (1930–1933). He observed the most commonly injured regions of the body (fingers, hands, ankles, muscles, knees) and offered recommendations such as warm-up exercises before games and the use of protective padding and Ace bandages.[6]

At Phillips Academy, an elite preparatory school in Andover, Massachusetts, school physician James Roswell Gallagher also reported on the athletic injuries he had seen. Based on data from 1940 to 1947, Gallagher found that varsity football had the highest incidence of major injuries per player, followed by junior varsity football. Combined, these two levels of football averaged more than twenty times as many major injuries per player as did soccer or lacrosse. Knee and head injuries in football were of particular concern. To prevent knee injuries, Gallagher suggested calisthenics, taping, and the exclusion of players whose "state of development and linear build" made them vulnerable. Head injuries, on the other hand, were more difficult to control. "The best in helmets and the proper fitting of helmets is the least, and perhaps the most, that can be done," acknowledged Gallagher.[7]

In this article, Gallagher insisted that he was not concerned with the "relative merits" of the particular sports he studied but rather with documenting the types of injuries one might expect.[8] In fact, however, he had previously expressed concern about football in school settings. By the 1930s, the rapid expansion of competitive high school sports had resulted in intense debates over the nature of interscholastic athletics. As Heather Munro Prescott observed in her history of adolescent medicine, Gallagher felt the physical education department at Phillips Academy was more preoccupied with creating a winning football team than fostering physical fitness among all its students. He therefore persuaded the headmaster to allow him to take control of the physical education department and in the early 1940s redesigned the program to provide each student with an individualized exercise regimen. The particular needs Gallagher observed among his teenaged patients, from athletic injuries to mental health concerns, eventually led him to become a central figure in the development of adolescent medicine.[9]

At the college level, Augustus Thorndike Jr., who served as physician to Harvard University's athletic department beginning in 1926, was one of the most prominent doctors to report his medical findings on the sidelines. His articles and monographs contributed to the development of sports medicine as a subspecialty. In a 1938 *New England Journal of Medicine* article, Thorndike wrote that he had observed the most serious injuries in informal games or individual recreation, such as skiing, baseball, and polo, rather than organized football. Even so, he wrote, more individuals were participating in sports, such that more injuries were to be expected. Doctors would need to be responsible for preventing recurrent minor injuries.[10]

In 1940, one week after Thorndike published another review of common athletic injuries, *Time* magazine profiled the doctor's work. While most sports injuries were slight, Thorndike acknowledged that "more accidents occur in football per playing hour than in any other game." Nonetheless, *Time* claimed, nobody was more vehement than this eminent physician, himself a former Harvard football player, about the physical benefits of athletics.[11] Rather than arguing for limitations on athletic participation, he supported medical supervision to protect athletes.

Thorndike's perspective was hardly unique. Doctors overseeing youth athletics typically promoted the overall benefits of organized contact sports. They saw their supervisory role as ensuring that participants could continue to enjoy the health benefits. Even those physicians without any athletic team affiliations, and those who were most concerned about the physical risks of football or boxing for young children, hastened to make clear that athletic competition could not and should not be eliminated. Following World War II, Cold War fears of socialism further amplified this belief: "Competition is part of our American way of life," emphasized pediatrician George Maksim in a 1958 *JAMA* article on youth athletics.[12]

Professional Responsibility and "Natural" Hazards

The belief in the value of organized sports was widespread in American society, including among medical professionals. Yet team physicians occupied a particularly ambivalent position, in some ways reminiscent of the dilemma that company doctors faced while studying occupational illnesses. Company doctors' duty to their employers was in tension with their duty to their patients.[13] But unlike company doctors, who were paid to be held accountable to corporate employers, most doctors and coaches serving youth football teams were volunteers. Their potential conflict of interest was not financial but rather ideological. The team physician's very role compromised the equipoise that would be needed to assess the real risks of the sport. In other words, doctors serving school athletic teams may have underestimated the risks of youth football because they believed a priori in the value of the sport.

In this sense, football coaches were in a similar position to medical doctors. Their role inherently involved both promoting football to the public and protecting players' well-being. Coaches naturally expressed faith in the value of competitive athletics. But amid public concerns over athletes' deaths and football's overall safety, coaches found it essential to demonstrate that they were addressing injuries. As a means of showing that football could remain beneficial, coaches sought to track deaths and severe injuries themselves through the AFCA.

In December 1921, college football coaches had formed the AFCA in part due to their alarm over the professionalization of the sport. As John Sayle Watterson recounts in his history of college football, coaches expressed moral opposition to students profiting from their football talents. But the coaches also feared the threat that the American Professional Football Association, recently established in 1920 and renamed the National Football League in 1922, posed to the college game. Ironically, in professing their disapproval of student athlete professionalism, American football coaches created their own professional organization, which functioned to legitimize their expertise and further professionalize football.[14]

AFCA members saw a need to formally address concerns about football's safety. At the association's 1931 annual meeting, renowned football player and coach John Heisman told the rules committee in an open discussion that football-related deaths occurred every year, "And what are you going to do about it? You cannot just laugh it off and you cannot just argue it off. That is not the way the public and the press are built."[15] In 1932, president Mal Stevens explained that the AFCA had deemed it wise to embark on a study of the sport's safety "so that we would be in a position to either answer the criticisms which have been directed at us, be able to refute them, or to acknowledge the criticisms as just and try to improve the game from a coaching standpoint." While in ensuing years the AFCA would make changes to the particular format of the survey, the organization would continue to collect information on football injuries and deaths every year.[16]

With the cooperation of the AFCA and NCAA, and the financial support of insurance underwriters, Stevens coauthored a 1933 text, *The Control of Football Injuries*, with Winthrop Phelps, an orthopedic surgeon at Yale University. Stevens and Phelps reviewed medical treatments for different types of football injuries and included appendices with several surveys of football injuries and deaths. Although their examination of Yale varsity football injuries revealed that "the per cent of football candidates injured is uniformly high," Stevens and Phelps hastened to clarify that not all of these injuries were "significant."[17] Moreover, they introduced their study by objecting to the recent "wave of public hysteria" over football injuries and contended that the "bumps and bruises" of football were worthwhile "in that they teach the youth of our country how 'to take it.'" Combining coaching and medical perspectives in response to public concerns, *The Control of Football Injuries* described football's physical risks, downplayed their severity, and reinforced beliefs about football's value in fostering toughness in boys.[18]

More broadly, coaches were responsible for serving as ambassadors for their sport while also overseeing the physical regimens of their players and maintaining the health of their teams. Coaches such as John Heisman, Vince Lombardi, and Pop Warner were celebrities in their own right. A photograph of Mal Stevens signing a football for two girls at New York's 1939 World Fair indicates the public profile that many football coaches enjoyed, particularly at the college level (see figure 11). The multiple roles that coaches occupied were further compounded when they had other careers as athletes, physicians, or both. Mal Stevens, a former football player as well as a coach, would go on to a career in orthopedic surgery treating sports-related injuries.

At the high school level, NFHS oversaw interscholastic sports, including football, in participating member schools across the United States. While the NFHS did not have its own separate survey of injuries and deaths comparable to the AFCA's, the organization did periodically share available safety statistics with its membership. At its December 1948 annual meeting, NFHS presented football injury counts from an insurance company study. The company reported these statistics according to several factors, such as player's position, age, date, and the nature of the competition (game versus practice).

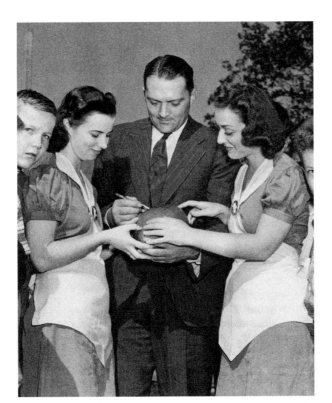

FIGURE 11 Mal Stevens, former president of the AFCA, signs
a football for two girls at the New York World's Fair in 1939.
Courtesy of Manuscripts and Archives Division, New York
Public Library.

But these numbers were useful neither for calculating rates nor for evaluating
whether any of these factors were meaningfully associated with injuries. For
example, the highest percentage of injuries occurred among seventeen-year-
olds (see table 1). However, the high percentage was "due to the fact that a
large majority of high school players are of that age." Without knowing how
many athletes of each age had played tackle football in total, and how many of
the players out of this sample had been injured, such numbers were not useful in assessing a meaningful indication of risk.[19]

Moreover, systematic epidemiological analyses to identify risk factors associated with football injuries and deaths remained limited to nonexistent. In
fact, the very notion of injury prevention as a field of public health inquiry
was new. An injury epidemiologist whose career began in the 1950s recalled
that "the literature on epidemiology and injuries before the 1960s was

TABLE 1 Football injuries by age, security life and accident company

Age	Percent of Total Injuries
Under 16	25.5
16 years	28.7
17 years	38.5
18 years	5.3
19 years	1.5
20 years	0.5
Total	100

Adapted from table in H. V. Porter, "National Federation Annual Meeting," *Scholastic Coach* 18, no. 6 (1949): 44–46; 60.

sparse."[20] Studying injuries systematically required a shift from a prevailing view of injuries as random or unpredictable "acts of God" to an understanding of injuries as predictable and preventable occurrences. The attitude that football injuries were "natural" mishaps that could not be avoided was even evident in some of the language used by doctors studying them. For instance, in a 1935 review of football injuries, New Orleans surgeon Lucian Landry cited an analysis finding that over a quarter of the more serious football injuries might have been preventable with greater attention to coaching, the players' condition, and the quality of the playing fields. Nonetheless, he concluded that the remaining majority of football injuries were "natural hazards": an inherent part of the game that one could not expect to prevent.[21]

A Kid's Sport: Sports Medicine and Pediatric Expertise

In the 1950s and 1960s, researchers increasingly began to attribute injuries to dangerous environments or poorly designed systems, rather than happenstance or the carelessness of individuals. Historian John C. Burnham has argued that the very term "childproofing," which emerged in the 1950s, illustrated this new understanding that engineering solutions could protect the safety of children.[22] The 1964 publication of *Accident Research: Methods and Approaches*, a new textbook devoted to the epidemiology of injuries, was an important landmark.[23] Another key development was increasing attention to preventing automobile-related injuries, highlighted by the 1965 publication of Ralph Nader's *Unsafe at Any Speed*.[24]

Doctors pointed to advances in other fields in order to call for similar organized efforts to address injuries among athletes. For example, Augustus Thorndike introduced a 1956 article on sports injuries with a discussion of James P. Mitchell, the U.S. Secretary of Labor. Mitchell had drawn public attention to the importance of preventing occupational injuries and deaths that affected nearly 2 million workers. Despite continuing "appalling numbers," the disability rate among American workers had declined from 1943 to 1954, a visible success for labor, industry, and insurance groups. Yet, Thorndike continued, in contrast with efforts to enhance worker safety, "one can observe little organized endeavor on the part of coaches, trainers, and others in the field of sport to institute training programs along the same lines."[25]

In conjunction with the growing prominence of injury prevention in workplaces and on the roads, sports medicine and related medical fields began to grow more organized and specialized. The National Athletic Trainers' Association was founded in 1950, and the American College of Sports Medicine (ACSM) was founded in 1954.[26] Historian Jack Berryman argues that the subspecialty of sports medicine had its origins in physical education, physiology, and cardiology, and was particularly influenced by military research and rehabilitation during World War II.[27] In 1960, the AMA developed a Committee on the Medical Aspects of Sports.[28] As the subspecialties of injury prevention and sports medicine developed, the issue of athletic injuries became increasingly visible.

The growth of sports medicine in the following decades also required its practitioners to confront the competing nature of their obligations. In 1975, several sports medicine experts participated in a roundtable discussion of the legal, ethical, and moral questions involved in their field. One panelist, a general surgeon and team physician for the Cleveland Cavaliers, observed that the team physician's first obligation was to the player. Even so, "the physician also has an obligation to the coaches, or in professional teams, the owners, because he must help obtain the maximum function of an athlete."[29] Expressing this perception more colloquially, one reporter would describe team physicians as "a combination of Dr. Spock and Dr. Feelgood."[30]

Sports medicine thus seemingly occupied a compromised position as a medical field. Its objectives included not only protecting player health but also improving sports performance. Nonetheless, the medicalization of sports-related injuries lent greater professional authority to trainers and doctors. A 1965 news story highlighted the increasingly scientific nature of athletic training. Whereas athletic trainers had once primarily dispensed aspirin and rubdowns, marveled a *Chicago Tribune* sports reporter, they now "bandied about and absorbed technical terms that would send Dr. Ben Casey scurrying for his medical dictionary."[31]

Despite this new scientific veneer, and despite the availability of some earlier survey data from insurance companies,[32] large-scale systematic studies of football injuries and injury prevention techniques remained rare. Doctors and coaches had repeatedly called for better data, but medical societies, funding agencies, and public health organizations had not developed formal centers or programs that would support systematic research on youth sports injuries. In 1959, George B. Logan, who would later serve as the president of the American Academy of Pediatrics (AAP), noted that "there is remarkably little factual material published on the injury rate among children engaged in various sports."[33] As late as 1964, the author of a *JAMA* article on high school football injuries observed that "no data have been gathered which demonstrate which parts of the game or equipment are responsible for the injuries."[34] A 1966 AAP report stated that sixty-five boys had died directly as a result of participating in high school football from 1960 to 1964, a figure that highlighted the need for research. "The actual amount of morbidity and mortality is unknown but is significant enough to raise serious questions about contact sports for youth who are too young, physically inadequate, or improperly protected by inadequate gear."[35]

Even without more in-depth data, such tabulations of deaths and severe injuries troubled many doctors and educators. Several leading medical and educational organizations already felt compelled to oppose football for prepubescent children. In 1953, the NEA hosted a two-day conference in Washington, D.C., on program planning in games and sports for young children. The forty-four delegates in attendance recommended banning football and other contact sports for children aged twelve and younger. Pediatrician George Maksim, representing the AAP, argued that "the risk of permanent bone and joint injuries is just too great." Joe Tomlin of Pop Warner football was the lone representative to vote against recommending a ban on football and other body contact sports. As the coordinator of the conference reported, Tomlin stated that he had founded Pop Warner "to get the children off sandlots and into a supervised program that stressed proper equipment and coaching."[36]

Leaders of youth football leagues naturally dissented from banning football, but leading medical organizations were not persuaded of organized football's overall benefits for youngsters. In the decade after the NEA conference, many doctors continued to object to football for young children. In 1957, the AAP's Committee on School Health, which had been founded in 1931, published a policy statement on competitive athletics for children twelve years or younger.[37] According to the statement, due to children's susceptibility to bone and joint injuries, "body-contact sports, particularly tackle football and boxing, are considered to have no place in programs for children of this age."[38] In 1960, *Time* magazine ran an article examining doctors' perspectives on organized sports and quoted several physicians who emphasized that collision sports such as football could not be made appropriate for young children. "Cutting down the field and changing the rules doesn't make football a kid's sport."[39] The November 1960 *Bulletin of Westchester County's Medical Society* published an editorial calling for limiting football among preadolescent children, stating that "one permanent deformity as a result of such activity is an unwarranted risk."[40]

Doctors and educators who believed that any permanent deformity resulting from youth football was unjustified had little data to indicate just how severe or minimal this risk might be. Yet during this period, medical concerns about football for growing children focused a great deal of attention on bone and joint injuries. Consequently, in addition to pediatricians, orthopedists were particularly vocal in their opposition to tackle football. Of 403 orthopedists who responded to a 1947 questionnaire on the safety of competitive sports, only 19 indicated that they considered football safe for participation for the junior high school age group. Yet 153 respondents considered boxing safe, and 235 approved of touch football.[41] One survey respondent observed, "I believe it is a tragic situation when any school permits the students to participate in football in the 10th grade or below."[42]

Indeed, doctors offered relatively few objections to the physical risks of high school football among older teenagers. The entrenchment of football in high schools likely influenced medical perspectives. At mid-twentieth century, it may have been more culturally feasible—or even merely conceivable—for doctors and educators to contest the novel expansion of football to younger ages, rather than challenging the widely accepted place of football in high schools.

Yet doctors' and educators' objections did little to stem the extension of little league football programs to include younger children. Competitions sponsored by private organizations proliferated. According to Hollis Fait, an instructor in physical education at East Oregon College of Education, "Almost without exception the literature which has appeared has been in opposition. Many physical educators and professional groups have gone on record opposing interscholastic competition for pupils below the tenth grade. Yet the practice continues."[43] Strikingly, the recommendations of professional societies such as the AAP against football among elementary and middle school aged children went largely unheeded. That pro-football arguments overshadowed the exceptional degree of cultural authority American physicians had attained at mid-twentieth century underscores the growing social power of competitive youth sports during this period.[44]

The Burden of Proof

Given the safety concerns, who had the authority to interpret the available medical evidence and evaluate the risks and benefits of youth football? A comparison of the perspectives of John Reichert, an assistant professor of pediatrics at Northwestern University Medical School, and Creighton Hale, the director of research and vice president of Little League Baseball, Inc., illustrates this contentious issue. In 1958 and 1959, Reichert and Hale each authored lengthy examinations of existing research on competitive athletics for young children. The contrast between their perspectives reveals a contest over which evidence was considered reliable, who had the authority to best interpret the evidence, and where the burden of proof ought to lie. It also indicates a growing divergence between pediatricians and academic physicians on one hand, and sports doctors, researchers and administrators on the other. The increasing professionalization of coaching and sports medicine introduced different professional imperatives in assessing the risks and benefits of youth sports.

As an assistant professor of pediatrics, previous chair of the AAP's Committee on School Health, and member of the city of Chicago's Board of Education, Reichert exhibited an extensive interest in school health. In 1958, Reichert characterized his perspective on the debate over competitive athletics for children younger than thirteen in *JAMA*. While acknowledging that the lines were not too clearly drawn, he nonetheless described two distinct groups as standing on each side of the issue. On one side, Reichert wrote, were people who believed that some limitations should be placed on competitive athletics for young children: "In this group are the majority of educators and physicians who have studied the issue." On the other side stood a group largely composed of "sports promoters, professional athletes, sports fans, and some coaches" who considered highly organized competitive sports desirable for young children.[45] Reichert observed that more research would be needed to clarify the long-term impact of athletic competition, but in the meantime, "one must doubt the claim that the stress of competition promotes optimum growth and development."[46]

In the face of scientific uncertainty, Reichert counseled that the preponderance of medical opinion favored a cautious approach. Much of this uncertainty specifically centered on tackle football. As safer alternatives, Reichert recommended touch or flag football for children. To support this opinion, he cited a personal communication from Eddie Anderson to Fred Hein, both physicians with interest and experience in youth health and fitness. In fact, Anderson was a successful college football coach at the College of the Holy Cross who had also earned a medical degree and who would later be inducted into the College Football Hall of Fame. These experiences lent him credibility as an authority on both football and health, and Anderson had observed that touch football would be a better training program for preteenagers than tackle football. Further citing an NFHS handbook, Reichert wrote that "about 60% of all injuries occurring in tackle football occur while tackling or being tackled," and that a switch to supervised touch or flag football would eliminate these injuries. He concluded that his recommendations were based on "the considered judgment of the majority of capable professional educators and physicians who have studied the problem."[47]

Not surprisingly, sports organizers disputed such assessments. Creighton Hale, vice president of Little League Baseball, characterized efforts to discourage competitive athletics for pre-high school age children as a "crusade." Hale, a prominent youth sports administrator, was also a physiologist with interests in sports safety research. A former athlete himself, Hale had attended the University of Nebraska on a track scholarship. Before joining the Little League organization as its director of research in 1955, Hale had earned a doctorate in physiology and conducted research at Springfield College. He would design a batting helmet to cover the full head and ears and would later serve as the president of Little League Baseball.[48]

Hale's 1959 article for the *Journal of Health, Physical Education, and Recreation* observed that medical professionals' studies had thus far been largely limited to opinion pieces and review articles. Hale criticized how "the armchair philosophers and the encyclopedic researchers, utilizing their intuitive knowledge and the crystal ball," had transformed competitive athletics for young children into the most controversial topic of the 1950s for the American Association of Health, Physical Education, and Recreation. Though he also noted that more studies were needed, Hale contended that the available research was favorable toward the educational value of athletic competition. He wrote that children who participated in competitive sports attained higher social status and prestige, and that they were more likely to exhibit many "desirable personality traits," such as cooperation, confidence,

leadership, sportsmanship, and sociability. While the children who participated in sports such as football and baseball were primarily boys, Hale also
cited research indicating that girls with athletic experience showed similar
social benefits, such as improved leadership qualities, greater activity in
clubs, and improved emotional stability.[49]

Hale further asserted that "normal" children would not be harmed by
strenuous physical activity. To support this claim, Hale largely sidestepped
concerns about physical injuries in contact or collision sports. Rather, he
sought to refute beliefs that strenuous activity might damage children's hearts
or hinder their growth. Hale cited several studies comparing the rate of physical growth in youth who participated in athletics with those who did not.
The findings of these studies were mixed. Hale acknowledged that differen-
tial rates of maturation in children of the same age meant that child athletes
needed to be carefully matched against competitors of a similar developmental stage to prevent injury. Nonetheless, for Hale, the existence of studies
finding that youth athletes were taller and heavier than their nonathlete
counterparts was sufficient to discount concerns about the impact of athletics on child development. "What is impossible to explain, if competitive athletics do retard growth, is why athletes are larger than nonathletes."[50]

Both Reichert and Hale, then, acknowledged a lack of research evidence
and critiqued the debate over competitive sports for youth as being based on
emotion rather than fact. Yet they reached very different interpretations of
the available research. At the outset of his article, Hale suggested that personal experience playing sports and male gender—two factors which were
certainly not independent of one another in the 1950s—lent those making
claims about sports safety greater authority and credibility. Hale implied that
those seeking to place limits upon competitive sports for children were bi-
ased against athletics. He cast suspicion on the basis for safety concerns in a
gendered fashion: "It has been established that women are less favorable
toward athletic competition than men and that people who have not had athletic experience are less favorable toward competition than those having this
experience." Hale's arguments were further based on the view that the burden
of proof lay with doctors and educators to clearly demonstrate detrimental
effects of competitive sports on children. He considered that the limited and
inconsistent medical evidence on the harmful health effects of youth sports,
even sports as seemingly dangerous as boxing, failed to meet this standard.[51]

Reichert, on the other hand, elevated the authority of medical and educational professionals to assess the health effects of sports over the views of athletes, sports coaches, or sports administrators. He recommended that children

should participate in safer, alternative sports in the absence of evidence demonstrating that full body contact sports were not harmful. Perhaps most strikingly, Reichert challenged not only claims in favor of the benefits of competitive athletics but also beliefs that adults could effectively mitigate the risks of injuries. Arguing that there were numerous fallacies in the notion that "injuries can be insignificant with adequate and intelligent adult supervision," Reichert asserted that children were susceptible to bone and joint injuries, as well as organ damage that might not be evident at the time of injury but could manifest itself weeks or even years later. Even the most careful adult supervision could not control such risks. Reichert concluded that immature children's bodies were too vulnerable to safely engage in body contact sports such as football or boxing and that "the burden of proof rests with those who disagree."[52]

A Supervisory Imperative

Among his arguments, Reichert had critiqued a prevailing assumption that adequate adult supervision of sports would reduce injuries. He likely emphasized this point in response to the widespread belief that adult-organized athletics were safer for children than unsupervised sandlot games. This notion underlay much medical and coaching advice and was often asserted as fact in medical and education literature without supporting data. For instance, in 1947 an orthopedic surgeon wrote that sandlot games were "far more dangerous than supervised school competition where children should be well matched and taught how to defend and protect themselves."[53] In this view, adults protected children by ensuring that only players of a similar age and size competed against each other and by instructing young athletes in football techniques. Such techniques included coaching children in how to fall so they would not land on their heads or necks, hitting other players with their shoulders instead of their heads, and keeping their necks straight (never bent up or down) as they hit.[54]

The emphasis on adult supervision was driven in large part by the perspective of those commenting on youth football safety. Personal involvement in football as a parent, coach, team physician, or trainer often motivated physicians to examine the sport's medical aspects and shaped their advice. A pre-existing involvement with the sport helped inspire physicians to consider football as an important and worthwhile subject of study. On the other hand, these physicians were unlikely to consider banning or limiting football. They instead generally regarded the sport as beneficial overall, with careful medical management sufficient to mitigate the risk of injuries.

Even in the decades before competitive youth sports expanded more rapidly after World War II, this perspective is evident. For instance, Joseph H. Burnett worked as a physician at Boston City Hospital and served as the attending physician for schoolboy games in Dorchester, Massachusetts, for many years. Players gave him the nickname "Hot Towels Burnett" for his standard treatment for bumps and bruises.[55] His research on football safety focused on high school and college players. In a 1940 article published in the *New England Journal of Medicine*, Burnett compared injuries among Harvard athletes versus Boston high school teams. He attributed differences in the percentages of injuries to the former having far more supervision than the latter, asserting that the worst injuries evidently occurred during unorganized games. "This type of play is unsafe, produces serious injuries and gives football an unjustified reputation as a dangerous game."[56]

Burnett therefore advocated for "a campaign of education and helpful advice" to respond to the risks of unregulated play, writing that adult supervision, adequate playing equipment, and removing injured or tired players from the game would help eliminate serious injuries. He extrapolated his findings and recommendations based on older players to younger ones. Burnett praised fathers in Belmont, Massachusetts, for organizing their eight- to fourteen-year-old sons into teams and supervising their matches as an ideal strategy for preventing injuries in this age group. He concluded that with such oversight, football was "certainly worth while." Burnett added that "young America will play football, with or without helpful supervision, so that it is the duty of their elders to help regulate the playing of juveniles."[57]

Among the elders regulating the youth game—coaches, parents, trainers, and doctors—doctors unsurprisingly argued that they should be the primary medical supervisors of the sport. Team physician duties included conducting physical exams before the season began, as well as observing and treating players as necessary throughout the course of the season (figure 12). Team physician James Daly argued that physical examinations were especially important because while all boys ought to have the opportunity to participate in athletics, tackle football was especially rough and dangerous. It would be "a serious mistake to include football for boys without real aptitude."[58] Physicians, then, would need to determine which boys possessed sufficient aptitude to safely participate.

Physicians also maintained that they ought to hold the final authority in diagnosing and treating any injuries that might arise. "The team physician's prerogatives of early diagnosis and treatment must not be usurped by coach or trainer, lest a minor injury become aggravated by continued play, causing a

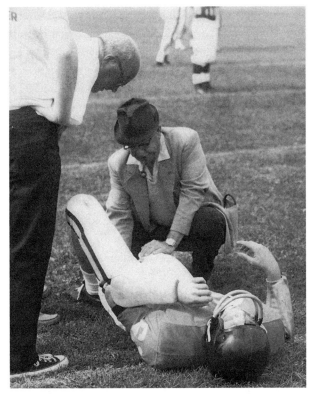

FIGURE 12 Dr. Raymond Hooper examines an injured
football player, 1960s. Photo by Oliver Warila, courtesy of the
Maynard Historical Society.

long period of disability," explained Thorndike.[59] He argued that doctors
were essential to early detection of injury, because coaches were necessarily
primarily interested "in the technical perfection of team and position play"
and thus could not be expected "to spot a limping or arm-weary player." Adult
supervision of youth football therefore required a clear division of labor, sep-
arating medical oversight from coaching responsibilities.[60] Coaches tended
to agree, although college football coach Clark Shaughnessy claimed in a
1966 article that many physicians failed to recognize that "well-conditioned"
athletes would recover more quickly than ordinary people. Shaughnessy contended that a team physician ought to be able to treat some football injuries
"for which he might hospitalize the average person, in a much different and
more practical way."[61]

In a 1957 article, orthopedist Rodney Atsatt described his twenty-five years
of experience serving as football team physician at Santa Barbara High School

in California. In addition to reviewing several kinds of specialized first aid involved in addressing football injuries, from treating a charley horse to taping ankles, Atsatt offered broader thoughts on the role, authority, and independence of a team physician. He also implied that the team physician might assist with the team's success on the field by advising the coach. Atsatt wrote that a football coach ought to have "complete confidence in the doctor's judgment," not only in deciding whether it was safe for a boy to continue playing but also in "matters of psychology." To address the latter issue, Atsatt described how he would observe the boys' attitudes while taping their knees and ankles prior to games and relay his impressions to the coach. He proudly noted that his observations would influence the coach's pep talk to the players. Atsatt provided an example of how, after he advised the coach to appeal to his players' pride after one game's disheartening first half, the team came back from a 20–0 deficit to win. Atsatt's oversight of youth football was clearly not limited to providing medical care.[62]

Atsatt's account also reveals how physicians functioned to reassure the spectators on the sidelines that potentially frightening injuries were being professionally managed. In his discussion of head and neck trauma during games, Atsatt advised that after a hard blow where a player emerged with "wooziness" but did not lose consciousness, the doctor ought to carefully observe the athlete but need not remove him from play. But if a player were "really out cold" on the field, he ought to always be brought off on a stretcher, Atsatt explained, in case the athlete had sustained a neck injury. Moreover, "it is very bad from the standpoint of the spectators to see a semiconscious boy walked off the field with his head bobbing from side to side, to say nothing of the possibility of further serious damage to the patient." In this way, a team physician not only worked to protect the health of football players but also to prevent the unfolding of an unpleasant and disturbing scene following a serious injury.[63]

The belief that adult supervision not only prevented physical injuries but also fostered moral development in boys further shaped medical advice. In a 1956 guest editorial published in *JAMA*, Allan Ryan characterized the AMA as working with educators and coaches to highlight "the character-building advantages of football" while minimizing "the danger of young boys playing too many games in one season." Ryan portrayed football as a healthy sport for building boys' bodies and promoting teamwork, but one that could be dangerous, even "a killer and a maimer," without medical supervision. He advocated for regular physical examinations of players conducted by physicians, properly fitting uniforms, and preplay warm-ups as effective means to preserve the assumed benefits of the "wholesome and valuable" sport.[64]

Coaches and league administrators defended the sport in very similar terms. For example, Don C. Osgood, president of the East Fullerton Midget Football League, told a *Los Angeles Times* reporter that football was "becoming a safe, wholesome sport for the grade school youngster" because games were "under the strict supervision and the safeguards imposed by the mothers and fathers themselves and by the Pop Warner Midget Football Association of America."[65] Indeed, promoters of Pop Warner and other youth leagues made remarkable claims about football safety. As Osgood continued in his remarks, "Unlike sandlot football in which injuries sometimes mar contests, Pop Warner League is amazingly free of mishaps. . . . When healthy boys meet in a body-contact sport such as football, there's not much chance of a serious injury."[66]

Not all doctors were convinced by claims that "the sport is as safe for youngsters as for their older brethren." Citing a study of high school football injuries, Dr. Fred Hein wrote that "the younger and greener a youth," the more likely he was to sustain an injury.[67] Still more doctors contended that football experience and skills did not appear to confer any particular protection. A 1962 examination of high school football injuries in California found that "head injuries occurred, for the most part, in players whose ability was considered excellent or good."[68] Others questioned the adequacy of physical examinations as a means to identify children who should not play the sport. An attendee at a 1962 conference on head injuries reported seeing 120 boys processed in the space of three hours and observed that this time was insufficient to thoroughly examine so many participants. Moreover, it was unclear whether physicians had effective methods to identify which boys were at greatest risk.[69]

But with the argument highlighting adult supervision as the key to safety, many parents increasingly insisted on supervision in order to protect their sons. Indeed, to some parents, only the presence of adults could make football suitable for the smallest boys. As one father told the *Chicago Daily Tribune*, "You hear a lot about these kids being too young for this game, but with the supervision and rules in Pop Warner football this isn't true."[70] This desire for supervision was not limited to the smallest players but extended through the high school level. For instance, in 1956, 300 parents signed a petition presented to the board of education in Los Angeles requesting increased coaching staff for the safety and welfare of high school football players.[71]

A Long Island youth football league kept its own statistics to reassure worried parents. The league collected and shared injury data not only to provide evidence of the sport's safety but also to reinforce the importance of supervision provided by organized leagues such as itself. In 1956, the league reported that in the previous year, among 288 players who had participated in a total of 9,706 boy-practice hours and 418 game hours, only eight injuries were reported. Neither the nature of these injuries nor the methods for data collection are described. Yet the *New York Times* journalist who reported these figures concluded, "It is reasonable to assume that many more injuries would have resulted if the same number of boys had played sandlot football on vacant lots, without proper supervision or equipment."[72]

Several historians and philosophers of medicine have discussed the notion of a "technological imperative" prevailing in medicine, particularly in the United States.[73] In youth football during this period, there might be said to exist a supervisory imperative: a prevailing belief that adult supervision was necessary and sufficient to provide for youth football safety. Such supervision was promoted as key to addressing injuries, especially as private football leagues for young children proliferated. The investment of coaches and team physicians in the sport of football influenced not only their understanding of risks but also the solutions they promoted to address safety concerns. Coaches and doctors recommended the involvement of more coaches and doctors, and the supposed need for supervision in turn justified the existence and expansion of organized youth leagues run by adults.

Moreover, adults' management of youth football represented a prism through which larger societal quandaries were being played out, from proper gender roles to racial discrimination. As protests over the Vietnam War and the civil rights movement took place in the 1960s, coaches and athletic administrators were often associated with more conservative-leaning politics. As American author James Michener characterized his own coach in his 1976 book *Sports in America*, "Like most coaches, he considered Democrats bad, and labor union people, and troublemakers, and college professors, and radicals, and anyone not wholeheartedly in support of the good society as he experienced it."[74] In the face of unrest and challenges to powerful institutions, coaches and athletic administrators promoted tackle football as a buttress against seemingly unpatriotic and undesirable behavior among youth. They argued that athletic programs in general and football in particular could foster in students a sense of loyalty to the United States and to traditional American values. In 1967, Art Baker, a football coach at Clemson University, summarized this perspective: "Perhaps never in the history of the United States have we needed to develop loyalty so badly as today. Everywhere we look it seems some group of American youth is demonstrating against something, often nothing worthwhile. . . . I am firmly convinced that if all American students were a part of a good athletic program we wouldn't have the draft card burnings, the long-haired beatniks, the burning of our sacred 'Old Glory,' or the waving of the enemy's flag in our streets."[75]

Baker's interpretation of the moral benefits of sports for American youth was addressed to physicians reading the *Journal of the South Carolina Medical Association*. An accompanying editorial comment noted that the state medical association was greatly concerned with safety in athletics and was consequently seeking to promote close relationships between physicians and coaches. As part of this effort, the chairman of the association's Committee on the Medical Aspects of Sports had submitted Baker's article for publication.

The ability of sports to foster American pride and loyalty in response to activism in the streets was thus foregrounded by a professional medical association as part of its examination of the medical aspects of athletics. Baker's article illustrates the close connections between coaches and physicians in framing the risks of youth football. Baker also included an extended reflection on the religious (specifically Christian) aspect of coaching, reinforcing the connections between American football, patriotism, and Christianity. The conceptualization of football injuries as a medical issue was thus deeply tied up with ideological, moralistic, religious, and even nationalistic beliefs about the role of youth sports, as well as the country's direction more broadly.[76] Cultural fears similar to Baker's persisted among physicians through the 1970s. In 1975, orthopedic surgeon Richard W. Godshall editorialized, "I would certainly rather have one of my children play football than smoke 'pot' in some dark room."[77]

Young America Will Play Football

By the mid-twentieth century, as organized tackle football expanded to increasingly include children younger than high school age, doctors and coaches asserted their authority on football safety in new and more professionalized ways. The way these men framed their expertise was decidedly gendered. Not only were sports doctors and coaches almost exclusively men, but their experiential knowledge of sports was valued as a key element of safety expertise. This largely excluded women's perspectives, especially mothers' concerns about the sport's safety for their sons, from being considered authoritative. Indeed, some sports administrators explicitly emphasized the importance of male athletic experience to credibility on matters of football safety. Moreover, male experts' experiential knowledge of football was associated with making boys into men. Their arguments for the benefits of organized youth football were based on the belief that men best knew how to impart desired values such as loyalty, patriotism, and discipline to young boys. Male supervision could most effectively transmit the sport's benefits to boys while minimizing its risks.

As sports medicine developed as a subspecialty, the attitudes of team physicians toward competitive youth sports increasingly diverged from those of pediatricians and educators. In the 1950s, the AAP and the NEA issued recommendations against football for children under twelve. These organizations' objections contributed to limiting tackle football programs within elementary and middle schools, though they did not stem the growth of privately sponsored leagues for young boys. By contrast, team physicians, sports researchers, coaches, and administrators highlighted the moral benefits of organized football and insisted that proper supervision and equipment were sufficient to protect young boys. While doctors and coaches who promoted organized youth football undoubtedly believed in the sport's character-building qualities, their arguments downplayed and sometimes even masked football's physical risks. Team physicians and coaches had a stake in the expansion of organized football to young children that pediatricians lacked.

That medical warnings against tackle football went largely unheeded while arguments in the sport's favor prevailed suggests that sports medicine had consolidated increasing professional authority by mid-twentieth century. But it also indicates the cultural meanings attached to organized sports that football coaches and sports doctors successfully tapped. Most Americans viewed football as a way to make boys into men with desired cultural traits. In framing the sport's health risks as manageable with adult supervision, team doctors and coaches played a crucial role in promoting the vision of American manhood associated with tackle football.

CHAPTER FIVE

The Rough and Tumble

What Counts as a Football Injury?

The enthusiast concedes that sports are hazardous. But too hazardous?
For whom? Under what conditions? Compared to what?
— Kenneth S. Clarke, 1966

On October 3, 1964, the Pop Warner youth football league saw its first re-ported fatality. During a practice session in San Jose, California, a fourteen-year-old player, Keene Mitsuru Yamamoto, complained of pain in the back of his head. His discomfort did not diminish even when his coach allowed him to remove his helmet and rest on the bench. Yamamoto lost consciousness and was taken to a hospital. The young teenager did not survive brain surgery for a blood clot. His family had him buried in a Buddhist cemetery.[1]

The AFCA's annual survey of football fatalities categorized Yamamoto's death as a direct fatality from brain injuries received at football practice. "Coach, I got it in the head," the boy reportedly told his coach. Yet the AFCA also mentioned unnamed newspaper reports suggesting that Yamamoto had been "hit in the head with a baseball some weeks prior to his death," raising the possibility that a prior brain injury may have been a contributing factor.[2] According to the *Los Angeles Times* story on the tragedy, doctors absolved Pop Warner organizers of blame for Yamamoto's death. They stated that the physical examination given to Pop Warner players prior to participation would not have shown Yamamoto's blood clot.[3] Newspaper accounts were unclear as to whether Yamamoto had a preexisting blood clot, and indeed, it may have been impossible from available medical records to tell.

Nonetheless, Yamamoto's death furnished an opportunity to consider argu-ments for and against organized youth football, "an activity in which miniature Jim Browns crash into miniature Sam Huffs while miniature pompon girls prance on the sidelines."[4] The comparison of young boys to two prominent NFL athletes underscored the extent to which youth leagues mimicked profes-sional football by the early 1960s. Subsequent reporting raised further ques-tions: What constituted a football injury or death? How did football's risks compare to other childhood activities? Were the sport's dangers an inherent part of childhood, or were there uniquely risky mechanisms in tackle football?

Whether a child's death or injury associated with playing football could be *attributed* to football was crucial in determining the risk the sport posed to participants. Popular beliefs about masculinity shaped answers to this question. In particular, medical and educational authorities stressed that boys inherently needed physical contact that only full-body collision sports like football could provide. Some acknowledged that additional physical dangers were a consequence of collision sports but argued that the benefits outweighed the harm. On the other hand, many football proponents contended that the sport provided an outlet for boys' energy without posing any higher risks of injury than they would experience in the course of an active boyhood. The belief that most youth football injuries were minor bumps or bruises facilitated this perspective. A child's death, however, had the potential to puncture the view that football did not pose unusually serious hazards. Determining whether football participation was fundamentally responsible for the deaths and injuries of young athletes, then, was key to evaluating the sport's risks.

Fatalities in Youth Football

Prompted by Yamamoto's death, the *Los Angeles Times* devoted a two-part series to examining both the popularity of youth football and controversy over its safety. Reporter Joseph Jares cited an official Pop Warner booklet stating that approximately 20,000 teams, with more than half a million players, played Pop Warner football throughout the United States and in several foreign countries.[5] In 1965, the journal *Physicians' Management* would estimate that 800,000 boys aged nine to fifteen participated in organized football leagues.[6] Moreover, the NFL was receiving greater television coverage and actively seeking to foster a youth audience. In 1961, the NFL had teamed up with Ford Motor Company to begin sponsoring a nationwide "Punt, Pass, and Kick" competition for children (see figure 13).[7] With corporate sponsorship of skills competitions, increasing youth tackle participation numbers, and the recent death of a participant, youth football safety debates were of great public interest.

According to Jares, football supporters asserted that the sport promoted academic achievement and improved moral character among young players and was no more hazardous than other activities. One parent, while acknowledging there was some danger of injury, felt the risk was "minimized by the fact that the kids that age are used to things like, oh, the rough and tumble, climbing fences and falling from trees." Jares also quoted Joel Adams, an orthopedic surgeon who had studied injuries in organized youth football and baseball, who recommended several safety rules to protect players. One was

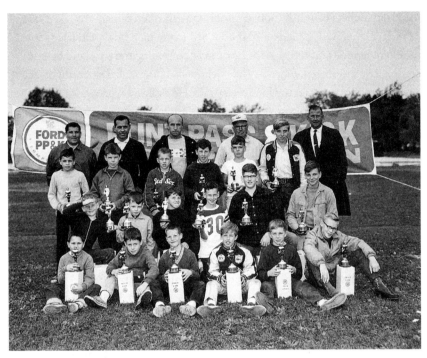

FIGURE 13 Football Punt, Pass and Kick Competition, Massachusetts, c. 1965.
Photo by Oliver Warila, courtesy of the Maynard Historical Society.

that: "Head injury with even momentary loss of consciousness automatically rules out the player for the remainder of the SEASON" (emphasis in original). This recommendation indicated that a number of physicians thought head injuries should be taken seriously and should not be treated as a minor matter of a player seeing stars or getting his head dinged.[8]

Elsewhere, critics would argue that youth football coaches rarely followed such cautious practices. As one reporter wrote in 1967, "How many young football players are pushed on to the field with broken or bruised ribs, wrists, arms, and minor head injuries? A shot of pain-killer and in they go. How many times do you see a young man knocked out on one play return immediately to action after a time out or brief rest?"[9] The 1964 *Los Angeles Times* series, however, conveyed that sponsors of youth football took medical supervision seriously, and that physical examinations and penalties for dangerous plays mitigated the sport's risks. "Pop Warner safety-first football generally lives up to its slogan," Jares reassured readers.[10]

Despite reports in the *Los Angeles Times* and other California newspapers, this 1964 Pop Warner fatality went unmentioned in medical literature examining the health effects of youth football. Just two years after Yamamoto's death, Fred Allman Jr., then vice president of the ACSM (for which he would later serve as president in 1968 and 1969), wrote an article examining the risks and benefits of competitive organized sports. While acknowledging that deaths might occur, Allman emphasized that they were very rare. He asserted that "one of the largest tackle football programs for youngsters, the Pop Warner program, has had over one million participants in the past 34 years without a fatality, a record that speaks well for the leadership and organization within the program."[11]

Moreover, the connection between Yamamoto's death and youth football was gradually erased in subsequent newspaper accounts. A 1974 *New York Times* examination of youth football referenced the death as having a distant association with the league: "In 45 years there has been only one fatality remotely connected with Pop Warner."[12] Four years later, in 1978, another *New York Times* story amended the claim to read that in almost fifty years of Pop Warner football, "there has not been one injury-related death."[13] This account implied that Yamamoto's death was not associated with any injury sustained while playing football. By the 1980s, Yamamoto's existence as a Pop Warner athlete effectively disappeared: news reports were claiming that in the history of Pop Warner youth football, "there have been no fatalities among more than 1 million participants."[14]

Moreover, Yamamoto's death was not the only instance of a child dying while playing Pop Warner football. In September 1971, a ten-year-old died after a head-on collision during a Pop Warner tackling drill in La Habra, California. Yet, as one of his teammates would later report, the brief news story on this fatality was strikingly scant: "No interviews with coaches, teammates, doctors. No analysis. Nothing." This child's death occurred during a football practice rather than a game, another factor that may have contributed to the relative lack of attention.[15]

Both deaths of Pop Warner players were treated as anomalies. This assumption made it possible for the claim that no fatalities had occurred in Pop Warner football to persist through the 1990s. In 1996, *Sports Illustrated for Kids* published a special supplement issue for parents on "how to help your kids get the most out of sports." An article focused on football asserted, "Pop Warner has never had a player fatality in its 67-year history."[16]

Putting the Risks in Context

The erasure of the connections between the deaths of Pop Warner players and football reinforced popular perceptions that tackling did not pose meaningful risks of severe injury or death for elementary and middle school aged children. But the dangers, particularly of less catastrophic outcomes and among high school students, remained a source of uncertainty. What exactly were the risks for boys playing tackle football on fields across the United States?

At mid-twentieth century, few epidemiological studies existed to answer this question. Instead, debates over the safety of football commonly featured efforts to place the risks in the context of other ubiquitous activities in American life. Despite little data to substantiate the comparisons, these analogies frequently featured in both defenses and denouncements of football. In fact, the lack of data may have facilitated the use of such comparisons and often made them more difficult to refute. These analogies also framed the risks in ways that the general public could more easily comprehend.

Drawing on their experiences and anecdotal observations, doctors and coaches portrayed football as a "reasonably safe" sport in the context of other American activities from horse racing to water sports. Boxing presented a particularly common foil to football. The risks of the ring often served to make football seem relatively tame by comparison, though they sometimes highlighted football's dangers. Given the discrepancies in the quality of available data on the sports' risks, the resulting claims could prove highly contradictory. For example, the author of a 1951 article decrying the dangers of boxing asserted without a citation that "professional boxing is 83 times more deadly than high school football and 50 times more deadly than college football."[17] A 1951 analysis published in *JAMA*, however, found that boxing competitions "produced far fewer deaths, in proportion to the number of participants, than occur in baseball or football."[18]

Boxing was also held up as a cautionary tale of what might befall youth football if the risks of injury could not be controlled. While historians have attributed the waning of professional boxing to economic factors rather than moral disapprobation, concerns over boys' physical and moral well-being undoubtedly surrounded the sport at the youth level.[19] As the author of an analysis of high school football safety equipment warned: "The sport of boxing is on the verge of being outlawed because of injury to the human body. . . . The sport of football could find itself in the same precarious situation in which boxing exists today if the coaching profession does not establish a philosophy of giving the player the greatest protection possible."[20]

To assert that football was not dangerous, orthopedic surgeon Mal Stevens made comparisons to boxing and a wide range of other popular activities. As president of the AFCA in 1931, Stevens had helped initiate the association's collection of data on football-related fatalities and catastrophic injuries. In 1962, he told readers of the *Boston Globe* that football was "safer than most water sports, less of a physical strain than basketball or tennis, less punishing than boxing. Football demands less stamina than soccer. There is more danger in being hit by a baseball, or being knocked from a racing horse, than being hit with a football or being tackled while running with one." Stevens further argued that while bruises and minor cuts were an inherent part of football, serious injuries and deaths were not, and they could be prevented.[21]

In both academic literature and newspapers, the risks of driving cars were a particularly common point of reference. Comparisons of the hazards of the road to those of the football field were almost always employed to portray football in a positive light. This argument had a long history. In a 1933 text on football injuries, Mal Stevens and another doctor claimed that "the inherent dangers of football have been greatly exaggerated" and reassured concerned readers that "the majority of coaches have never seen a football fatality. . . . In our experience it is definitely more dangerous to drive to the Yale Bowl as a spectator than it is to play football the entire season."[22]

In the 1950s, driving was often highlighted as particularly hazardous for teenage boys. Lou Little, a former AFCA president and a Columbia University football coach, asserted that "the injury rate for the millions of boys who play football is very low, and the fatality rate is 15 times smaller than that from walking around outdoors and driving in the family car."[23] While the original source for this figure remains unclear, the "15 times safer than driving" claim circulated among football coaches. In an article arguing that the advantages of football heavily outweighed the dangers, high school football coach Charles Mather asserted that for teenagers it was "approximately 15 times safer to play football than to be a pedestrian or driver of an automobile!"[24] This figure bolstered the argument that if parents allowed their boys to drive a car, or even to ride in one, they could not reasonably oppose their sons' participation in football. An article in *Athletic Coach* even more dramatically claimed that motor vehicles were "180 times more dangerous than football" based on fatality statistics from a five-month period.[25]

A more precise comparison of the fatal risks of driving and football was later published in the medical literature. In 1964, Floyd Eastwood, who chaired the AFCA's survey committee on football fatalities from 1942 to 1964, reported the results of the annual survey in the *New England Journal of Medicine*. In addition to comparing football fatalities with deaths from firearms and drowning, he specifically noted the number of motor vehicle deaths among teenagers and young adults. "It has been estimated that for the group fifteen to twenty-five years of age there is approximately 1 football fatality for 265.5 deaths associated with motor vehicles (August to January). . . . This relative comparison indicates that other activities are more hazardous (fatal) than football."[26]

These figures did not, of course, capture the potentially catastrophic non-fatal hazards of football, such as spinal cord injuries or even paralysis. Furthermore, without a denominator, the raw numbers did not represent the level of risk relative to the number of participants or time spent engaged in the activities being compared. Other researchers, however, did seek to calculate fatality rates using the number of high school students participating in football and driving. Using data from the 1963 football season, orthopedic surgeon A. Ross Davis estimated 1.5 deaths per 100,000 high school students playing football, compared to approximately 21 deaths per 100,000 high school students from automobile accidents. Davis interpreted these rates as meaning that the numbers of deaths in football were "less alarming" than they might otherwise appear.[27]

Doctors communicated these comparisons to major American newspapers. With similar figures for football but a higher rate of deaths among teenaged drivers than Ross had reported, team physician Stephen Reid told the *New York Times* that the fatality rate in high school football "was only 1.62 per 100,000 players compared with 57 per 100,000 for male automobile drivers between 15 and 19 years of age."[28] These various claims made by medical professionals, football coaches, and sports administrators circulated in the media and influenced public perceptions. Parents who allowed their sons to participate in tackle football echoed the driving comparison. The *Los Angeles Times* noted, "A father reflects the sentiments of other dads when he says 'they're safer than if they were in an auto on a highway.'"[29] In 1962, high school football coach Fred Parks of Oak Lawn told the *Chicago Daily Tribune*, "As a father and as a coach, I would a million times rather have my son on the football field than riding around in an automobile."[30]

Such comparisons, whether made by parents, coaches, or doctors, relied on a false dichotomy: playing football and riding in a car were not mutually exclusive options for boys. The quality and sources of the data used in making these comparisons were also questionable. In a 1966 *JAMA* article, Kenneth S. Clarke of the AMA's Department of Health Education critiqued the careless use of statistics in debates over the safety of youth sports. He sought "to bring more professional sensitivity to this concern" by more judiciously tabulating outcomes and incorporating key variables, such as the number of participants in the activity and how often they were exposed to the risk.[31]

TABLE 2 Number of accidental deaths due to football, Metropolitan Life, 1965

	Direct Causes		Indirect Causes	
Type of Game	1955–59	1960–64	1955–59	1960–64
Sandlot	19	13	4	10
High School	49	66	18	34
College	6	12	4	7
Professional and Semi-professional	4	4	1	2
Total	78	95	27	53

Data source: Committee on Injuries and Fatalities, AFCA. Table adapted from table 2 in Metropolitan Life Insurance Company, "Competitive Sports and Their Hazards," *Statistical Bulletin of the Metropolitan Life Insurance Company* 46 (1965): 1–3.

In particular, Clarke observed that the AFCA and NFHS relied on counts of football fatalities that distinguished between direct and indirect football-related deaths. These organizations considered fatalities caused by injuries sustained while playing football to be direct, whereas football-related deaths attributed to systemic failure, such as heat stroke, were categorized as indirect. These counts were widely promulgated. In particular, a 1965 *Statistical Bulletin* published by the Metropolitan Life Insurance Company, relying on the AFCA's counts, drew media attention. This report observed that the overall number of deaths directly associated with football among high school and college players had increased between 1955 to 1959 and 1960 to 1964 (see table 2).[32]

Yet on top of these fatalities, a spate of football heat-related deaths in the early 1960s drew attention to the issue of whether such noncontact fatalities should also be considered directly attributable to the sport. As one commentator pointedly asked in 1962 after the death of a fourteen-year-old football player, "The boy was examined by a doctor a week ago and was pronounced in good health, but do we have to accept the viewpoint that the child might have died anyway if he had not gone off to a training camp in the heat of August?"[33]

Clarke observed that "few would argue that the heat stroke deaths in the first week of football practice are not 'directly' related to going out for football." He considered distinctions between direct and indirect football deaths to be misleading, especially because they were also strongly "influenced by the specificity of information provided by a voluntarily returned questionnaire" sent to coaches or athletic directors.[34] Rather than focusing merely on the counts of deaths sustained while playing football as compared to other activities, Clarke suggested the actuarial question: "Does a young male increase his statistical risk of death by announcing his candidacy for football?"[35]

After reviewing significant pitfalls in interpreting the available statistics, Clarke sought to build a different model incorporating exposure estimates based on a range of assumptions (specifically a high school football season lasting eleven weeks, with two-hour-long practices scheduled five days per week, and further accounting for periodic player absences due to injuries). He compared the resulting fatality rate per hours of football exposure to the fatality rate associated with daily living and with motoring; he found that the football fatality rate was higher in both cases. Clarke did not use his analysis to advocate for or against youth football but rather to argue that such calculations of fatality rates did not indicate whether the hazards outweighed the benefits of any of the examined activities. He added that one could not know what a football athlete might have otherwise chosen to do had he not participated in football. But "certainly, he would not choose football over riding in a car on the basis of the relative risk of death resulting from this exercise."[36]

Proponents of youth football who continually pointed to the risks of driving were certainly not alone in attempting to compare the sport to other dangerous activities. To portray football in a less favorable light, one doctor turned to occupational hazards. In a 1963 paper provocatively titled "High School Football: Valuable Sport or Sado-Masochistic Excess?" physician Frank Tabrah examined the risk of disabling injury in high school football as compared to underground coal mining. As suggested by the paper's title, Tabrah employed the coal mining comparison to contend that football was not a valuable sport given the risks. In his analysis, he compared 1962 data on football injury rates in two Hawaiian high schools with injury rates in high-risk occupations such as logging, mining, and construction. Tabrah made the incredible claim that the frequency of injuries in football was nearly 14,000 times greater than in underground coal mining, the most dangerous American industry.[37]

In addition to asserting that the hazards of football outweighed the benefits, Tabrah argued that football was not worthwhile because so few athletes continued to play the sport past their school years. "Astonishing amounts of time and effort are expended on a sport skill that virtually no one utilizes after high school or college age." Tabrah contended that activities in which people might engage throughout their middle age and older years, such as tennis or swimming, should be prioritized over football and other risky sports predominantly played by adolescents and young adults.[38] This notion that lifetime sports should take precedence over youth-oriented collision sports would continue to feature in debates over the safety and value of tackle football.

A Boy's Right to Physical Contact

Yet Tabrah's view was a distinctly minority opinion. Claims about the moral benefits of football's aggressive physical contact were related to a host of prevailing beliefs about freedom and masculinity in American society that shaped interpretations of football's risks. One important and persistent view was that boys had an extraordinary amount of youthful energy that could only be satisfied by physical contact. According to this belief, alternative non-contact sports, even ones that might require significant physical exertion, simply would not suffice. As one Ohio high school football coach put it, football provides "a wholesome outlet" for the "tremendous energy" of boys. "You can't channel this sort of energy into passive pursuits such as chess or stamp-collecting, and the explosive urge cannot be completely satisfied by such otherwise wonderful sports as golf and tennis."[39]

This belief in football as an outlet for the physical instincts of boys was long-standing. In 1931, team physician Joseph H. Burnett wrote that properly supervised football "gives boys a natural outlet for their nervous energies and keeps them off the streets, thereby avoiding many mishaps, such as automobile, motor-cycle and trolley car injuries, and others too numerous to mention." On this view, if boys did not play a collision sport like football, they would simply be at risk for injuries in other settings.[40]

Even educators concerned about the hazards of football shared the assumption that noncontact sports could not satisfy boys' physical needs. In response to a high incidence of serious football injuries, educators at Purdue University sought an alternative, less hazardous sport, while "realizing that a successful program of intramural sports needs at least one contact game." To address this requirement, assistant professor George Haniford advocated "American ball" as a suitable and safer alternative. This sport was created in 1934 as a combination of elements of baseball, basketball, and football. Writing for the journal *Recreation*, Haniford acknowledged that American ball was not well known but encouraged readers to consider it.[41] Emphasizing that this purportedly safer sport nonetheless fulfilled players' need for physical contact, a quote from military psychiatrist William C. Menninger introduced the article: "Competitive games provide an unusually satisfactory social outlet for the aggressive drive. The most aggressive outlet is seen in those sports in which there is bodily contact."[42]

The assumption that competitive contact sports filled a biological necessity for men was generally conjoined with the view that women did not experience such needs. This belief permeated not only defenses of football as
necessary for boys and men, but furnished an explanation as to why such
sports were not desirable or appropriate for women and girls. As philosopher
Paul Weiss would write in a 1969 examination of sports, "Most women do not
make the effort to train or to participate because they are not subject to the
tensions that young men suffer. . . . The women have already achieved a satis-
fying integration of mind and body."[43]

A 1958 *Athletic Journal* article on how coaches should respond to parental
resistance to football emphasized the importance of contact in terms of both
mind and body. The author, a youth football coach, explained that a boy prevented from playing football "is being deprived of his right to physical contact and loses certain benefits to his total personality." Furthermore, the coach
argued, football developed a mental toughness "born of a burning desire to
exceed and excel. This quality must conquer all of a boy's weaknesses, if he is
to be victorious." While girls might not be expected to conquer weaknesses
popularly associated with femininity, boys were expected to overcome perceived mental vulnerability to become successful and strong men. On this
view, boys were not only entitled to the physical contact football offered, but
benefited psychologically as well as physically.[44]

Coaches and educators also argued that the sport in some sense protected
boys. Football fit in with broader efforts to use organized activities to prevent
juvenile delinquency or street crime. For instance, in 1948, surgeon Walter
Boyd organized the Long Beach Junior Football League for boys aged fourteen and under in order "to get the boys off the streets."[45] In 1955, the deputy
commissioner of New York City's police department lauded the city's Police
Athletic League's youth programs as "typical of the work done by crime-
prevention agencies across the United States."[46] Rough bodily contact at
younger ages was also justified in preparing boys to continue to play sports as
they grew older. "The body contact actually makes the youngsters better
equipped for play in interscholastic and collegiate competition as they attain
maturity."[47] An improved ability to successfully compete in high school and
college football, then, was considered a worthwhile goal in itself.

Many medical professionals endorsed the notion that the risks of serious
injury or death were small compared to the social benefits. Orthopedic surgeon A. Ross Davis reviewed athletic injuries in the Houston Independent
School District, where football commanded the largest number of participants among the sports on offer. Acknowledging that some athletic injuries

were inevitable, Davis concluded that overall, the harms were "not so severe as to negate the obvious advantages of participating." The particular advantages Davis highlighted included that children were participating in organized activities "rather than spending their afternoons in leisure and in the corner drug stores."[48]

Writing for the *Journal of the Medical Association of Georgia*, orthopedic surgeon Fred Allman highlighted similar moral advantages by contrasting the value of organized athletics with alternative activities for boys younger than fifteen. Allman wrote that, in 1965, a ten-week YMCA tackle football program served 1,450 boys in grades two through seven, with just thirty-one recorded injuries, of which only six were fractures. During the same period, Allman asserted, a similar number of boys would have surely been injured falling from trees, riding bicycles, or even being hit by a car. Furthermore, "some might have even had time to engage in a mischievous act or embarked on a career in crime." He approvingly quoted former U.S. President Herbert Hoover as stating, "Next to religion, sports are the greatest developer of morals."[49] Tackle football was surely worth the risk if the alternative was for boys to embark upon a life of crime. To some extent, then, the belief in football's moral benefits rendered concerns about the sport's physical risks moot. Few physical costs could outweigh the perceived social benefits when football was framed as a fundamental defense against delinquency and immorality among boys.

Parental Responsibility and Player Attitudes

In highlighting football's benefits, news stories also conveyed the idea that it was up to parents and players to minimize the risks. In 1962, the *Chicago Daily Tribune* examined high school football safety by surveying 160 Illinois high school coaches. Addressed to parents, the article explicitly characterized the question as a matter of weighing the physical and moral benefits of football with the potential for injury. "Will the bone-crunching game of football make a man or a cripple out of your high school age son?" the newspaper asked its readers. "The answer, Mom and Dad, is very much up to you."[50]

Thus, it was parents' responsibility to realize football's unique ability to safely transform their sons into men. Reporting that most football coaches did not think that injuries were increasing, despite "scare statistics," most of the *Tribune* article consisted of advice to parents to keep their sons safe. The list of rules included making sure their sons reached peak physical condition before the football preseason, checking their sons' equipment for proper fit, not pampering their sons "over minor bruises," and not seeking to advise the coach or school's athletic director. While parents were expected to investigate any possible injuries their child may have sustained, one coach advised that "players and parents not be so injury conscious that they regard every hangnail as a catastrophe." Instead of overly fretting about minor injuries, players and parents needed to take responsibility for learning the basics of the sport.[51]

In another article, Columbia University football coach Lou Little similarly advised fathers that a little home coaching on their part would prevent injuries. "Football's safety principles are so few in number and so easy to grasp that it's foolish for a boy to be hurt for lack of knowing them."[52] Meanwhile, the president of a youth football league in California claimed that injuries were highly unusual, suggesting that those that did occur were attributable to the poor physical condition of individual players. He told the *Los Angeles Times* that "the rare instances in which injury has occurred have been traced to a team permitting an overweight boy to play."[53] Such articles minimized the potential risks of football and largely transferred responsibility for addressing these risks from sports organizations and coaches to the parents and even the players themselves. The 1962 *Chicago Daily Tribune* article concluded that tackle football could be "just about as safe as Mom and Dad care to make it."[54]

Despite the prevailing emphasis on the relatively minor hazards of football, some doctors and coaches examined whether the sport posed unique risks. Several physicians questioned whether specific football techniques might be contributing to especially severe injuries. In a 1959 *JAMA* article, orthopedist Donald Slocum wrote that medical professionals had paid only scant attention to the mechanics of football injuries, but that "a small corps of active observers—the team physicians, the coaches, and the trainers" had observed recurring patterns of situations that were especially risky.[55]

Yet such observations were hampered by a lack of data. Acknowledging that "no accurate statistics are available as to how these injuries have occurred," Slocum speculated "that the most lethal weapon in football is the oncoming knee." He highlighted the force of on-field collisions, providing a "rough example" of a 185-pound varsity-level fullback who could run a 100-yard dash in 10.5 seconds. This athlete could kick 500 pounds with his knee while standing, 625 pounds with one step, 725 pounds with two steps, and so on. Noting how much farther football players ran during actual play and adding the formula "momentum equals mass times velocity," Slocum left it to his readers to imagine the real-life risks.[56]

Were such dangers inevitable and inherent to athletes running into each other at high speeds, or did the players themselves bear some responsibility for the risks? Slocum suggested that whether and how a player was injured or caused harm to another player might be attributed to their personality and approach to the sport. "An aggressive, alert player may receive a serious head injury, and the fatigued, weak or 'loafing' player may be doubled up in flexion and receive serious spinal trauma." Doctors particularly suspected players who were unskilled or reluctant to participate in football as prone to exaggerating their injuries. As several team physicians explained in 1959, "A boy may use the injury as an excuse. . . . He may not have any real desire to play football, but feels he should because of his size; his family, or fraternity brothers may have encouraged him to go out for the team. This boy may not want to heal his injury. A surgeon cannot put desire into a knee joint. We have been impressed with how few injuries we have seen after a winning ball game."[57]

Other medical experts agreed that there were athletes whose personality or player types left them especially susceptible. In response to the question, "Is there such a thing as the injury-prone player?" at a 1962 symposium on football injuries, neuroscientist Richard C. Schneider responded in the affirmative. "Yes. The boy who does not actually wish to play football but is under pressure from his family or from his schoolmates to participate tends to have a high incidence of actual physical injuries as well as a slow rate of recovery. In addition, he may be subject to other symptoms, such as headaches which may be due to psychic tension."[58] None of these doctors provided data to support the claims that there were certain loafing or otherwise injury-prone types of players who suffered higher rates of injuries or recovered more slowly than other athletes.

Player attitudes and characteristics were blamed in part for injuries even in discussions centered on the importance of improving coaching techniques. Coaches had consistently acknowledged responsibility for teaching their players how to play more safely. In fact, every AFCA fatality report from 1931 to 2008 mentioned improving coaching methods as a preventive measure to reduce football injuries and fatalities.[59] In the 1950s, two journals aimed at coaches, *Scholastic Coach* and *Athletic Journal*, often featured articles on football that suggested improving various conditioning techniques and fostering sportsmanship and better player attitudes. Such recommended techniques were often relatively generic and intersected with beliefs about fearful or reluctant football players being prone to injury. For example, to minimize injuries purportedly associated with boys' attitudes, one former trainer advised scrimmaging during practices where boys would be hit by their teammates. In this way, "the boys receive that 'first shot' which seems to cause so many injuries. But they receive it in a different manner. There is no tenseness and the boys are more relaxed . . . . that fear of the 'first shot' is gone." Eliminating fearful attitudes was thus promoted as a means to enhance safety.[60]

In the early 1960s, concerns over coaching methods increasingly focused on players' use of their heads, notably the technique of spearing. Concerned doctors were uncertain precisely where and how the technique had spread in popularity. As Schneider observed, "It is *alleged* that 'spearing,' i.e., a tackler using his head as a weapon, planting it in the ball carrier's midsection without attempt to tackle with the arms, is more frequently taught the further westward one travels. This is purely hearsay and requires confirmation." Whatever the geographic origins and distribution of the technique, football players' use of their heads as weapons was undoubtedly facilitated by the increasing use of plastic helmets.[61]

Herbert Crisler, chairman of the NCAA's rules committee, drew attention to the need to potentially restrict the use of the head in blocking and tackling if injuries persisted. He pointed to a survey conducted for a sports equipment firm found that head, neck, and spinal injuries were not declining. Crisler blamed these injuries on "spearing and goring," and attributed these risky techniques to the advent of helmets with face masks which "give a player the confidence to drive in on an opponent with his head." Consequently, either the design of the helmets or the practice of spearing, which was then perfectly legal, would have to change. "Unless we can find new equipment to reduce head and neck injuries, we may have to do something about these new techniques."[62]

Doctors took note of the risks of spearing as they began to conduct large-scale studies of youth football injuries. A 1964 study of more than 19,000 high school players in Southern California found that about 61 percent of the 203 players who had sustained head injuries had been taught to spear. The authors did not argue that the dangerous technique ought to be removed from all levels of play but instead focused objections on youth players. Children who were not yet fully developed seemed particularly vulnerable to a technique in which the head was used as a weapon. "One must question the place of spearing in high school football. A man who plays football at a university is quite different from a boy playing at the high school level."[63]

At the 1963 NFHS meeting, Thomas Shaffer of the AMA warned attendees of the dangers of spearing and poorly made helmets. Both issues had drawn much media attention in the early 1960s. While there was "great hazard" in the use of inexpensive, poor-quality helmets, Shaffer emphasized that the problem of spearing was not fundamentally a matter of equipment but rather of "coaching ethics." The face guard provided players with essential face and mouth protection and should not be eliminated from the game or used as a weapon. Shaffer cautioned that as long as spearing was employed as a technique, injuries would persist.[64] A spokesman for the AMA's Committee on the Medical Aspects of Sports blamed athletes, stating, "Anyone who would deliberately set out to injure his opponent, by spearing, while at the same time endangering his own life must be lacking in moral values and intelligence."[65]

Contact Builds (Male) Character

Doctors and coaches attributed significant responsibility to boys learning to play football. Young athletes were expected to eliminate their fear of contact. Their desire to hit one another would not only develop their character and keep them from a life of crime but would also physically protect them from injury. At the same time, if boys engaged in improper techniques such as spearing, with the intention of injuring themselves or others, they would cross the line from moral to immoral forms of full-body contact.

Attitudes toward moral character and physical contact thus profoundly shaped perceptions of youth football injuries and deaths. Two key and related assumptions underpinned mid-twentieth century efforts to characterize the health risks of organized football. First, doctors, parents, and educators promoted the view that boys had a unique need for physical contact that only a collision sport like football could satisfy. Second, if boys did not play football, they would get injured anyway in the rough and tumble of other childhood activities. Younger boys might fall from trees; older teenaged boys might crash a car. As a result, the perceived social benefits of football in promoting morals and preventing crime far outweighed the risks.

These prevailing beliefs about boyhood also influenced discussions of unique mechanisms of injury in football, such as spearing, by suggesting that player attitudes were in part to blame. Physicians who studied youth football regarded reluctance to tackle as an indication of a boy's injury-prone nature. If contact built character, fear of contact revealed moral and physical weakness. If the hazards of football were no greater than any other boyhood activity, then any major injuries or deaths said more about a boy's character than the sport of football. In both the medical literature and in public perceptions, beliefs about masculinity, physical contact, and moral character influenced whether injuries and deaths were attributed to football.

Part III
Risk and Responsibility

CHAPTER SIX

Controlling Hazards

Insurance, Data, and Consumer Product Safety, 1930–1974

Before we can decrease football injuries we have to have a hell of a lot more
knowledge about them than we do now.

— James Garrick, 1975

It looked as if the 1930 high school football season in Nashua, New Hampshire, might be the town's last. The Great Depression had diminished ticket
receipts at games, making financing the sport challenging enough. But far
worse, that season the team's young players suffered an unusually high and
expensive number of injuries. Between doctors' bills, x-rays, and hospital attention, medical expenses came out to $800. The city solicitor announced
that the city could not cover this cost, an enormous sum amid a nationwide
economic crisis. Many local parents, in turn, responded that they would not
allow their sons to play if the city could not foot the bills for injuries. The following year, only eight boys turned out for the team, not even enough to fill
out a full squad.[1]

Fortunately for school football fans, local businessman Frank A. Mac-
Master "dug down into his own pocket out of civic pride and love of sports" to
save the program. To cover the team's players, MacMaster decided to sponsor
an insurance policy with the Vermont Accident Insurance Company. After
the announcement of his largesse, forty-six boys turned out with their cleats
to play for their school's 1931 team. MacMaster was hailed as a hero; "the boys
and girls nearly raised the roof" from the school auditorium in celebration.[2]

But not every football town had a sports-loving benefactor who was willing and able to bail out youth teams after a financially calamitous season. In
addition to the potential for steep medical bills, school football programs
regularly faced more predictable expenses, such as outfitting players with
equipment. The Great Depression only heightened the need to control football's financial risks.

In the 1930s, state athletic associations began developing insurance programs to manage medical expenses. The operation of these programs resulted
in the collection of large sets of data on football injuries, information that
further motivated coaches and administrators to examine how to prevent

injuries and minimize costs. Although insurance data were not collected for the purposes of epidemiological research, they furnished an important information source for doctors and educators seeking to study the scope of youth football injuries. In the 1950s and 1960s, as injury epidemiology and sports medicine emerged as specialized fields, injury researchers often turned to insurance data.

As researchers undertook larger and more sophisticated epidemiological studies in the 1960s, they identified concerning patterns of football injury. Their findings suggested that not even the best equipment could prevent frequent and serious injuries. By this period, however, youth football was even more entrenched in American schools and communities. Fundamentally altering the sport to prevent injuries was not treated as a serious option. Instead, in conjunction with a growing consumer safety movement, researchers and policymakers identified football helmets as a potentially hazardous consumer product in need of study and regulation.

By the 1970s, youth football teams generally no longer needed to rely on local businessmen such as Frank MacMaster to control the financial hazards of football injuries. Insurance programs had helped spread the costs. Preventing injuries from occurring in the first place, however, proved a more challenging matter. Yet, to control football's risks, communities and researchers prioritized strategies that would not alter the collision nature of the sport.

Developing Athletic Insurance Programs

In the early decades of the twentieth century, largely without insurance coverage, local schools, coaches, and families typically shouldered the burden of medical expenses for sports injuries. A 1936 study found that only four of twenty-five insurance companies surveyed offered athletic insurance. The authors recommended that state high school athletic associations and college conferences take full charge of athletic insurance for member schools. Group insurance would reduce expenses and substantially relieve parents and coaches of the financial burden of caring for sports-related injuries.[3]

This recommendation was consistent with an emerging trend already under way. Beginning in the 1930s, a number of state athletic associations began developing insurance programs to cover medical bills for injuries that students sustained while playing high school sports. In 1930–31, the Wisconsin Interscholastic Athletic Association (WIAA) became the first state athletic association to inaugurate a self-administered insurance program. The WIAA developed its plan under the supervision of the state insurance commission, which had first approached insurance companies about the possibility of coverage for athletic injuries only to find them reluctant. Insurers believed the cost to be prohibitive; one company reportedly indicated that $14 per participant would be necessary to provide coverage of football alone.[4]

Wisconsin schools were offered the choice of two possible benefit plans, as well as two payment options: either purchasing blanket coverage based on student enrollment or offering policies to individual athletes at a higher cost per student. Notably, in either case the policy premium more than doubled if football coverage was included. In its first year, the WIAA's benefit plan paid out $5,330 to cover 101 claims, including broken legs, arms, and collarbones. In the 1967–68 school year, the same program would cover 36,000 claims for a total of $875,000.[5]

In the fall of 1932, the New York State Public High School Athletic Association similarly put an experimental athletic protection plan into effect. That season, sixty-six schools registered for football, with the fund covering 1,255 student athletes. The program proved a success and was extended to other sports. As with Wisconsin's plan, New York's program continued to grow in the ensuing decades. In the 1949–50 academic year, the association's executive secretary reported that the plan covered over 48,000 student athletes and had paid over $65,000 in claims.[6]

State athletic associations across the country began adopting similar programs in the 1930s and 1940s, often modeled after the plans developed by Wisconsin, New York, or other "mother states." Texas, for instance, adopted a schedule of benefits similar to New York's protection plan in 1940. Often, schools contributed part of the cost while parents of players put up the rest in individual payments. The risk of injury was typically rated higher in contact sports as compared to noncontact sports, and fees were set accordingly. In 1945, for instance, New York charged $2.50 per player for football and wrestling, $2.00 for hockey, lacrosse, and skiing, $1.00 for basketball and soccer, and $0.50 for track, tennis, baseball, golf, and cross-country.[7]

While state athletic protection programs became increasingly widespread, they did not necessarily cover all football-related injuries. Many continued to rely on "self-insurance" rather than purchasing a broad-based external plan. A 1951 *Scholastic Coach* article warned coaches and administrators that interscholastic programs did not provide unlimited funds to defray the expenses of treating injuries, and that they could not rely on the *pro bono* work of neighborhood doctors to make up any potential difference. The article advised on factors to consider in choosing benefit options, such as nonprofit versus commercial plans, and whether plans included coverage for such extras as transportation to and from out-of-town games. Furthermore, coaches were reminded that parents—especially parents in lower income brackets—were concerned about the economic risks of football. Controlling financial expenses was evidently crucial to gaining many parents' consent to allow their sons to play football. A coach who could clearly inform parents what insurance plans covered "is sometimes able to add extremely valuable manpower to his varsities and various intramural sports."[8]

Both the cost of insurance and the documentation of injuries from claims prompted some coaches and administrators to reevaluate ways to reduce injuries and expenses. After Texas's Interscholastic League adopted its benefit plan in 1940, the Texas High School Football Coaches Association met over the summer to discuss the causes of injuries and possible prevention strategies. Their recommendations were consistent with the long-standing emphasis on adult supervision discussed in chapter 4. They urged complete medical examinations for all players, three weeks of conditioning before boys were permitted to play in games, enhancing the availability of first aid, ensuring proper equipment, scheduling interschool contests with institutions of a similar size to avoid lopsided matches, and an emphasis on "football fundamentals" over the course of the season.[9]

Although insurance claims forms were designed to collect data for the primary purpose of providing insurance coverage, such data also provided some of the earliest and most extensive available information on causes and rates of morbidity and mortality.[10] This included data on sports injuries among large populations of Americans. Indeed, in the absence of large-scale epidemiological studies, insurance companies represented one of the only available sources of such data.[11]

Once state athletic associations developed their own benefit plans, administrators could use this information to compare rates of injuries among different school sports. For instance, the New York State Education Department, in collaboration with an education professor at New York University, used data from New York State's Athletic Protection Plan to study accidents among schoolboys. From February 1958 to January 1959 when schools were in session, they collected data from ninety-six secondary schools in New York State, excluding New York City. The study found that interscholastic athletic competition accounted for two-thirds of all accidents. Of the sports included in the study, tackle football represented both the highest gross number and the highest incidence of injuries (see table 3).[12]

Examining the causes of injury identified in insurance claims, the researchers found that "tackling in football was the skill or activity most frequently

TABLE 3 Top five activities by gross accidents, New York State, 1958–1959

Activity	Number of Accidents	Percentage of Total Accidents	Exposures	Incidence per 1,000 Exposures
Football	542	38.5	258,453	2.1
Basketball	224	15.9	515,300	0.43
Wrestling	108	7.7	216,567	0.5
Soccer	85	6.0	175,975	0.48
Track and Field	79	5.6	310,986	0.25

The 96 schools from which these data were derived were selected by a proportional, stratified random sampling technique. An exposure was defined as "participation by a boy in a class or extraclass activity during a school day." New York State Bureau of Physical Education, *Safety in Physical Education.*

engaged in at the time of the accident." Football injuries also represented the highest dollar value of claims, accounting for well over half of all interscholastic athletic claims paid in 1961–62. Considering that football was clearly the most hazardous sport based on insurance claims data, the study concluded by questioning whether it should continue to be considered "a desirable educational offering in the secondary school athletic program."[13] Yet tackle football was already entrenched as one of the most popular sports in American high schools. In the 1960s and in the decades to follow, recommendations that questioned the sport's fundamental educational value were not seriously pursued.

The Limits of Protective Gear: Knees and Legs

Methods of sports injury data collection before 1960 typically did not allow investigators to clearly calculate the *incidence* of football injuries, meaning the number of new injuries occurring over a defined period of time in a defined population. Instead, injury reports generally involved simple retrospective counts, lacking the data about the total number of participants needed in order to calculate the rate of injury. Researchers who did report an incidence of football injury typically conducted their studies on a small scale, such as school physicians who had documented the injuries they treated among students at the single high school they served. Insurance data sometimes made estimating incidence possible, but such data had significant limitations because they were not collected for the purposes of scientific research.

By the 1960s, however, medical societies and athletic associations started to conduct larger prospective studies of injury incidence among youth players. The emergence of sports medicine and injury prevention as specialized fields, as described in chapter 4, helped enable this research. In 1966, the AMA published its first standard nomenclature of athletic injuries, "so that meaningful records and statistics concerning sports injuries and their causes" could be maintained. Efforts to treat athletic injuries as worthy of systematic study, like other forms of injury and disease, helped promote epidemiological research on football injuries. Insurance data facilitated some of these early studies. Such research, in turn, raised questions about the extent to which football equipment served as a protective or even a risk factor for injury.[14]

Some of the first large-scale football injury research happened at the state level, as state medical societies formed athletic subcommittees that provided greater institutional support. For example, the Athletic Medical Advisory Committee of the Academy of Medicine of Cincinnati, Ohio, tracked football injuries among 2,846 students at thirty-one high schools from 1962 to 1964. The Ohio researchers shared their data with orthopedic doctor William Garrahan, who had started tracking injuries at twenty-five Rhode Island high schools, and added eight more by 1965. While the Ohio study had sent out questionnaires to schools, Garrahan instead relied on insurance claims forms to obtain injury data.[15]

Garrahan reported that approximately one out of five high school football players sustained some kind of injury, a similar result to the Ohio study. Dental injuries had decreased after mouth guards became mandatory in 1962 (see chapter 3), suggesting the effectiveness of the equipment. Other types of injuries remained relatively stable. Garrahan further reported that only about one out of thirteen players had sustained a "potentially serious" injury, which he defined as "injuries to vital parts of the body, but not necessarily serious because of the force involved." Concussion, for example, did not constitute a serious injury according to this definition. Garrahan observed that the incidence of concussion remained high throughout the study, but that "there were no serious head injuries during the six year period." Despite this relative lack of clarity in defining categories of injury and other limitations, the studies in Ohio and Rhode Island nonetheless represented some of the first attempts to document the incidence and nature of high school football injuries among a large group of students in a prospective, multiyear study.[16]

State athletic organizations studied football injuries primarily in order to improve player safety by modifying rules or equipment, rather than reconsidering the value of the sport. For example, in response to the New York

State Education Department study finding that football was the most dangerous school sport, the New York State Public High School Athletic Association (NYSPHSAA) did not drop football. Instead, it initiated a conditioning program and began to conduct its own studies of injuries.[17] Its research program and publications illustrate how one such association worked to collect data to improve athlete safety in the 1960s. Discussions at medical conferences at which researchers shared their data also reveal how beliefs about the value of football constrained the interpretation and application of these research findings.

In August 1963, NYSPHSAA's State Football Committee began a voluntary, experimental preseason football conditioning program. The program was intended to minimize injuries and improve athlete fitness and was open to any school interested in participating. The NYSPHSAA allocated funds to track injuries and evaluate the program's effectiveness. In conjunction with this effort, the association initiated a series of studies intended to identify the major causes of injury among interscholastic youth football players in New York State. In May 1966, a report evaluating the three-year experimental program showed a reduction in football injuries.[18]

In addition to continuing this successful conditioning program, in 1967 the NYSPHSAA leadership decided to undertake another study of head, thigh, knee, and ankle injuries, for which they received a grant from the state education department. Ultimately the association sponsored two studies, one large and one small, examining whether equipment modifications could prevent injuries to players' legs. Orthopedic surgeon Murle Laurens Rowe of the University of Rochester led the smaller study of 1,235 high school varsity football players at forty-four schools. He hypothesized that football cleats might contribute to injuries that occurred when players cut or pivoted on their feet. Using multiple combinations of shoe and cleat types, Rowe found that low-cut shoes with plastic disc heels were associated with fewer injuries as compared to the conventionally cleated football shoe. In 1969, he reported his results to several New York State-based conferences and journals.[19]

In 1967–68, the NYSPHSAA also undertook a much larger statewide study of lower extremity football injuries, with the support of the New York State Education Department. This study included more than 17,000 varsity high school football players, representing over 90 percent of such players in the state. The authors asserted that the program was "unparalleled in scope" and "the first statewide survey in the nation designed to catalogue such injuries, in a standardized and medically acceptable manner, by type and severity."

In 1967, the first year of the study, the researchers largely failed to control for key variables, such as equipment worn and the number of games played. Consequently, the authors could not draw many conclusions from the data they had collected about whether different types of equipment were associated with injuries.[20]

The next year, researchers adjusted their study design to include data on several experimental variables, such as player's conditioning, experience in sports, and type and extent of injury. Physician members of the Committee on Medical Aspects of Sports of the New York State Medical Society developed a system of injury classification, including a four-point scale to assess seriousness of injury. They also incorporated several checks of the reliability of the data, such as checking 10 percent of injury notations against school health and/or athletic department records.

Based on the 1968 data using this stronger study design, the researchers advised that football players ideally be outfitted with low shoes and some form of disc or flat heel, or short cleats, similar to the results of Rowe's smaller study. The clearest finding, however, was that a previous knee injury made players far more likely to be seriously reinjured. The authors' primary recommendation, then, was that players with a previous knee injury should undergo a planned program of rehabilitation before being permitted to return to football. Furthermore, physicians should thoroughly examine such players before the start of each football season to evaluate the athletes' fitness to participate.

Yet even with such modifications, the association's final report emphasized that the majority of knee and ankle injuries would not be prevented. Out of the 328 total serious knee injuries recorded, their estimates suggested that only some ten or twenty cases would be reduced even if all players were outfitted with ideal shoes. And even if all players with a previous knee injury were completely rehabilitated prior to returning to play, the total number of knee injuries would be reduced by only forty or fifty cases.[21]

Based on these numbers, the report cautioned that further research on shoe equipment was unlikely to be productive. Instead of focusing on protective equipment, the study suggested the nature and conduct of football should be examined, especially in order to eliminate dangerous situations caused by such tactics as players piling on each other and "spearing" (using the head as a weapon). The researchers concluded that various rule changes, such as restricting players to blocking one another above the waist, needed to be attempted and evaluated, "regardless of whether they change the 'traditional' nature of the game."[22]

In addition to supporting football injury research, the New York athletic association also sponsored conferences in collaboration with doctors and educators to examine player safety. In 1968, the association cosponsored its first symposium on the medical aspects of sports along with the Medical Society of the State of New York and the Health, Physical Education and Recreation Association. At the symposium, researchers described the preliminary results of some of the youth sports injury data that had been collected over the previous five years in New York State. Every year, Rowe stated, about one-third of New York State high school football players sustained a reportable injury. Of these injuries, about one-third affected players' legs (16 percent were knee injuries, 13 percent ankle injuries, and 4 percent affected other parts of the leg). Rowe asserted that both this preliminary data and his experience made clear that preventing knee and ankle injuries "in a running, heavy contact sport like football" would be very difficult.[23]

Anthony J. Pisani, an orthopedic surgeon who served as team physician for the New York Giants, shared Rowe's concern about the vulnerability of players' knees. "It is my opinion that mechanically the human knee was not meant for football. . . . Cleats or type [*sic*] of footgear variation certainly are a boon to the manufacturers or the sporting goods houses, but play little or no part in the prevention of knee injuries." If equipment was not a promising solution to preventing knee injuries, Pisani instead suggested that athletes could best protect themselves with their style of play. He cited advice from coaches and athletes that football players should keep their legs moving at all times, even if they were not directly involved in action on the field. In this way, even if they received a blow to their legs, it would be "a glancing type of force rather than a square impact." He added that one college football coach had claimed that thanks to this approach, none of his players had sustained knee injuries requiring surgery. Pisani concluded, "Constant movement of the legs during the actual play sets up a moving target that affords the best chance of survival to play another day."[24]

Both Rowe and Pisani communicated to the popular press their concerns about the difficulty of preventing football injuries. They were both quoted as sharing the view that "the knee is not meant for football" in a 1968 *Chicago Tribune* article on professional football injuries. Rowe supported better officiating and leg conditioning but concluded "that there is no real solution to the knee injury problem."[25] Their skepticism of equipment as a preventative strategy was similar to the conclusion of the 1969 New York study, which had found that focusing on shoes and cleats did not seem a promising route for preventing knee and ankle injuries.

If better shoes or cleats were not the solution, two alternative options seemed to present themselves: recommending particular playing techniques to athletes that might best protect them (and thereby making players responsible for their own safety) or altering some of the rules of football. Pisani's advice that players constantly move their legs at all times during football matches fell into the former category. Meanwhile, the 1969 NYSPHSAA report advised the latter strategy. The association's researchers recommended revising even the most seemingly traditional rules of football and evaluating whether such changes could eliminate some of the most dangerous situations that occurred in the sport. While no real solution was apparent to the problem of knee injuries, none of these experts suggested that tackling should be eliminated or football banned outright.

Helmet Design Controversy

In the late 1960s, protective equipment did not appear to be the most promising option for reducing football-related leg injuries. The effectiveness of helmets in preventing head injuries also represented a source of uncertainty. In 1969, researcher and Northwestern football team physician Stephen E. Reid argued for doing away with football helmets altogether to prevent players from using their heads as weapons. Eliminating the equipment, he believed, would result in less head contact in the game—but, he acknowledged, it would interfere with the techniques of the sport as it was then played.[26]

And again, the option of drastically altering, let alone banning, football was not on any influential table. Suggestions to eliminate football helmets or otherwise "interfere" with the sport were largely sidelined in favor of improving headgear. Despite uncertainty over the fundamental benefits of football equipment, the 1960s saw an increasing emphasis on improving equipment, particularly football helmets.

Some of the impetus for initiating football helmet research had its origins in automobile safety. In 1956, a popular racer, William "Pete" Snell, died of head injuries he sustained in an amateur auto racing collision in northern California. Because his helmet failed to protect him, several physicians who were also fellow amateur racers decided to work on improving head protection in Snell's honor. They established the Snell Memorial Foundation in 1957.[27]

The foundation's helmet test facility was set up at the University of California's Davis campus, and its resources provided the opportunity to

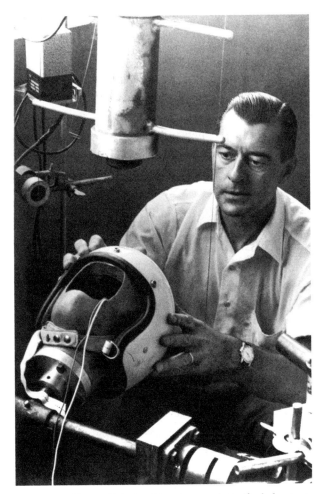

FIGURE 14 George Snively with swing arm tester for helmets at
the UC Davis testing facility. Undated photo c. late 1950s or early
1960s. Courtesy of the Snell Memorial Foundation.

study football helmets as well as racing crash helmets (see figure 14). George
Snively, a physician at Sacramento County Hospital, collaborated with two
researchers from UC Davis's physical education department who were concerned about head injuries among the school's football squad. With funding
from the National Institutes of Health, they obtained eleven different models
of helmets from the open market. They compared these against a prototype
helmet with a fiberglass outer shell that covered a foamed, nonresilient plastic lining. Finding that the prototype helmets performed better under high
impacts in the lab, they provided several of these fiberglass helmets to UC

Davis football players for use in field trials during football practices and games.[28]

Orthopedic surgeon and team physician Harold Fenner was similarly motivated by Snell's death. Fenner had raced cars professionally in the 1950s and would later serve as president of the board of directors of the Snell foundation. He began to study football helmet safety in his own practice, and observed deficiencies in the helmets used by student athletes on the local high school football team in Hobbs, New Mexico. Due to a weakness of the then-available plastic shell helmet, he found that an object could make solid contact with the shell against the wearer's head, particularly below the headband level of the helmet. To address this defect, Fenner argued that a much more rigid shell, such as fiberglass, was necessary. In March 1960, Fenner obtained a prototype fiberglass helmet from Snively, made some modifications in consultation with the Hobbs High School coaching staff, and began to use this redesigned headgear among the school's team. Despite initial concerns that the inner liner would need frequent replacement due to damage, Fenner reported that after four seasons of use at Hobbs High School, it had not been necessary to replace any of the liners.[29]

Physicians were thus experimenting with different helmet designs among students playing on high school and college teams with which they were affiliated. Such unsupervised experimental research took place in an era before institutional review boards were established to oversee the ethics of research on youth. At the time, these physicians felt they were meeting an urgent need of developing more effective equipment for their players. They hoped their innovations might provide a model for the type of equipment all football players ought to wear, and they urged the need for standardization. "It is apparent that the time to establish minimum standards for football helmets is not only here but has passed," Fenner insisted after documenting the "alarming variance in the performance of energy absorption among different brands of helmets." Only three of the sixteen major brands of football helmets on the market provided adequate protection, he warned. Fenner concluded his 1964 report by recommending that the sale of plastic helmets for small children be banned. At the time, such helmets were used not only in football but also in soapbox derbies, go-cart racing, and baseball.[30]

In addition to efforts to identify more effective materials for use in the construction of football helmets, the recently added face guard was a source of contention. This problem was the focus of a 1965 study conducted by neuroscientist Richard Schneider and ophthalmologist Bartley Antine. The physicians found that face guard innovations with the potential to enhance the overall protection afforded by football helmets would constrain players' visual fields. In grappling with this trade-off, the authors stated that even a transient limitation on players' vision might not only hamper their success on the field but could increase their risk of injuries. While they acknowledged that no design was without its limitations, Schneider and Antine recommended face guards with "J shaped" lower bars as the most promising option to protect players' faces without overly constraining their vision.[31]

To address such difficulties involved in improving equipment, in 1968 several doctors, academics, sports administrators, and sporting goods manufacturers organized a national conference on protective equipment in sports. The members of the planning committee included Creighton J. Hale, then the director of research and vice president of Little League Baseball, as well as team physicians, professors of physical education, safety education, and engineering, and the vice president of research and engineering of sporting goods manufacturer Riddell.[32]

The concerns that prompted this 1968 conference included identifying where equipment would be of value in sports and ways to improve currently available equipment. There were also questions about which newly available materials from the decade's "scientific explosion" might be incorporated into protective gear and how to set equipment standards. The introduction to the proceedings highlighted an overarching need for a more systematic approach, contending that sporting goods manufacturers' efforts "have been guided more by individual suggestions from coaches, athletes and other interested persons and by deficiencies or failures of existing items rather than by a planned approach to the problems of protection in sports."[33]

University of Wisconsin team physician Allan Ryan contributed a conference session examining the fundamental question of what injuries might be preventable with protective equipment, particularly in contact or collision sports. "Studies of the forces involved when today's fast and heavy athletes collide have raised serious doubts in the minds of some as to whether any type of protective equipment we can provide within the limits of practicability can decelerate these forces rapidly enough to prevent injury." Furthermore, he continued, if equipment was effective, this might cause athletes to act in "careless disregard of injury," taking risks that they might not have taken otherwise. Even worse, they might use their equipment to deliberately injure another player. In making this point, Ryan was likely referring to the ongoing issue of "spearing" in tackle football.[34]

Despite these caveats, conference attendees did not propose removing any piece of equipment from any sport. Rather, they focused their recommendations on how to improve existing equipment. They called for establishing uniform injury reporting techniques and the use of standard nomenclature for athletic injuries to improve the accuracy of injury data. They further recommended the formation of a "Committee for Protective Equipment in Sports" that would include representatives from a wide range of fields and encompass equipment in a variety of sports: football, ice hockey, baseball, wrestling, basketball, soccer, lacrosse, and rugby. While not as far-ranging as the committee envisioned in these recommendations, the forthcoming establishment of the American Society for Testing and Materials (ASTM)'s F-8 committee on sports equipment and the National Operating Committee on Standards for Athletic Equipment (NOCSAE) in 1970 (see chapter 7) would in many ways resemble this description.[35]

Consumer Product Safety Movement

By the late 1960s and early 1970s, researchers were increasingly applying epidemiological methods to the study of athletic injuries.[36] Yet, as one researcher complained, there remained a relative "paucity of published information" because "the design and construction of protective equipment, particularly for American contact football but for other sports too, has unfortunately followed a general pattern of consumer suggestion, generational development of prototype devices, and, what for the most part appears to be outright 'divine guidance' in lieu of controlled field testing."[37]

But a shift from "divine guidance" to controlled testing was beginning to occur. Two key developments contributed to increasing systematic study and standardization of football equipment. First, changes in tort law meant that a new strict liability standard was increasingly applied in legal cases involving defective products, including lawsuits related to sporting goods. Previously in American law, plaintiffs needed to be in a contract relationship (in "privity") with defendants as a necessary condition of liability. But a number of court cases chipped away at this requirement throughout the 1940s and 1950s.[38]

Then, in 1963, the Supreme Court of California held in *Greenman v. Yuba Power Products, Inc.* that manufacturers would face strict liability for injuries to human beings caused by defects of their products. This new standard meant that plaintiffs would not need to prove negligence or intent to cause injury, only that the product had caused a person harm. Furthermore, the weakening of the privity requirement meant that courts could find manufacturers legally responsible for the harms caused by defective athletic equipment beyond the individuals who had purchased the product. Courts would go on to recognize three general types of manufacturer conduct that might make a product unsafe: defective design of product, defective manufacture of product, and inadequate marketing or failure to warn.[39]

Strict product liability quickly swept across the United States, a movement one legal scholar described as "the most rapid and altogether spectacular overturn of an established rule in the entire history of the law of torts." In 1964, the American Law Institute approved the *Restatement (Second) of Torts* § 402, highlighting the national shift to strict liability. In addition, by the 1960s and 1970s the notion that the threat of increased liability could help prevent accidents "became a standard feature of tort theory." The shift toward strict liability motivated manufacturers to support equipment standards and certification that would reduce their liability for harm caused by defective products.[40]

Secondly, broader consumer product safety concerns contributed further attention to protective equipment in sports. One of the most prominent developments in injury prevention in the 1960s was more active federal involvement in automobile and highway safety. Following the 1965 publication of Ralph Nader's landmark book *Unsafe at Any Speed*, in 1966 President Lyndon Johnson signed the National Traffic and Motor Vehicle Safety Act. This act created the National Highway Safety Bureau, whose first director was William Haddon Jr., a pioneer in the field of injury prevention. The bureau, which would later become the National Highway Traffic Safety Administration (NHTSA), adopted an epidemiological approach to preventing highway injuries. Rather than focusing on modifying driver behavior, regulators were authorized to set minimum safety standards for automobiles in the United States.[41]

Michael Pertschuk, the consumer counsel for the U.S. Senate's Commerce Committee, later recalled how this federal legislation on automobile safety influenced efforts to address the dangers of consumer products more generally. After the passage of the National Traffic and Motor Vehicle Safety Act, Senator Warren Magnuson and his staff began exploring "what seemed to be the next logical step, omnibus product-safety legislation covering other potentially hazardous manufactured products." They decided that an independent national product safety commission was not yet politically ripe. Instead, by introducing legislation to create a temporary National Commission on Product Safety (NCPS) to study the issue, the senator and his staff hoped to focus public attention on product safety and to develop a record of evidence on the hazards of consumer products. In this way, NCPS was designed to foster the familiarity and legitimacy needed for the formation of a new regulatory commission.[42]

Following the formation of the temporary commission, the U.S. House of Representatives held hearings that addressed the dangers of a wide variety of consumer products. Football helmets featured prominently. At hearings held in February 1969, the testimony of several lawyers, members of the public, and a professional football player focused on youth football injuries and the effectiveness of youth helmets. The variety of testimony presented at these hearings demonstrates how different groups framed the issue of protective equipment and football safety, and why football helmets remained on the commission's agenda as a product of public concern.

The testimony began with several personal stories from members of the public. Larry Csonka, a fullback with the Miami Dolphins, testified that even with his experience as a professional football player, he would not be able to determine which of two helmets in a sporting goods store would provide the greatest safety. While Csonka believed that safe helmets were available, a consumer's ability to evaluate helmet effectiveness was the essential missing factor. He emphasized that the key issue was the protection of youth football players, such as his own two sons.[43]

Next, two parents, Mr. and Mrs. McLelland, each testified about a catastrophic football injury their eighth-grade son, Michael, had suffered despite wearing a helmet. Following a collision with another player during a blocking exercise overseen by two coaches, Michael collapsed, went into a coma, and ultimately required five brain surgeries. At twenty, the young man was partially paralyzed, had a speech disorder, and was unable to care for himself. Mr. McLelland indicated that he and other parents had all been aware of and would be willing to accept injuries such as broken arms and broken legs. But based on Michael's experience, he argued that parents around the country needed to consider whether they would be willing to consent to brain injuries of this nature.[44]

Lawyer Harry M. Philo, whom the American Association for Justice would later describe as "one of the giants of plaintiff trial law," proceeded to testify that helmet makers needed to be held liable for the injuries that football players sustained while using their products. Philo blasted manufacturers for their role in serious and fatal football head injuries across the United States. He dubbed the injury toll from tackle football "a national disgrace that has been hidden from the public." Makers of football helmets, he claimed, had failed to heed calls from doctors and coaches for the development of adequate standards of protection. Pointing to the research conducted by

Snively and Fenner, Philo argued that helmets with a fiberglass shell offered greater protection; he claimed the main reason manufacturers had not switched to fiberglass shell helmets was that plastic helmets could be made so cheaply.[45]

Philo noted that, in addition to failing to adopt more effective materials, helmet manufacturers had never once tested the safety of the 125,000 helmets they sold each year. Instead, he contended, executives had "pleaded ignorance of the deficiencies in their helmets" and "put their heads in the sand." As an example of the data the manufacturers were ignoring, Philo cited a 1967 study on the incidence of concussions among football players at sixty-three colleges. He warned that "the new knowledge of bizarre personality changes caused by microscopic brain damage from subfatal acceleration injuries should cause society great concern over the inadequacy of football head protection."[46]

David Rust, an attorney representing the major sporting goods manufacturer Rawlings, disputed Philo's claims. Rust asserted that Philo was exaggerating the numbers of injuries and deaths, that the statistics had not been hidden, and that the industry was working to understand what impacts helmets could absorb. Not only did helmet manufacturers face the challenge of how to improve helmet design, Rust added, they also had to grapple with the trouble of players who preferred "a light helmet because they have a severe sweat problem." Rust's argument that athletes' sweat represented a significant hurdle to improving protective equipment did not appear to impress the commission. Commissioner Emory Crofoot drily retorted, "Well, we can put a man on the moon, it would seem to me that we can overcome this problem."[47]

As an industry lawyer, Rust sought to portray football injuries as unpredictable and random occurrences. Even if helmets could protect users from any head injury, he noted that manufacturers could not control for all circumstances: "We might also end up ruining the few boys who get socked with that helmet." He cited documents from the 1968 Conference on Protective Equipment in Sports to demonstrate the difficulty of protecting against injury in football and the progress manufacturers had nonetheless made in improving equipment. He portrayed sporting goods manufacturers as providing the best possible helmets given the constraints of design and technical challenges. While granting that any single player's death was of course important, Rust deftly minimized the concession by adding "as well as any death in the hundreds of thousands that we are losing in Vietnam." He further insisted that "it is a physical impossibility to design a football helmet in the state of the art now or in the foreseeable future that will totally prevent death in a football game."[48]

Both Philo and Rust thus drew on medical literature to make conflicting arguments about the effectiveness of available football helmets. Despite Rust's testimony contending that manufacturers were designing the best possible helmets while forced to accommodate athletes' inconvenient sweat problems, the NCPS continued to include football helmets among their list of dangerous products under review. At another 1969 hearing, Representative Joshua Eilberg of Pennsylvania asked whether manufacturers should continue to have exclusive power to set standards for "football helmets that do not prevent brain concussions" along an array of other dangerous products, from charcoal lighters to floor furnaces with grills that could burn toddlers.[49]

In 1970, the National Commission issued its final report to the president and Congress, arguing that there was no justification for exposing an entire population to risks of injury or death that were not apparent to consumers. "Such hazards must be controlled and limited not at the option of the producer but as a matter of right to the consumer." The report specifically identified sixteen consumer products as "unreasonably hazardous," including football and motorcycle helmets in the category of protective headgear.[50] After describing the severe injury suffered by eighth-grader Michael McClelland, the report noted that "no industry standard whatever has been developed for protective headgear." Furthermore, buyers were completely dependent upon manufacturers, because a superficial inspection of a helmet was not sufficient to determine its strength and effectiveness.[51]

The final report described the need for government action. In addition to football helmets, a long list of household and consumer products had prompted extensive concern, from fireworks to infant furniture. Major newspapers reported on the commission's key findings and recommendations: No government agency had general authority to ban dangerous products or require that consumer products meet minimum safety standards. Existing authority over particular categories of products was scattered across agencies and hampered by "bargain-basement budgets" and enormous bureaucratic hurdles. The federal government did not systematically collect or disseminate data on product safety and thus had no "early-warning system" of potentially hazardous products, nor could it mandate the recall of dangerous products.[52]

Following the National Commission's recommendations, in October 1972, Congress passed the Consumer Product Safety Act. This act created the U.S. Consumer Product Safety Commission (CPSC), an independent federal agency to protect Americans from dangerous or defective consumer products. The agency was granted the authority to set mandatory safety standards and to recall or ban products, among its other powers. To address the absence of injury data, Congress also gave the CPSC a major nonregulatory responsibility: the establishment of an "injury information clearinghouse to collect, investigate, analyze, and disseminate injury data."[53]

The CPSC would primarily meet this responsibility through the National Electronic Injury Surveillance System (NEISS), a system originally designed in 1970 to obtain injury data from a sample of 119 representative emergency rooms. The NEISS became the core data system of the CPSC's Bureau of Epidemiology once the agency was activated in 1973, forming one of the major mechanisms for the CPSC to collect injury statistics. A 1975 CPSC brochure, "Together We Can Reduce Injury," emphasized the NEISS as a key part of CSPC's work and a source of reliable information about product safety. The development of the NEISS was hailed as part of a broader movement toward a scientific approach to tracking and reducing injuries.[54]

In 1974, the CPSC published an analysis of football injuries based on NEISS data, as well as an assessment of the efficacy of football equipment. The report estimated that 300,000 football injuries were treated annually in hospital emergency rooms nationwide, a figure extrapolated from the 14,280 injuries reported in the NEISS data set for the 1973 calendar year. Over 80 percent of these football injuries affected children aged five to nineteen years. The majority were strains, sprains, contusions, and abrasions. Only 1 percent of the reported injuries were concussions, "a diagnosis which can be quite serious," observed the report. It seems probable that concussions were vastly underreported in this data set, given that football players were unlikely to go to the emergency room for treatment for a concussion during this period unless they had been severely and obviously injured.[55]

The CPSC also assessed the effectiveness of protective equipment by conducting in-depth investigations of 112 of the reported injuries. This subset of injuries was not randomly selected; investigators focused on the most severe injuries documented in the emergency room records. Investigators assigned an evaluation of "Protective Equipment Not Effective" to cases where injuries occurred underneath protective padded covering (see table 4).

Most of these injuries occurred after contact or tackling and included cases of concussions that occurred despite athletes wearing a helmet. Investigators found that when safety equipment was involved in injury, the equipment tended to be ineffective rather than defective. Most injuries were not life-threatening, the CPSC report observed. Nonetheless, the report concluded, "No single act, short of prohibiting football, could have a dramatic

TABLE 4 Sample of CPSC case reports of football injuries

Age	Precipitating Event/Activity	Description	Result (Diagnosis)	Disposition	Product Make/Composition
15	Hit in head	Victim was tackled in a high school game. The coach said, when he fell, his chin hit the ground and the tackler's jaw bone hit the victim's temple.	Concussion, head	Treated and released	Face guard
13	Hit in head	After he was tackled in a junior high game, victim's helmet was struck by another player's knee.	Concussion, head	Treated and released	Riddell football helmet
16	Elbow in face	After making a tackle during practice, other player's forearm struck victim's nose, breaking it. All of the players were practicing in full football protective equipment. Face mask had a single bar.	Fracture, nose	Treated and admitted (1 day)	Single bar face mask
10	Hit in head	Victim was tackled in midget league practice. "After the play was over, several other players piled on."	Concussion, head	Treated and released	Wilson football helmet F 2043 (D)
16	Tackling	This was the first day of contact during preseason practice. During one-on-one tackling the victim was struck by the head and shoulders of the other player, on helmet and upper trunk. He was lifted up and back falling on his buttocks. He suffered a mild concussion in October 1972.	Subdural hematoma	Hospital (28 days) Expired	Helmet MacGregor 100MH

This is a sample of injuries included in the "Organized Football (Protective Equipment Not Effective)" chart reported in the CSPC's 1974 analysis of football hazards. For the purposes of this sample of injuries, case numbers, dates, and sex were all removed. All included cases affected males, and all injuries occurred in 1972 or 1973. U.S. CPSC, *Hazard Analysis: Football*.

effect in reducing the injury rate." Despite this striking conclusion, the agency did not regard prohibiting football as a viable option. Even where the limitations of helmets were most acknowledged, the perpetuation of youth football was taken as a given.[56]

Permitting a Hazardous Activity

The high costs of injuries in the Great Depression did not put an end to youth football. Neither, several decades later, would the accumulation of evidence indicating that only prohibiting football could significantly reduce injuries. Instead, doctors, researchers, and sports administrators chose to manage the sport's physical and financial risks by shifting the focus to the quality of protective gear and the adequacy of insurance coverage.

Despite substantial and ongoing challenges in keeping expenses low, large athletic insurance programs offered families and schools a greater degree of financial protection against the risk of football injuries. The development of these programs also had the important side effect of influencing football injury epidemiology. Insurance claims represented one of the only sources of large-scale data on injury rates at mid-twentieth century. Even if limited by the design of insurance claims forms, these data nonetheless proved important in early football injury studies. More sophisticated systems to control financial costs of injury thus contributed to more sophisticated approaches to tracking injuries.

A number of doctors, state athletic associations, and prominent safety organizations conducted studies based on large-scale data. Medical opinion and research findings pointed to the limits of football equipment, from Pisani's opinion that "the human knee was not meant for football" to the 1974 CPSC report's conclusion that no act short of banning football could dramatically reduce injuries. A few doctors and researchers suggested removing helmets or making fundamental rule changes. But most did not countenance such drastic changes to the sport.

A businessman such as Frank A. MacMaster stepping in to save a high school football team might represent local support for football. But prominent doctors and researchers with national influence also used the resources at their disposal to "save football" when evidence of the sport's injury risks threatened the game. The efforts of laypeople, as well as the experts responsible for protecting youth health, represented a broad cultural investment in preserving the sport. As the CPSC noted, "Frequently, one can seek to prevent the potentially hazardous event, thereby preventing the injury. In football, we must reduce the risk of injury but permit a potentially hazardous activity to occur."[57]

Yet knee and ankle injuries were acknowledged to be an inherent part of tackle football in a way that head injuries were not. As the testimony of two parents about their injured son at the 1969 NCPS hearings indicated, parents were not willing to accept catastrophic brain injuries in the way that they might accept broken legs or arms. Consequently, football helmets proved to be the source of greatest debate and concern. A broader consumer product safety movement and the shift toward strict liability in tort law helped motivate a focus on football helmet standardization and evaluation. Addressing youth football safety as a consumer rights issue shone a spotlight on the limitations of equipment but also hindered bigger questions about more sweeping changes to the sport.

Thus, even when recognizing that they lacked sufficient knowledge of how to reduce football injuries given the rules of the game, most researchers chose to focus on improving football equipment. Their efforts were consistent with American faith in science and technology to control hazards. Coaches wanted to preserve football and protect their players, and furnishing athletes with the most modern equipment seemed to fulfill both these goals. By the early 1970s, the most influential sports and research organizations had zeroed in on setting standards for football helmets as the most important technological strategy needed to control the sport's hazards.

CHAPTER SEVEN

A Clear Conscience
Setting Helmet Standards and Legal Responsibility for Injuries, 1960s–1970s

All current methods of testing the effectiveness of headgear are somewhat unsatisfactory. . . . The single most important fact to remember is not what happens to the helmet but what the effect is upon the underlying brain.
—Glenn W. Kindt, Elwyn R. Gooding, and Richard C. Schneider, 1973

He wasn't a large or imposing athlete, but he was fast. As a teenager growing up in Rio Linda, California, Ernie Pelton avidly participated in multiple high school sports: wrestling, basketball, track, and football (figure 15). But Ernie particularly dreamed of earning a college football scholarship. His high school football teammates called him "Puffa Puffa," after a popular breakfast cereal featured in 1960s television commercials. The rice cereal was small but "shot out of a cannon," recalled his sister-in-law.[1]

On November 10, 1967, at the start of the second half of Rio Linda's match against Elk Grove High School, Ernie and his teammates lined up to return a kickoff. Ernie caught the ball out of the air and carried it for forty-five yards before being tackled near his team's sideline. When the players huddled up, Rio Linda's quarterback Mike James realized something was wrong. Mike noticed Ernie standing too far inside the huddle, with his hands holding both sides of his helmet. Then Ernie collapsed.[2]

Despite wearing a Rawlings protective helmet, Ernie had suffered a severe brain injury that put him in a coma for months. Less than two weeks after celebrating his eighteenth birthday, Ernie was rendered quadriplegic. In 1968, his father sued Rawlings on his son's behalf, as well as the store in which the helmet was sold and the school district in which the game had been played. Ernie's lawyers contended that Rawlings could have made a safer helmet, while Rawlings argued that Ernie's brain injury had been caused by a hit to the chin, and that the helmet was not to blame.

By the time of the trial, the linebacker who had tackled Ernie was a Marine serving in Vietnam. He nonetheless managed to give a deposition describing the fateful hit as "head-to-head, straight on." Although this testimony supported the Pelton family's case, Rawlings had lined up a football celebrity on

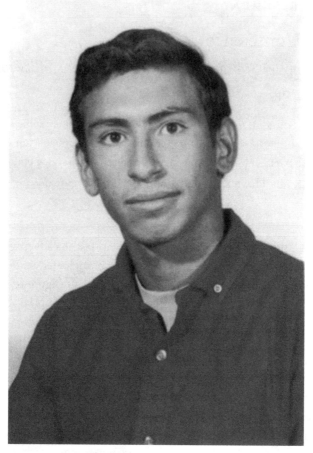

FIGURE 15   Ernie Pelton yearbook photo, Rio Linda High
School. Courtesy of Virginia Pelton.

its side. In March 1970, the sporting goods manufacturer called in NFL star
running back O. J. Simpson to testify. "I believe in this helmet," Simpson told
the Sacramento jury, which sent a note to the judge asking for the star's autograph. After an 89-day hearing, the jury cleared the manufacturer of any responsibility for Ernie's injury. The president of Rawlings not only celebrated
the outcome for his company but also suggested the future of the sport had
turned on the case. "Football was on trial at Sacramento." Meanwhile, Ernie
would never walk again.[3]

Ernie Pelton's injury, and the subsequent lawsuit, came at a time when attitudes toward both football helmets and legal responsibility for youth sports
injuries were in flux. By the 1960s, long-standing criticisms about the lack of

football helmet standards had become complementary to broader calls for government product safety research and regulation. Several nonprofit voluntary standards associations formed by scientists and engineers began devoting attention to protective football gear. Ultimately, however, a new organization funded by sporting goods manufacturers would prove most influential in establishing football equipment standards.

Manufacturers' influence on the development of helmet standards was spurred by changing ideas about who could be held responsible for harms caused by consumer products. New legal principles had increased the number of lawsuits against football helmet manufacturers. The sporting goods industry, in turn, sought to limit its liability by framing football injury prevention as the responsibility of individual players, parents, and coaches. Manufacturers insisted that their voluntary adoption of helmet standards, and their avoidance of government interference, would save football. But the industry's efforts to limit its liability made families like the Peltons responsible for managing the consequences of devastating, lifelong injuries.

Setting Helmet Standards

In the 1960s, the American Standards Association (ASA) led one of the earliest efforts to set football helmet standards. Originally established in 1916 by several professional societies of American engineers, this nongovernmental association set voluntary national standards for a range of products. In 1961, ASA established its first committee on protective headgear. Its initial focus was road user safety. Committee chair George Snively, a physician and amateur race car driver, was particularly motivated to address this issue after the 1956 crash death of fellow auto racer Pete Snell. The committee's membership also included the U.S. armed forces, motor sports associations, the National Safety Council, insurance associations, law enforcement agencies, helmet manufacturers, and independent experts. The committee developed its first standard for headgear for vehicular users in 1966.[4]

Snively's interest in improving protective headgear went beyond car racing. He had also used his research lab to test football helmets with fiberglass outer shells (see chapter 6). In November 1967, the ASA committee considered broadening its scope to include the development of standards for helmets used in sport and began by drafting its first football helmet standard. Yet at congressional National Consumer Product Safety (NCPS) hearings in 1969, Snively testified that all such "voluntary standards" suffered from a lack of enforcement. He pointed out that, despite the existence of the vehicular headgear standard, "many manufacturers are far from the upper limits of the present state of the art with respect to their product." Snively concluded that external quality control enforced by an agency or other source independent of helmet manufacturers appeared necessary.[5]

Around this time, another voluntary standards organization, ASTM, also became involved in studying football helmets. As with ASA, manufacturers could determine for themselves whether or not their products met any standards ASTM promulgated. ASTM announced in an October 1968 newsletter that, at the request of representatives of organized football and of the American College of Surgeons, they would be sponsoring a conference on ways to reduce athletic injuries. They invited all interested parties, from players, trainers, and doctors to design experts and sporting goods manufacturers, with the hope that "a re-examination of the entire football contact environment in such a multidisciplinary organization as ASTM can achieve beneficial results."[6] As so many other professional organizations had done, ASTM noted the need for more research on football's health risks. The conference announcement cited the Philadelphia Eagles' team physician on the inability to evaluate theories about the causes behind football injuries: "Until data can be gathered and studied, it simply won't be possible to reach valid conclusions."[7]

Following the conference, ASTM staff sent out thousands of invitations to interested individuals and organizations to establish a new, broad-based technical committee on sports equipment and facilities. Designated as Committee F-8, this group first met in September 1969. Its goals were to establish standards for sports equipment and related materials and to minimize injuries "with initial emphasis on football." Creighton Hale, vice president and director of research for Little League Baseball, was elected chairman. A physiologist and promoter of youth sports, Hale had previously argued that research favored competitive sports as being beneficial for young children (see chapter 4). Now he would chair a committee intended to write minimum standards for protective equipment to reduce sports injuries.[8]

With an initial focus on football helmets and preventing head and neck injuries, Committee F-8 soon expanded its work to include a range of other sports and activities, from skiing to trampoline use.[9] In 1971, Hale delivered a lecture at ASTM's annual meeting in which he discussed the committee's work on helmet standards. He emphasized that the committee faced significant challenges: "Unfortunately, sufficient knowledge of human tolerance of impacts to the head is not available in a form that can be applied directly to the design of helmets." Hale further highlighted the difficulties of conducting experiments that would show how the human brain actually responded to the forces to which players were subjected on the field. He concluded that the primary obstacle to improving protective equipment was not the sports in which people engaged but "the fact that we are working with humans," including all the complexity of human bodies and human behaviors.[10]

Media characterizations of these challenges were at times more sanguine. Hale's statement "What F-8 must accomplish can be stated very simply" was apparently rephrased by one reporter to read, "Basically, it's very simple to set standards for football equipment." Beyond the alteration of meaning involved in such a translation, the portrayal of the existing evidence also downplayed the risks of tackle football. "Some claim that professional football players get punchy from too many blows to the head, but there is no factual evidence to prove that claim now," Hale was quoted as saying. The absence of evidence was construed as an absence of harm. Despite acknowledging the engineering challenges, Hale concluded his address with confidence that ASTM would successfully set effective helmet standards to minimize injuries and deaths.[11]

In 1974, ASTM published a helmet test method supported by laboratory data from seven laboratories, "none of which is a football helmet manufacturer." By 1976, Committee F-8 boasted a roster of 263 members serving on 15 subcommittees that addressed such issues as biomechanics, facilities, and headgear. ASTM further expanded its work on sports-related standards by developing a new subcommittee focused on female athletes.[12]

Yet neither ASA nor ASTM would have the influence on football helmets of the National Operating Committee on Standards for Athletic Equipment (NOCSAE). NOCSAE was similar to ASTM's committee in that it was created as a multidisciplinary group with an initial focus on football helmets. But the organizations differed in several key ways that help explain why NOCSAE's certification standards ultimately proved most influential for football equipment.

First, leading sports organizations, notably the NCAA at the college level and the NFHS at the high school level, joined together to form NOCSAE. As exercise researcher J. Nadine Gelberg has observed, these organizations' involvement in NOCSAE was intended to ensure that they could retain control over sports standards, rules, and regulations. Neither college nor high school athletic associations paid any membership dues. Instead, all of NOCSAE's financial support came from the Sporting Goods Manufacturers Association (SGMA).[13]

Furthermore, ASTM's committee emphasized expertise in standards writing and explicitly sought to limit the influence of vested interests in sporting goods manufacturing. In fact, ASTM had a rule that the committee's chairman could not be an equipment producer, hence the selection of Creighton Hale of Little League Baseball as chair. Another ASTM rule required that the number of producers could not exceed nonproducers of sports equipment on the committee. But with the logistical clout and financial support of leading sporting goods manufacturers and organized football organizations, NOCSAE standards were more readily available to be adopted by the rules committees of leading football associations.[14]

Finally, ASTM operated as a "consensus" standards organization. This meant the society was required to follow a set of due process standards until "substantial agreement is reached by concerned interests." This was "the prime difference between a NOCSAE standard and an ASTM voluntary consensus standard" explained an ASTM representative in 1976. ASTM defined this due process as involving eight points, including in part the opportunity for all interested parties to participate in meetings, the publication and distribution of meeting minutes, adequate notices of proposed standards and actions, reports on balloting results, and attention to minority opinions throughout the process. ASTM committees were open and any interested party could participate in meetings. By contrast, NOCSAE was composed of organizations and its membership was closed.[15]

Sports safety researcher Kenneth S. Clarke later recalled that the formation of NOCSAE was prompted by the determination that ASTM's "consensus" process for developing standards "would be too time-consuming to rely on for the earliest possible resolution" of the football head injury problem.[16] This desire to swiftly establish helmet safety standards was in turn connected with a fear of potential lawsuits. In 1970, *NCAA News* described the formation of NOCSAE as part of an article announcing the jury decision—a victory, from the NCAA's perspective—to clear Rawlings of any legal responsibility for a catastrophic football injury. It was the case of Ernie Pelton, the high school player who had been left quadriplegic "from a violent twisting of the head" after being tackled.[17]

Manufacturers and sports administrators emphasized the importance of legally protecting themselves in such cases, while contending that helmets were not at fault for injuries. David Rust, counsel for Rawlings in the Pelton case, testified at the 1969 NCPS hearings in support of the manufacturers' perspective. Rust explained that his legal team had needed to show that the helmet had nothing to do with Ernie's injury, because helmets could not protect players against rotational forces. "The only way to protect against this is to encapsule the person—but then he couldn't play football." As Rust had successfully argued in court, the serious risks associated with twisting or rotational forces could not be prevented with protective gear. But limiting boys from playing football was seemingly not an option open for consideration. Consequently, brain injuries presumably needed to be accepted by youth football players and their parents as an inherent risk.[18]

The NOCSAE Seal of Approval

Despite this particular victory, sporting goods manufacturers and sports organizations remained concerned about the legal responsibility they might face down the road for injuries. The *NCAA News* warned readers that "vindication proved expensive for Rawlings," with a price tag of $500,000 for legal fees and other expenses. An NCAA staffer and secretary of NOCSAE stated, "A very grave danger to intercollegiate—and all other—athletics does exist concerning protective headgear."[19]

Administrators and manufacturers framed the Pelton case as representing an existential threat. They contended that future lawsuits might not only ruin football and the business of protective gear, but even sports more broadly. A NOCSAE committee member told *NCAA News* "the future of athletics is in jeopardy because of potential lawsuits relating to injuries received in sports."[20] One former sports marketer later contended that "court dockets were beginning to be inundated with liability litigation," and characterized the late 1960s as the period when football faced "the greatest danger since the warnings of President Teddy Roosevelt." NOCSAE was presented as a solution to this danger.[21]

Planning for NOCSAE began in 1969, and the organization's first formal meeting took place on April 8, 1970, one month after O. J. Simpson testified in the Pelton case. Representatives from sporting goods companies (Rawlings, Wilson, MacGregor, Spalding, and Riddell), the NFHS, the National Junior College Athletic Association, Oklahoma State University, the Big Eight Conference, the NCAA, and the National Athletic Trainers Association were all in attendance. The committee unanimously agreed that creating NOCSAE as a permanent committee, with the goal of establishing minimum standards for athletic equipment, was in the best interests of interscholastic and intercollegiate athletics.[22]

In 1970, NOCSAE awarded its first research grant to the department of neurosurgery at Wayne State University in Detroit for a one-year study of football head impacts. In 1971, research led by engineer Voigt Hodgson began at Wayne State's Gurdijan-Lissner biomechanics lab; the university had also been selected to develop NOCSAE's voluntary football helmet standard. Hodgson wrote that the first problem he confronted was devising a more realistic head model for use in testing. He used measurements from cadavers to develop a synthetic head model and devised a test method based on a cerebral concussion tolerance curve that had been developed in 1966 by Charles Gadd of General Motors.[23]

Critics had already urged caution in using such popular head tolerance criteria because it was based on translational motion instead of rotational motion. Translational motion, or linear motion, refers to movement in a single direction, whereas rotational motion refers to movement around an axis. Rotational movements of the brain could occur in cases of "whiplash" with no direct impact to the head, for instance. Notably, in 1970, participants in the Fourteenth Stapp Car Crash Conference observed that rotational motion appeared to be more critical than linear motion to the production of human brain injury. Nonetheless, the development of NOCSAE football helmet standard was closely connected with 1960s car crash safety research based on linear impacts.[24]

In 1973, NOCSAE promulgated its first helmet standard. Leading football organizations at both the youth and college levels quickly adopted it. By 1975, all new helmets in high school and college football would be certified by the NOCSAE standard. After a "grandfather" period for older helmets, NOCSAE-certified helmets became mandatory in 1978 for NCAA college players and in 1980 for high school players competing under the auspices of the NFHS. Hodgson expressed confidence that the replacement of older helmets with NOCSAE-certified helmets would significantly reduce head injuries.[25]

While ASTM continued to work on developing a standard, the adoption of NOCSAE's helmet standard got under way. Football coaches and administrators were eager to obtain the most effective equipment for their players. At times, they were also understandably confused and even frustrated by the apparent proliferation of standards without a clear indication of which specific helmets offered the most protection. A 1976 national conference on sports safety included a session on sports equipment and facilities standards with extensive presentations from both NOCSAE and ASTM representatives. When the floor was finally opened for a question and answer period, the very first questioner inquired, "We spent a lot of time and energy to improve our football program for next year. Despite all our efforts, we could not find anyone to tell us what was the best kind of helmet to buy. Is there any possibility that at some point these helmets will be ranked in order according to safety and/or will anybody who is in a responsible position come out and give us a definite answer as to what is the safest helmet to put on a youngster's head?"[26]

Hodgson responded that he did not want to endorse any particular helmet at the moment, and that defining the "best helmet" was difficult. Instead of ranking helmets, NOCSAE was offering a minimum standard for helmets to meet. Helmets that met this standard would be granted NOCSAE's certification and seal of approval, he explained. In advance of making NOCSAE-certified helmets mandatory in 1980, the NFHS prepared a set of "NOCSAE Questions and Answers" to clarify the requirements for its members. The handout indicated that referees would not be expected to inspect helmets to see whether they carried the NOCSAE seal. Instead, each team's head coach, along with the school's trainers and equipment managers, would be responsible for ensuring their players were wearing proper equipment. Explaining that no waivers for uncertified helmets would be permitted after 1980, the handout reiterated the view that the adoption of the NOCSAE test standard was associated with fewer football head injuries and fatalities.[27]

NOCSAE's helmet standard was swiftly adopted amid ongoing uncertainty about how effectively lab-tested standards might translate into on-field protection, particularly with regard to preventing concussions. As Hodgson acknowledged in response to a question about higher helmet standards, "We just don't know that much and we're kind of feeling our way along . . . . It's not pure science that we are dealing with here."[28] In fact, in a 1977 review of NOCSAE's program, Hodgson expressed the hope that one of the more counterintuitive ways NOCSAE's helmet standard would decrease football injuries would be by increasing awareness of the limitations of equipment.[29]

As it turned out, the promulgation of NOCSAE standards not only raised questions about equipment limitations but also about the limits of NOCSAE's standards themselves. In 1984, researchers G. Rex Bryce and Ruel M. Barker at Brigham Young University called into question NOCSAE's "woefully inadequate" testing policy of sampling a single helmet in order to determine whether a set of refurbished helmets was acceptable. To evaluate NOCSAE's approach, Barker and Bryce had obtained thirty helmets from three different schools that had been furnished by three different manufacturers. After randomizing the helmets, they sent them to Don Gleisner of the All American Company, a company that reconditioned football helmets and shoulder pads.[30]

Gleisner was a former football player who had signed with the Chicago Bears but never played again after sustaining an injury in a preseason exhibition match. Though he had helped form NOCSAE, he proceeded to question the value of setting the new NOCSAE standards "without including helmets that went through the reconditioning process after being worn for a season." Gleisner went on to start the National Athletic Equipment Reconditioning Association in 1975.[31] For this study of refurbished helmets, Gleisner enlisted Hodgson's help to test the helmets according to NOCSAE standard testing procedures at his Wayne State laboratory. Based on the results of these tests, Barker and Bryce found that both the testing variability and the helmet-to-helmet variability were much larger than expected. This meant that helmets could frequently be found in compliance with the NOCSAE standard without actually meeting it. They concluded that "the current recertification standard established by NOCSAE will do little to protect players if it is followed to the letter by refinishing firms."[32]

But even before later studies identified such flaws, NOCSAE had its critics. Lawyer Harry Philo was particularly severe in his characterization of NOCSAE standards and the process by which they had been created. Philo had testified at the 1969 NCPS hearings on the inadequacy of football head protection and had represented Ernie Pelton against Rawlings. According to Philo, helmet manufacturers had resisted meaningful standards and helped form NOCSAE as a more "compatible" organization for the interests of the industry. Members of the committee "quickly gave their NOCSAE seal of approval" to an ineffective standard and

> just as quickly eliminated the independent scientists and critics—men such as Dr. George Snively and Dr. C. D. Chichester of the prestigious Snell Memorial Foundation; Dr. Verne Roberts and Dr. James McElhaney of the Highway Safety Research Institute; Dr. Harold Fenner, pioneer in football helmet and head protection; Marshall Irving, helmet test engineer, and others. The resistance to meaningful criticism and the desire of NOCSAE to meet in secret continues today; conferences and seminars are only open to invitees. . . . Most (but not all) helmet manufacturers are still making tens of thousands of helmets each year that will not even meet the NOCSAE approval level. If coaches are willing to buy inferior products, then industry stands willing to participate (for profit) in the crippling of our youth.[33]

Such biting critiques were not widely discussed in popular media outlets, however, and thus did not appear to influence public perception of helmets. Instead, NOCSAE standards were largely celebrated as scientific efforts to prevent injuries. For example, John Friend, a high school football coach, athletic director, and national football chairman of the National High School

Athletic Coaches Association, argued in a 1979 *Chicago Tribune* article that NOCSAE played a major role in football safety. He cited statistics showing a decline in catastrophic head and neck injuries and told readers that football was becoming "safer and more skillful each year as coaching technique improves and equipment is researched and upgraded." Sporting goods stores advertised their NOCSAE-approved helmets. Helmet safety testing and NOCSAE-approved equipment reassured coaches and administrators that they were appropriately managing the risks of youth football to the best of their abilities. As one high school football coach, a self-described "safety kook," put it, "I feel that if every kid has his equipment checked by a professional, if something happens to the kid, I'll have a clear conscience."[34]

Many sports medicine professionals shared this confidence. A 1980 article coauthored by a certified athletic trainer and a physician in the *American Journal of Sports Medicine* claimed that "today's modern equipment provides adequate protection," and "all helmets with the NOCSAE seal provide adequate protection if properly fitted." The culprit for injuries was not the equipment itself but overconfident athletes playing with "reckless abandon" or using improper or ill-fitting equipment. To address the latter problem, a problem particularly in evidence at the high school level of play, the authors furnished a fitting guide for various types of football equipment.[35]

By 1980, equipment standards organizations, medical professionals, and coaches had endorsed the belief that modern, standardized equipment, when correctly fitted and worn, provided youth football players sufficient protection against injuries. The publisher of the coaching magazine *Athletic Journal* held up the development of NOCSAE helmet standards as a watershed moment in the history of American football. He lauded the committee for averting the threat of government intervention, commending the NOCSAE members who "have served notice that never again shall a President or agency of the United States have to issue a warning . . . 'Clean up your sport or we will shut it down for you.'"[36]

The Assumption of Risk

Despite the *Athletic Journal*'s depiction of NOCSAE's efforts, manufacturers were not motivated to develop helmet standards by the U.S. government threatening to shut down football. Rather, standards were largely prompted by a shifting legal landscape that increased manufacturers' risk of liability. Federal agencies were not threatening the existence of football, but legal trends were threatening the industry's profits.

Sports injury lawsuits had not always been a common occurrence for potentially vulnerable parties, such as school districts, coaches, and sporting goods manufacturers. School boards typically protected themselves legally by requiring parents of prospective student football players to sign release forms. For example, in the early 1960s, the Houston Independent School District's approval slip for participation in competitive sports asked parents to sign "with the distinct understanding that the Houston Board of Education and the employees of the Houston Board of Education assume no responsibility for any accident or injury as a result thereof." The district also required parents to sign a statement that they would agree to use their own family health and accident insurance to cover the expenses of any medical or hospital bills associated with interscholastic sports.[37]

Furthermore, courts typically applied a legal doctrine known as "assumption of risk." This principle held that athletes playing competitive sports knowingly and voluntarily assumed the risks by participating, and could not recover damages from sports-related harms. As a result, plaintiffs rarely won the limited lawsuits resulting from sports injuries prior to the mid-1960s.[38]

The case of *Vendrell v. School District No. 26C, Malheur County* exemplifies the application of this doctrine. In 1953, fifteen-year-old high school football player Louis Vendrell suffered a broken neck after being tackled by two members of the opposing team. Vendrell testified that "I put my head down and just ran into 'em and that is when I heard my neck snap." The injury resulted in permanent paraplegia. In his suit against the school district, Vendrell claimed that he had not received "proper or sufficient instructions" in the techniques of football nor had he been provided "the necessary and proper protective equipment."[39]

Vendrell's case reached the Supreme Court of Oregon in 1962. But the court found neither his coaches nor the school district negligent, explaining that no prospective football players, including children, needed to be warned that they might sustain an injury. While not explicitly characterizing permanent paralysis as an inherent part of the game, the court nonetheless indicated that coaches did not have a duty to warn athletes of potential injuries, because no warning should be necessary. "Body contact, bruises, and clashes are inherent in the game. There is no other way to play it. No prospective player need be told that a participant in the game of football may sustain injury. That fact is self-evident. It draws to the game the manly; they accept its risks, blows, clashes and injuries without whimper. No one expects a football coach to extract from the game the body clashes that cause bruises, jolts and hard falls. To remove them would end the sport."[40]

The court's reasoning reframed boys as adults; indeed, the court's very language suggested that the essence of football was to attract "the manly" and transform boys into men. The risks of football, and the willingness to sustain these injuries "without whimper," were treated as intrinsic components of this vision of masculinity. Removing those risks "would end the sport," a scenario the court's language presented as flatly unacceptable. The court further dispensed with Vendrell's argument that his coaches had not taught him to avoid using his head, stating that "one of the first lessons that an infant learns when he begins to toddle about on his feet is not to permit his head to collide with anything." Vendrell was thus found to have assumed all the risks of tackling. These risks were so obvious, the court indicated, that even infants ought to be aware of the potential dangers of subjecting one's head to blows.[41]

Several years later, the Supreme Court of Oregon similarly ruled against another football injury plaintiff. In 1972, the court heard the case of Robert Whipple, a fifteen-year-old boy who had played with the Salvation Army Boys Club youth program in Medford, Oregon. Whipple sustained a knee injury while being tackled immediately after he had jumped and caught a ball. His allegations against the Salvation Army included inadequate supervision and allowing untrained boys at an "excessively early age" to participate in tackle football. The court held "as a matter of law, that a 15-year-old boy, without evidence of mental deficiency or untoward seclusion from life's experiences common to boys of that age, sufficiently appreciates the dangers inherent in the game of football so that he assumes the risk thereof when he plays."[42]

Such rulings meant that even catastrophically injured child athletes were unlikely to find success in the courtroom. As lawyer Samuel Langerman observed in 1964, "Litigation seldom arises from a sports injury." Furthermore, he explained, many schools and institutions were exempted from tort liability under legal doctrines of sovereign immunity or charitable immunity. These doctrines exempted from private suit most public schools, universities, nonprofit groups (such as the YMCA), and other types of organizations that typically sponsored youth athletic programs. Beyond the legal challenges, injured players or their families often had a "natural hesitancy" to sue their own coaches or schools. Given the reluctance of many injured parties to bring suit, and the significant obstacles to succeeding if they did, sports injury lawsuits were relatively rare.[43]

Yet just a decade later, Langerman, a law partner noted for his experience in handling sports injury litigation, would revise this opinion. In 1977, writing for *Trial* magazine, Langerman and his colleague Noel Fidel argued that new legal trends were clearing the traditional roadblocks to sports injury litigation.[44]

The move toward strict liability, as discussed in chapter 6, was one of the legal developments that made school districts and sporting goods manufacturers increasingly vulnerable to product liability lawsuits after the mid-1960s. Langerman and Field argued that the duty to warn in the products liability field established basic principles that also applied to coaches, teachers, and athletic program managers. "Does the football player who makes a head-down charge with an ill-fitting helmet, or the trampolinist who works out with a headache or cold, comprehend and appreciate the magnitude of the risk of a lifetime of quadriplegia? Not unless his coach has met his educational responsibilities."[45]

In contrast to the 1962 *Vendrell* decision, then, courts might no longer consider the risks of permanent paralysis to be obvious to prospective football players. Adult coaches and trainers were increasingly treated as having a "duty to warn" prospective players, especially children, of the potentially devastating risks of athletic participation. This transition toward a coach's duty to warn was connected to a broader rejection of assumption of risk in occupational as well as recreational settings. By the mid-twentieth century, many industry leaders acknowledged that they had a responsibility to inform their employees of the dangers associated with their work, and that strategies such as the use of warning labels could protect industry from lawsuits in the event of harm.[46] Administrators of youth football programs increasingly saw themselves as legally vulnerable. A 1974 reference manual for Pop Warner coaches warned that even volunteer coaches might be "held liable for physical harm incurred by players in their charge" if proven negligent.[47]

The landmark 1982 case of *Thompson v. Seattle Public School District* signaled this changing legal landscape. In this case, a Seattle jury awarded Christopher Thompson $6.3 million for the 1975 high school football injury that left him quadriplegic. Thompson argued that his coach had not warned him of the dangers of putting his head down while tackling. Meanwhile, the school district sought to characterize the injury as a freak accident, arguing that students must assume the risk when choosing to play football. Following the verdict in favor of Thompson, the school district's athletic supervisor warned that the case could potentially affect athletic programs nationwide: "If we're doing it wrong, all districts in the country are doing it wrong."[48]

In 1983, two professors of physical education at Washington State University pointed to *Thompson v. Seattle Public School District* as a sentinel case. They argued that the court appeared to be "placing all responsibility for the prevention of injuries and therefore, blame for injuries, on the coach or supervisor of an activity. . . . The fact that a participant may be injured in a sport is no longer considered self-evident." In shifting the responsibility for the risks of football and other sports from players to coaches and administrators, this precedent-setting case weakened the long-standing "assumption of risk" doctrine. Courts were increasingly limiting the amount of risk that a sports participant should be expected to assume, particularly when athletes were young and had less extensive athletic experience prior to their injury.[49] A 1986 *Athletic Business* article claimed that with the *Thompson* decision, the concepts of "failure to warn" and "failure to instruct" had become "enshrined in the legal lexicon, adding new definitions to the definition of negligence."[50]

Following the *Thompson* case, the *Los Angeles Times* reported that the Seattle school board considered a resolution suggesting the elimination of football. The injured student had been awarded more than $6 million in damages, and the district had been insured for $5.5 million. Ultimately, the Seattle School District developed a lengthy list of recommendations, including that students and their parents be required to sign an assumption of risk form, that coaches be required to have CPR training, and that coaches inform participants of the types of catastrophic injuries that could occur and how to avoid them.[51]

Sports programs across the country responded to legal concerns by reading additional warnings to players and placing labels on helmets. In 1986, the NFHS's Football Rules Committee stated that beginning the following season, "each player's helmet must have a visible exterior warning label regarding the risk of injury. Although most schools complied previously, the label will now be required."[52] Thomas Appenzeller, a professor of sport management who was a high school football coach in North Carolina in the 1980s, recalled, "In the mid-season my principal called me in there. He said, 'We just got these stickers and you've got to put one on every helmet and you've got to read this statement before every football game.' And it was a warning and it resulted from a lawsuit out in Seattle, Washington, where a high school player had broken his neck. . . . I remember for the next game I actually read [the statement] and before every game that year I read it. Then after that we just had to read it before the season started as a warning that you weren't supposed to use your head to ram or to lead with it and that there was a danger of serious injury with head and neck injuries."[53]

Sporting Goods Manufacturers and Legal Responsibility for Injuries

In addition to school districts and coaches, sporting goods manufacturers were also becoming increasingly vulnerable to lawsuits. Plaintiffs contended that manufacturers had a duty to warn prospective consumers that football helmets could not protect against particular head and brain injuries. For instance, in 1974, a Texas high school football quarterback, Mark Daniels, sustained a head injury in a collision with a teammate. The force of the impact left an indentation in his helmet. Daniels, subsequently diagnosed with a subdural hematoma that left him with severe and permanent brain damage, sued Rawlings Sporting Goods. The Twentieth Judicial District Court of Robertson County, Texas, awarded Daniels a $1.5 million judgment, a decision which Rawlings unsuccessfully appealed. In upholding the ruling, the court of appeals of Texas's Tenth District explained that while all evidence suggested that the primary purpose of a helmet was to protect its wearer against head and brain injuries, nonetheless, "Defendant [Rawlings] admitted that it never made any attempt to warn potential users of the limitations of its helmets; that it had known for a long time that helmets will not protect against brain injuries; that it made the 'conscious decision' not to tell people the helmet would not protect against subdural hematomas; that the company 'elected' not to warn that the helmets would not protect against head injuries, in spite of the knowledge that laymen believe that the purpose of the helmet is to protect the head."[54]

In addition to arguing that manufacturers needed to warn of the inherent limitations of helmets, plaintiffs contended that manufacturers should be held liable for defective helmet designs. In 1975, the successful suit of Greg Stead against prominent football helmet manufacturer Riddell was based on the argument that the helmet's improper design had contributed to Stead's catastrophic injury. More broadly, *Stead v. Riddell* emerged as a landmark case to which both manufacturers and lawyers would point as representing trends in product liability law. In numerous settings, from congressional hearings to medical journals, these groups deployed *Stead v. Riddell* to advance their preferred framing of legal responsibility for youth football injuries.

Stead was paralyzed from the neck down due to an injury he sustained on the opening kickoff of a high school football game on September 30, 1971. Stead's attorney argued that after a player on the opposing team kicked Stead, causing his client's head to jerk backward, Stead's neck was broken between the fourth and fifth vertebrae by the unpadded back of the Riddell helmet he was wearing. By the time of the trial, Stead was twenty years old and sat through the five-week proceedings in a wheelchair. A jury awarded him $5.3 million in damages.[55]

Sporting goods manufacturers and their lawyers depicted *Stead v. Riddell* as heralding an impending wave of lawsuits threatening their ability to do business. Riddell lawyer Richard Lester would later characterize this 1975 case as the beginning of an "onslaught" of damage suits filed against manufacturers. Although the multimillion-dollar award was unusual, *Stead v. Riddell* was certainly consistent with broader legal trends. Examining products liability law through 1990, two legal scholars found that beginning in the mid-1970s and through the early 1980s, courts "seemed to compete with each other to see who could make it easiest for plaintiffs to reach juries with claims of defective product design."[56]

Manufacturers turned to *Stead v. Riddell* as the perfect example of litigation run amok in efforts to minimize their susceptibility to such suits. Notably, in 1976, the SGMA formed the Multi-Association Action Committee (MAAC) to address product liability. The committee included 119 leaders from a range of industries, such as aircraft, cast metals, recreation vehicles, and small farm implements. MAAC's stated goals included "to call attention to the plight of industry manufacturers in product liability suits and costs for defense" and "to notify Americans that we have unleashed a wave of <u>un-founded</u> suits and attendant <u>unprecedented awards</u> that guarantee inflation for the next decade" (underline in original).[57]

At MAAC's SGMA-sponsored conference on liability reform in 1976, SGMA president Harold J. Bruns referenced the *Stead* case. "Did you know that a football helmet manufacturer lost a $5.3 million lawsuit to an injured player while the defendant's attorney contended there was no proof that the injured party was even wearing the defendant's helmet?" Bruns asked. He further alluded to Stead's presence in the courtroom throughout the trial as unjustly swaying the jurors. Although jurors were charged to render decisions based on fact and fairness, Bruns complained, they "instead must view a paraplegic in a wheelchair which conjures irresistible emotion and remorse." Consequently, "a sports equipment manufacturer is made to pay a fortune out of sympathy rather than neglect." Depicting such cases as frivolous and opportunistic, Bruns suggested that justice was being "outwitted by lucid trial lawyers." Manufacturers were forced to pay extravagant sums as "a sacrifice to ease the social conscience." Bruns hastened to clarify that he was certainly not blaming "the paraplegic doomed to a life of thinking," nor the judges and juries doing what they believed to be right. Instead, he contended that the legal system was at fault.[58]

Bruns urged reform of the tort system as the ultimate solution. In 1977, he explained to the *Chicago Tribune* that SGMA's goal was to return the law of the land "back to where it was prior to 1964, when the doctrine of strict liability was adopted." In the testimony he submitted to the U.S. Senate's Select

Committee on Small Business, Bruns laid out SGMA's objectives: public awareness of the problem, statute of limitations on manufactured products, limitation of awards, plaintiff to assume responsibility for all defendant's costs related to unfounded suits, limitation on contingency fees, state of the art at time of manufacture as a defense, and elimination of punitive damages. Without such reforms, he threatened, "next year may well be the last year for the Super Bowl." The notion that lawsuits threatened the very existence of football would persist in SGMA's policy arguments through the 1980s and early 1990s.[59]

The specter of lawsuits putting an end to football was repeatedly disseminated at conferences and in journals aimed at sports medicine specialists. "The whole existence of contact sports as we know them is being threatened," said one speaker at the American College of Sports Medicine's 1977 annual meeting. A 1985 *Physician and Sportsmedicine* article promulgated the view that manufacturers had made football helmets safer, and in "reward," they had become subjected to increasing liability for injuries. This analysis cast the sporting goods manufacturers as victims suffering the toll of multimillion-dollar lawsuits. A 1987 *Physician and Sportsmedicine* article, whose very title signaled the dangers to "the American way of sport," opened with the image of a high school football game under way in "Anytown, United States." The author, a contributing editor of the journal, suggested that this scene, "as American as apple pie," was in danger of disappearing. She cited sporting goods manufacturers as a source of the concern. Sports medicine physicians, whose work was fundamentally tied to organized sports, were thus encouraged to share SGMA's framing of product liability law as posing an existential threat to sports.[60]

The example of *Stead v. Riddell*, as well as liability concerns faced by sporting goods manufacturers more generally, featured prominently in debates over federal legislation. In April 1976, President Gerald Ford established a Federal Interagency Task Force on Product Liability to study ways to stabilize recoveries and insurance premiums. The task force continued its work under President Carter and ultimately recommended the drafting of a model uniform law for use by all states. The task force also recommended federal legislation to allow small businesses to form self-insurance pools; such legislation would ultimately become law in 1981 as the Product Liability Risk Retention Act.[61]

But before the passage of this act, in 1977, the U.S. Senate held hearings to consider an earlier version of product liability legislation. The bill, proposed by Senators John C. Culver (D-Iowa) and Gaylord Nelson (D-Wisconsin), would have established a national product liability insurance administration and arbitration program, as well as a product liability insurance pool to increase the availability of coverage. The perspective of manufacturers featured in these hearings in the form of letters submitted by William C. Merritt, who had defended Riddell against the lawsuit brought by Stead. Merritt's arguments illustrate how sports manufacturers sought to frame product liability lawsuits and to deflect responsibility for football injuries away from themselves.[62]

Merritt drew on social prejudices to argue that the Florida jury that had ruled against Riddell was largely composed of "middle class people of not high intelligence." He noted the inclusion of a black maid, the wife of a civil servant, an Italian terrazzo and tile man, a Cuban postal clerk, and a retired man. Not only did the judge ask questions during the *voir dire* to play upon the sympathies of these purportedly simpleminded jurors, Merritt suggested, but the judge also failed to understand the suspension system of Riddell's helmet and its complete irrelevance to a neck injury case. Merritt emphasized the testimony of the assistant football coach at the high school where Greg Stead had played. The coach stated that he had specifically and repeatedly instructed Stead that "you stick a man with your helmet and you're going to break your neck."[63]

Merritt further questioned the credibility of plaintiff witness Harold Fenner, who had testified that the helmet's ability to attenuate the impact of blows to the head could contribute to the plaintiff's neck injury. Merritt repeatedly emphasized that Fenner was not board certified as an orthopedic surgeon and that other experts disagreed with Fenner's assessment. "Medical research has shown that the helmet has no relationship to the injury," Merritt would continue to insist in the following years. Lawyers and the sporting goods manufacturers they represented thus argued that well-meaning but relatively uneducated jurors were unduly swayed by the sympathy-inducing presence of catastrophically injured athletes, that these athletes had been sufficiently warned by their own coaches of the risk of injury, and that medical testimony about the possible role of the helmet was uncertain and suspect.[64]

Beginning in the 1970s, a number of manufacturers ceased making football helmets. Remaining manufacturers claimed that lawsuits were driving them out of the business. In 1970, there were eighteen football helmet manufacturers in the United States; by 1994, there were only two. In 1977, Frank Gordon, the president of Riddell, told the *Chicago Tribune* that manufacturers were toying, half seriously, with the notion of "going on strike" and not producing helmets for a year or two, to draw public attention to the legal crisis. While

such a strategy was not particularly realistic, suggesting the threat of a football helmet manufacturing strike to a major American newspaper was in itself
a means of raising public concern. A 1979 *Los Angeles Times* article claimed
that "making football helmets can be as potentially risky as playing the game
without any."[65]

While manufacturers blamed product liability laws, consumer groups
such as the National Insurance Consumer Organization, the Consumer Federation of America, and Public Citizen contended that insurers were charging
exorbitant premiums to compensate for poor risk judgments in previous
years. The president of the National Insurance Consumer Organization told
the *New York Times* that while the courts had expanded the concept of liability, that had nothing to do with insurance rates. "The insurance problem
shouldn't be used as an excuse to take away victims' rights to sue."[66]

Despite—or perhaps thanks to—the emphatic alarm that sporting goods
manufacturers continued to sound in the press, in legislative hearings, and in
medical journals, ultimately not many multimillion-dollar cases were settled in
favor of plaintiffs. In fact, in 1979, the chief financial officer of Wynn's International Inc., which had recently acquired Riddell, observed that despite a spate
of lawsuits following *Stead v. Riddell*, "since then, we have not had any large
adverse jury awards or large settlements." He characterized *Stead v. Riddell* as
an anomaly.[67] In fact, by the late 1980s, the legal trend was instead moving
toward limiting plaintiffs' rights to recover damages for product-related injuries. Two legal scholars suggested that this "quiet revolution in products liability" might be attributed to the success of tort reformers in linking product
liability cases to the insurance crisis of the mid-1980s. In the area of athletic
equipment, they found that plaintiffs had a success rate in two-thirds of cases
from 1979 to 1984, which decreased to less than half of cases from 1985 to 1989.[68]

But perhaps the manufacturers' most notable strategy was their argument
that the fundamental responsibility for football injuries should rest with the
players, their parents, and coaches. This argument fit in with broader, prevailing American beliefs about individual responsibility for addressing health
problems. For instance, in a widely cited 1977 article, physician and president
of the Rockefeller Foundation John Knowles argued that educating individuals about health risks, from cigarettes to lack of exercise, and promoting a culture which encouraged individuals to assume responsibility for their
behaviors, were the keys to improving health. By making legal arguments that
emphasized the personal responsibility of individual child athletes and their
parents to assume the risks of football, sporting goods manufacturers drew
on wider beliefs about who should be held responsible for health problems.[69]

An SGMA-funded coalition advanced this perspective in a strategy reminiscent of other industry-sponsored front groups. In 1990 hearings before the U.S. Senate, SGMA described their public education operation, the Coalition of Americans to Protect Sports (CAPS), as being founded in 1986 as "a grassroots organization whose purpose is to inform coaches, schools, and the general public about the detrimental impact liability is having on manufacturers of sports equipment and programs across the United States." Rather than a broad-based grassroots movement, however, CAPS was primarily an arm of SGMA. Lobbyist Richard Feldman recalled that he and other SGMA leaders renamed the group CAPS in 1988 in order to make it sound more like a united national organization.[70]

As part of its goal to minimize the potential for liability litigation, CAPS asserted that better equipment and personal responsibility would address the issue of safety in sports. For instance, Sharon Lincoln, the communications director of CAPS, argued that lawsuits discouraged people "from accepting the rational, logical, and foreseeable risks of their own behavior." She singled out football as essential to American culture and education. Although football was particularly vulnerable to liability lawsuits and thus more costly to play and to insure, Lincoln argued that "many school administrators would laugh at the idea of doing away with it. Football is financially critical to schools." Instead of filing lawsuits, players and coaches needed to accept the risks and take responsibility for preventing them. CAPS developed a risk education program aimed at sports administrators and coaches that emphasized the ways such "frivolous, nonsensical" lawsuits could be avoided.[71]

In the *Journal of Physical Education, Recreation & Dance*, Lincoln promoted the *CAPS Sports Injury Risk Management Manual* and other CAPS materials "to help the sports community maximize athlete safety while minimizing the potential for litigation." CAPS artwork included an image of a dejected youth baseball player sitting under a sign that read, "Field closed due to lack of insurance." These materials were disseminated in manuals, videos, and clinics.[72]

Similar to the public relations strategy of big tobacco companies and fast-food industry groups of shifting responsibility for risk away from themselves and onto consumers, CAPS sponsored a vision of individual responsibility for the risks of competitive athletics. CAPS presented its safety promotion strategies as essential for avoiding lawsuits and high insurance premiums. In the form of educational resources to protect player safety, SGMA shared a message of personal responsibility that obscured the involvement of industry interests.[73]

A Clear Conscience

The goal of preserving youth football amid safety concerns, in conjunction with sporting goods manufacturers' efforts to reduce their liability for injuries, prompted the development of football helmet standards. NOCSAE standards were mandated by the most influential organized football associations. The committee's rush to develop and adopt helmet standards ironically occurred in the context of significant uncertainty over how to effectively test helmets. Nonetheless, the industry's efforts not only reinforced the centrality of protective gear to sports injury prevention but also bestowed a scientific and medical imprimatur upon helmets. The use of standardized equipment could even provide adults involved in youth football a "clear conscience": if injuries did occur, the adults had done everything possible to protect their players. But the function of equipment in providing reassurance—and absolution in the event of injury—highlighted one of the most important ongoing tensions in the debates over protective football equipment: whether even the best equipment could effectively compensate for the limits of the human body.

Manufacturers continued to market their protective equipment as central to athletic success as well as safety. Yet in defending themselves against product liability lawsuits, they emphasized the lack of relationship between helmets and the injuries of individual plaintiffs. Manufacturers further argued that individual coaches, parents, and children should take responsibility for preventing football injuries because they had voluntarily chosen to assume the risks of the sport. The industry threatened that lawsuits would doom football by rendering sports equipment manufacturing and insurance prohibitively costly. Sports medicine journals and conference speakers promoted manufacturers' framing of injury risks to physician audiences, while coaching manuals and videos targeted coaches and educators. Ultimately, manufacturers largely succeeded in framing football safety as a matter of individual responsibility.

The success rate of plaintiffs in product liability lawsuits related to athletics declined in the 1980s. Athletic administrators, coaches, and the general public largely maintained their beliefs in the importance and efficacy of protective equipment. Schools prioritized investing in equipment above other potential football-related expenses. If anything, buying the latest and best equipment became an even greater priority for legal as well as safety reasons. As an athletic director told the *Los Angeles Times* in 1990, "The way lawyers are today, if a kid gets hurt wearing a helmet that's five years old, you won't have a leg to stand on legally."[74]

Part IV
Whose Bodies, Whose Brains?

CHAPTER EIGHT

It's All We've Got

Community, Education, and Youth Football

Football is "the pretty girls, the gay flags and that awesome, incomparable sound of roaring thousands in some Saturday stadium. Football is a spectacle as much as it is a contest; an occasion of social and community importance apart from its sporting significance."

— Lamont Buchanan, 1947

In 1958, Henry Steele Commager, a renowned American historian, assessed trends in American high school education. Commager sharply critiqued an overemphasis on competitive athletics as failing to meet or even hindering the educational goals of sports. He singled out tackle football as an example of how competitive athletic programs failed to offer equal opportunities to all students. "A system where a handful of boys devote most of their energy to football, while five thousand students sit in stands and watch them, is not designed to provide sound bodies to go with sound minds."[1] Such a system was at odds with the purported ideals of American public schools—and tackle football itself—to democratically provide students of all backgrounds access to the benefits of physical education.

Commager contended that the most dangerous aspect of embedding competitive sports, particularly football, in high schools was the relationship between youth athletics and the community. Child athletes, he said, were being exploited at nighttime athletic contests "for the convenience, the entertainment, or the profit of adults. We would not expect or permit our high-school daughters to entertain the community in a night-club or burlesque show; there is no reason why we should permit our high-school sons to entertain the community by what are, in effect, burlesque performances on the playing field."[2]

Commager homed in on a persistent, fundamental debate: whether football's association with education and its function as a major community spectator event benefited young players. Over the twentieth century, as the demographics, tactics, equipment, and many other aspects of youth football changed, the relationship between football, schools, and local communities persisted as a key feature of American life—and as an ongoing source of concern. In addition to individual character building, youth football was also perceived to offer improved social status to athletes and success to their larger communities. Indeed, sociologist Gerhard Falk has observed that American football was not only a sport but "an alternative status system."[3]

Ideas about football's perceived social benefits circulated among different levels of play. Notably, football's status in high schools and local communities contributed to its expansion at the little league level. Football for elementary and middle school aged children increasingly served as a feeder system for future high school play. Yet little league football also acquired particular meanings of its own, as examined in this chapter in a case study of a local youth football organization in King of Prussia, Pennsylvania. In addition, the appeal of future access to social and financial resources, including the hope of landing a college scholarship, influenced how parents and players weighed the costs and benefits of youth football.

Football's association with access to higher social standing and higher education contributed in part to its changing demographics. The face of football changed enormously after the early 1900s, a period when it was associated primarily with the white Anglo-Saxon protestant college students of elite schools such as Harvard and Yale. By the end of the twentieth century, tackle football became predominantly associated with working-class and disproportionately minority youths, particularly African American boys. Debates over the risks and benefits of football thus became debates over the safety of a largely more economically and socially vulnerable set of young bodies. Meanwhile, the growing prominence of the NFL in America's media landscape and sportscasters' glorification of "big hits" fostered celebrations of football's physical dangers even as administrators claimed both educational and health benefits for the youth sport.

While physical activity was certainly valued, the primary advantages of tackle football were above all framed as social benefits, carrying particular meaning for vulnerable, marginalized groups. The racial and ethnic composition of youth football, and the geographic and economic conditions of communities where school football rose to greatest prominence, raise the question of whose bodies were at risk and for which athletes and communities the social benefits of football carried the greatest significance.

The Feeder System of Football from the Cradle

In 1961, *Sports Illustrated* profiled Massillon, "a rugged steel town in northeastern Ohio." The immense popularity of Massillon's high school football team had already gained substantial national media coverage in the late 1940s and 1950s; the city was dubbed "Touchdown Town" in a 1951 newsreel.[4] This 1961 article emphasized that football dominated the lives of boys in the town even from their births. The local booster club presented boys born in area hospitals with footballs, and young boys were encouraged to begin playing the sport in anticipation of a potential high school career. "By fifth grade he is playing organized football. When he enters one of Massillon's three junior high schools, he learns the formations and plays that the high school varsity uses. . . . There's no time for tears in Massillon's football program. The young boy with the professional-looking helmet may privately wonder if football is really for him, but in Massillon he has little choice. . . . With his mother and father and the Boosters shouting encouragement from the sidelines, with a small army of coaches studying his actions and with a large mechanical board to suggest what play he should run, there is nothing the boy need decide for himself."[5]

This profile illustrates a number of recurrent themes in organized youth football: the dominance of adults, including coaches, parents, and the community booster club; programs for elementary and junior high school students in preparation for high school football; equipment that mimicked the gear used by professionals; and the promotion of a tough, unemotional form of masculinity ("there's no time for tears"). The profile expressed ambivalence over whether the boys themselves were willing participants, but it made clear the immense value that the broader community placed on football. Beyond the parents and coaches on the sidelines, other adults throughout Massillon were deeply involved, including a group of "Side-liners" who "adopted" players each season and treated them to dinner and the movies the night before each game.[6]

Community booster clubs and other local supporters were often instrumental in lending necessary material and financial support. In a 1967 examination of high school football in Ohio, Carl Benhase recounted how the athletic department was $10,000 in debt when he took over as football coach at Circleville, Ohio. Because the football team lacked the funds and the approval of the athletic board to purchase the equipment they wished to obtain, the team improvised with the help of local businesses and parents. For example, local merchants donated old mattresses to be used as fillers for standup blocking dummies, the equipment used to help players practice blocking techniques. Benhase also helped reactivate the local booster club, which in his first year of coaching at Circleville "raised enough money to purchase new varsity football game uniforms, sponsor a post-season banquet, and finance several other athletic activities."[7]

Similarly, a 1979 examination of Texas football highlighted the wide range of financial support such clubs offered athletic programs. "Calling themselves the Bobcat Boosters or the Bay City Quarterback Club, they organize caravans to out-of-town games, welcoming committees for home games, team banquets with guest speakers; they pay for tutors or surgeons for dull or injured players, for various kinds of fancy equipment—prostyle Riddell helmets, say, or sideline headphones for the coaching staff—things the local school board can't find any way to finance or justify."[8]

Booster clubs also reinforced coaches' efforts to instill particular values in players, notably ideals of aggression and masculinity. In examining the "psychological approach to football," Benhase detailed how the booster club of Sandusky, Ohio, assisted the coach in "the subtle art of 'needling'" the football team. The illustrations of "needling" that Benhase included as models for other coaches to follow primarily played upon stereotypes of gender and sexuality. "On one occasion several years ago, Coach Tom Griswold of Deer Park High School aroused his boys to perform in a more aggressive manner by sending them each a pink powder puff in a plain envelope." On another occasion, the town's club sent a flock of chickens to the locker room just prior to a game. As Benhase explained, "There had been some uncomplimentary talk about several players being 'chicken.' Rather than single out those individuals, the chickens were sent to the team with the implication the team was 'chicken.' The team got fired up and won a tough game."[9]

Community members were motivated to "fire up" child athletes in part because high school football was a major event in many regions of the United States, particularly in the Midwest and the South. Several towns in northeastern Ohio drew media attention in the 1960s for demonstrating particularly strong interest in the sport.[10] A 1962 *Life* magazine profile of Martins Ferry, Ohio, reported that on each Friday night in the fall season, about 8,000 people out of the town's population of 12,000 enjoyed the entertainment provided by the town's high school football team. Gene Minder, a millworker, stated, "I told my two boys that if they wanted to amount to something better than their dad they would have to play football."[11]

This depiction of Martins Ferry proved highly controversial among locals. Many residents were proud of their town's football heritage and dismayed by the seemingly unflattering portrayal. As one Martins Ferry native recalled, "People took exception to *Life*'s selection of pictures to use in the issue as well as some of the quotes depicting Ferry and surrounding areas as grimy mill towns. . . . This resulted in many subscriptions ending up in the annual (fall) bonfire."[12]

Indeed, several weeks after the profile's 1962 publication, the magazine published a number of letters from residents of Martins Ferry registering their objections. The mayor of Martins Ferry declared that residents were shocked and hurt. A resident dubbed the profile in *Life* to be "the most slanted, distorted and disgusting article I've ever read. . . . There is no depressing atmosphere in our town. And above all, football isn't the only means for a person to leave his home town." Despite controversy over this national media portrayal, the immense popularity of football was unquestioned. To many locals, this popularity ought to have been portrayed in a more positive light. They disagreed with the implication that large-scale community involvement in high school football was an indicator of blight or a lack of other options in a "grimy mill town."[13]

Sportswriter Taylor Bell's examination of the history of high school football in communities across Illinois similarly depicts locales where the sport represented a major focus of community life and aspirations. Particularly in small towns and rural areas, local high school football matches emerged as a source of large-scale entertainment. Al Martin, who began coaching high school football in Du Quoin, Illinois, in 1988, stated, "The streets are decorated with jerseys hanging on telephone poles. Everyone is at the game. You might not appreciate it as much as we do if you are from a big suburban school in Chicago. But it's a big deal in Du Quoin. It's all we've got." Martin further observed that in their rural community, where some children were homeless and some parents unemployed, football represented a particular source of pride and motivation for youth living in adverse circumstances.[14]

High school football players were often heroes to younger children aspiring one day receive similar acclamation for their exploits on the field. A former coach in Geneseo, Illinois, another small town of several thousand people, recalled that each Friday night, "as we waited for the sophomore game to end, a number of little kids would be standing around the back door of our locker room."[15] From the other direction of the age spectrum, adults also placed pressure on the high school football players for whom they cheered. This aspect of youth football was perhaps most compellingly and famously depicted by H. G. Bissinger in *Friday Night Lights*, a work of nonfiction that followed the story of a 1988 high school football team in Odessa, Texas. Bob Rutherford, a local realtor in town, casually told the author, "Life really wouldn't be worth livin' if you didn't have a high school football team to support."[16]

Not all community members readily embraced football, requiring some coaches and administrators to address parental skepticism. When Ron Jones took over a relatively new high school football program in Piketon, Ohio, he faced difficulties in recruiting players: "Coach Jones' problem was typical of that in a new school where football has not been previously played. Most of the parents felt that football was a brutal sport, and there was little or very limited value of a boy participating in it." The community's embrace of football was far from assured; it would need to be fostered by coaches and administrators.[17]

Jones responded to parental reluctance by arranging home visits with prospective players and their parents in order to "sell" the program to them. Other coaches took different approaches. As discussed in chapter 2, mothers were often perceived as the barrier to their sons' participation. Thus, coach Tony Mason at Niles-McKinley High School in Niles, Ohio, initiated a football class for women in the community to teach them the rules and strategies of the game. With attendance reportedly numbering more than 100, this class resulted in a Mothers' Club to aid in preparing the team banquet as well as raising money for other team needs. Building football programs involved reassuring parents that the risks of the sport were minimal and that participation would confer valuable physical and social benefits.[18]

The intensity with which many American communities embraced high school interscholastic athletics generally, and football particularly, influenced football's expansion at the junior high school level at mid-twentieth century. A 1958 survey of interscholastic programs in junior high schools found a pronounced trend in some states toward formalized football for eighth and ninth graders. A common complaint was that senior high schools composed of tenth, eleventh, and twelfth grades were at a competitive disadvantage if their students were not exposed to organized football while enrolled in junior high. Furthermore, the report noted that youth football leagues outside the jurisdiction of state athletic associations (such as Pop Warner leagues) were making inroads in a number of states. Out of 1,968 junior high schools across the United States responding to the survey, 1,384 schools reported having tackle football teams. This made tackle football the third most commonly reported sport on offer, after basketball and track.[19]

The report's authors compared the number of principals who responded saying they favored interscholastic athletics with the number of junior high schools that offered these activities and concluded that "it is evident that a greater number of schools *have* interscholastic athletics than the number that *favor* them" (italics in original). This suggested that broader community pressures and values, not merely administrators' views, were fostering the growth of interscholastic athletics among younger students. The report noted the danger that sports "which promote a high degree of spectator interest" would dominate physical education programs. "Even in the earlier grades the influence of the high-school interscholastic program may be so great that the physical education instruction becomes primarily a 'feeder' for high-school athletics and thereby neglects activities more suitable to the growth and development of the younger children."[20] As discussed in chapter 4, in this era, medical concerns about the physical risks of football for prepubescent children were particularly focused on how injuries might harm bone growth and physical development.

In 1963, a committee of representatives of medical, educational, and recreational associations similarly characterized a harmful relationship between social pressures and the physical risks of tackle football at the junior high level. They argued that the use of junior high school athletics as a "farm system" for developing high school prospects intensified the physical dangers and the emotions associated with competition. "Unless these factors can be controlled—and the kind of equipment, facilities, health supervision, coaching, and officiating that are necessary for the optimum safety of the participants can be provided—tackle football should not be included in the junior high school athletics program."[21]

Yet successful high school football programs more commonly inspired increased participation in programs for younger children. One such example occurred with a string of high school football victories and state championships under Bob Reade, the head coach at J. D. Darnall High School in Geneseo, Illinois, from 1962 to 1978. The program's success "really gave the community something to hang its hat on" recalled Reade's statistician, who later served as principal of the high school. Moreover, the victories "trickled down to the youth football league. From fifth grade on, half of the boys in every class, 50 or more, would try out for football."[22]

Reade later wrote a book entitled *Coaching Football Successfully*. Famed Penn State coach Joe Paterno, who would be dismissed in 2011 due to a sex abuse scandal associated with his football program, contributed a foreword. Reade emphasized the importance of promoting participation before high school: "The real key is that the kids coming into the program have all had an opportunity to play." He recommended that high school football coaches building their programs attend as many games at lower levels of play as possible. "The head coach must show the young people participating in the program he is interested in them."[23]

By the 1950s and 1960s, the extent to which high school football was entrenched as part of school and community life shaped understandings of the sport's effects on student well-being. Leading educators took as a given that football conferred social and educational benefits to students. At the same time, they expressed concern about the increasing use of youth football as a feeder system and uncertainty about what precisely constituted the educational value of contact sports. In a 1967 interview, the supervisor of athletics for the New York State Department of Education stated that the department believed strongly in the benefits of contact sports: "They have special values that other activities don't." Yet he also asked, "What's educational? Are eighteen games more educational than twelve? Where do you reach the limit? . . . We don't know what is soundest educationally in terms of boys' learning a sport and milking it to its maximum for his own educational use and use after graduation."[24]

A 1969 master's thesis in education by Richard Stuetz, who would go on to coach football at Saddleback College, is a particularly instructive example of efforts to evaluate youth football's educational benefits. Stuetz examined the Pop Warner football league in Orange County, California, which at the time had about 1,200 boys enrolled, playing on around sixty teams. Stuetz remarked that one of the greatest selling points of the program was its "amazing lack of injuries" and its use of safety equipment. Yet whether such youth football leagues promoted values consistent with broader educational objectives was unclear, he argued, and needed to be assessed.[25]

Stuetz's chosen methodology to answer this question—asking several coaches to fill out a questionnaire indicating whether they believed each of their players had evinced particular values—appears highly subjective and susceptible to individual bias. Stuetz's analysis nonetheless reveals the types of community and educational values that physical educators associated with football. The objectives Stuetz evaluated at the Pop Warner and high school levels of play included loyalty, living and working with others, appreciating "the significance of the family as the most important unit in a society," and understanding the rights and duties of a citizen in a democratic society (see figure 16).[26]

Based on the coaches' responses, Stuetz reported that "the high school is doing the best job here of promoting both pride in the community and promoting fair play." Stuetz identified two major negative factors at the Pop Warner level: parental pressures and untrained coaches. Addressing these problems, he argued, was not only important for improving the experience of the youngest players but also for ensuring that they would continue to play

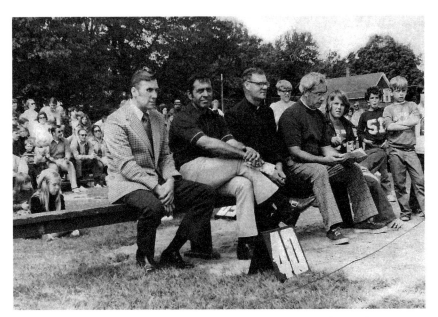

FIGURE 16 Opening day, Pop Warner football, c. 1966, shows both adults and children watching the game from the sidelines. Photo by G. B. Williams Jr., courtesy of the Maynard Historical Society.

the sport. A successful experience at the Pop Warner level "will give a boy the desire to continue on in the high school program and remain involved in healthy activity."[27] Thus, high school football was in many ways treated as the "gold standard" of youth football. Where little league organizations fell short, Stuetz argued that they needed to adopt the positive aspects of high school football.

Many communities, coaches, and parents believed youth football participation was crucial to boys' future success in school and in life. Such justifications, the explicit involvement of high school football coaches in encouraging younger players, and the belief that participating at younger ages would increase athletes' chances of playing for their high school teams, all pushed younger children to participate in football leagues not associated with schools.

King of Prussia Indians, Pennsylvania

In addition to operating as feeder systems for high school football, little league teams acquired their own status as centers of community life. The growth of the King of Prussia (KoP) Indians youth football team in King of Prussia,

Pennsylvania, exemplifies the transition from informal sandlot games to adult-organized league play. The heavy involvement of adult leaders in supervising boy football players and girl cheerleaders also illustrates the importance that football could attain in local communities for even elementary school aged players.

In 1956, starting with twenty-two young boys, Alan Richter founded the KoP youth football team in the small Pennsylvania town. Practices took place in a local cow pasture. Shortly thereafter, Dave and Mary Vannicelli joined as adult volunteers and would remain prominent leaders for several decades. Dave Vannicelli had played college football at Widener University, then known as the Pennsylvania Military Academy. He transitioned to coaching after seeing an advertisement seeking an assistant coach. In 1958, the KoP Indians became charter members of the Bux-Mont League of southeastern Pennsylvania, and in 1959 the KoP team came in third place in the nationwide Pop Warner Conference Little Scholars program, losing to an All-Star team in Cape Canaveral. A thirty-year retrospective on the team kept by the Vannicellis proudly noted that the KoP team had thus gone "from cow pasture to Cape Canaveral" in the space of three years.[28]

The KoP Indians became formally organized as the King of Prussia Football Association (KPFA) in 1960, and in 1963 they were legally incorporated. The Vannicellis' daughter Sandy recalled that Mary Vannicelli was named as one of the three incorporators, because her husband Dave was a team coach. The couple wished to avoid a possible conflict of interest, a worry which suggested the great seriousness with which the adult supervisors treated youth football.[29]

By this time, the KoP Indians had uniforms, equipment, fundraisers, and local media coverage. For example, in 1963 the *Valley Forge Sentinel* covered the team's games, fundraising efforts, and the ways parents and community members supported the league. One issue included a photo of the football players and the team's cheerleaders at a fund drive. The caption noted: "The King of Prussia Indians and their cheerleaders boarded a fire truck Sunday and toured Upper Merion on a house-to-house fund drive. The players' fathers, mothers and sisters pitched in for sideline and grandstand chores" (see figure 17). The Vannicellis submitted the results of the team's games to local newspapers, which reported on the scores of the matches of even the youngest football players.[30]

In 1964, Dave Vannicelli wrote a letter to the national Pop Warner office describing the amount of volunteer time he and his wife had dedicated to the KPFA in the previous year. Tasks included "coaching, committee work such

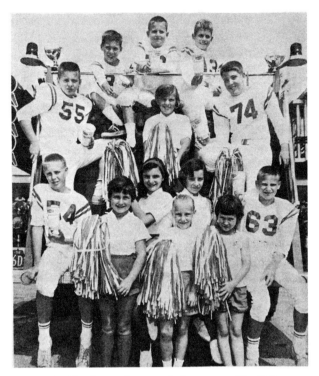

FIGURE 17 The September 12, 1963, front page of the *Valley Forge Sentinel* described these child football players and cheerleaders posing on a fire truck during a fund drive as "injuns on an engine." Dave and Mary Vannicelli Collection, KPHS, King of Prussia, Pennsylvania.

as equipment, banquet, trophies" as well as "meetings, mailing of information, preparing and reproduction of all paper work, establishing and maintaining a League player registration file, correspondence, etc." He estimated that throughout the year he had devoted about 700 hours to KPFA, while his wife had given about 350 to 400 hours of her time. While the Vannicellis may have been particularly dedicated volunteers, these estimates nonetheless suggest the level of involvement that running a youth football association entailed.[31]

The adult leadership of the KoP Indians emphasized that their primary objective was fostering moral character in young athletes and shaping future adults according to community values. This mission was made clear in the KPFA's constitution, which stated that the association's goal was "to implant firmly in the boys and girls of our community, the principles of good character development, i.e., courage, responsibility, sportsmanship, fair play, leadership, and respect for rules and regulation, as well as to foster higher achievement in scholastic activities." These goals "shall be achieved by providing supervised competitive football games and related activities within a program that fosters favorable character development . . . the molding of future men and women is of prime importance."[32]

An undated Q&A on the history of the KPFA from Dave and Mary Vannicelli, likely from the late 1980s or early 1990s, noted that at the time of its writing, the league had twelve football coaches, ninety-five "young men" aged six to thirteen years old playing football in four different weight-class teams, fifty-six cheerleaders, three adult sponsors, and forty-five adults "engaged in administration including officers, board members, team mothers, business managers, and equipment personnel." With varying degrees of involvement, a large number of adults volunteered their time with the league.[33]

The division of labor among these numerous adult supervisors remained heavily gendered throughout the final decades of the twentieth century. A 1999 KoP information packet for new and returning members distinguished between the responsibilities of "team moms" and "business managers (team dads)." The duties of the team moms included keeping the children orderly on the bench, arranging snacks for game days, signing up parents to work in the teen activity center on practice nights and at home games, working to promote fundraisers, relaying organization communications to the parents, and arranging the team party. Meanwhile, the team dads were expected to "help to keep order on practice nights and games days; assist in relaying organization communications to parents; conduct weigh-ins prior to the start of each game; check that players have necessary protective equipment; carry medical cards at all times; provide write-ups of games to the Publicity Director and provide scores of all home games to the Publicity Director."[34]

Team fathers' duties thus explicitly encompassed oversight of youth safety by assisting with practices and games and checking player equipment and medical cards, whereas mothers managed social events and oversaw player behavior on the sidelines. Identifying fathers as "business managers" also had the effect of distancing fathers from their more personal, parental role as dads. Their contribution as adult supervisors was instead framed as providing professional, managerial, and athletic skills rather than nurturing or social skills.

The Q&A response to a question on how the league ensured the safety of its players emphasized the adult supervision that was primarily furnished by coaches and fathers. Men matched children according to age and weight so that players would not be overmatched physically. They also ensured that all athletes received quality protective equipment, including NOCSAE-approved helmets that were regularly inspected by an outside agency. In addition to overseeing physical conditioning and training, the league required game day medical coverage, which was provided by medical personnel from the Lafayette Ambulance Squad in Upper Merion, Pennsylvania.[35]

The supervisory imperative, as described in chapter 4, is clearly evident in the structure of the KPFA league and the strategies the league employed to provide for its players' safety. With coaches in charge, fathers directly involved on the field, and mothers assisting on the sidelines, the adults overseeing the sport believed that football offered significant social and moral benefits to children and that their involvement minimized the risks. In fact, the community's response to those youth football injuries that did occur was characterized as exemplifying the virtues of teamwork and caring. In a 1996 letter to the president of the KPFA, a board member noted that families from the fifty-five-pound team and others within the KPFA organization had expressed concern about a knee injury that a young player, Robert, had sustained. She noted that her phone had been ringing off the hook with inquiries. Young Robert had received several visitors at the hospital as well as follow-up phone calls asking how his orthopedic exam had gone. She requested that the KPFA president convey to the board "that even if nothing else we are teaching these kids what a team is and what it means to be part of that team including caring enough to show it when someone is hurt." It was understood that some injuries would occur even with adult supervision. Yet provided they were not too serious, the injuries that players sustained carried redeeming moral value: the response to football injuries could be the source of the types of social lessons the adult organizers were seeking to impart to young athletes.[36]

Board meeting minutes, mainly available from the 1990s, document significant attention by the league's leadership on how to best ensure medical supervision of youth games. For instance, in October 1997, the board noted that providing coaches with CPR training would be less expensive than paying emergency medical technicians to cover home games. In November 1997, three parents from the fifty-five-pound team attended the meeting to discuss apparently inadequate medical coverage at games. When a KPFA representative asked a "medical person" to provide identification, they were given a blank form. Without identification of the attendant's medical training, they did not let the game continue. In addition, the opposing team "introduced a man who never came on field when a boy was hurt. Parents questioned the league's ability to enforce coverage." The KPFA board decided that they should not play against this team given this failure and that the following year coaches and dads would enforce this policy. Ensuring trained medical supervision was evidently an ongoing challenge with which the adult men associated with the league were tasked.[37]

KPFA's leadership also included a groundskeeper and equipment director who supervised the fields used by the team, as well as the provision and recertification of protective helmets. In 2000, KPFA member Bob Gray held this position, and his notes on the status of the association's helmets indicate the logistical and legal complexity of maintaining this single piece of equipment. Gray kept a detailed list of helmet sizes and dates purchased. He noted that two-thirds of the association's inventory had been purchased between 1990 and 1992, making most of the helmets nearly a decade old. While other helmet models had a mandatory discontinuance of use policy after the eighth year from date of manufacture, this was not the case for the helmets in use by KPFA. Additionally, at the high school level, Gray noted, all football helmets were required to be recertified annually, but this was not mandatory at the youth level. Unlike the high school level of play, which was overseen by the NFHS, leagues for younger children were overseen by a variety of private organizations that set their own policies.[38]

While particular policies varied at different levels of play, it is clear that the institutionalization of football safety practices in little leagues, junior high schools, and high schools all resulted in an emphasis on a large number of technical requirements and safety boxes to check. These ranged from documenting the presence of medical personnel at games to notifying football league commissioners that all the players' helmets had been certified by NOCSAE.

Despite these forms of oversight, parents remained concerned about injuries through the latter decades of the twentieth century, as suggested by the effort that leagues and sports organizations invested in reassuring parents that tackle football was indeed safe for children to play. The KoP football archives include a 1996 article by reporter Kent Hannon entitled "Is Football Safe for Kids?" Published as part of a special supplement of *Sports Illustrated for Kids,* this issue was intended for parents, advising them on "how to help your kids get the most out of sports." KoP football organizers had most likely saved this article for use as a reference for coaches and parents about football safety.[39]

The article opened by illustrating concerns over an apparent head injury which purportedly proved to be unfounded. It recounted the story of Brent

McEwan, then 10, who was playing linebacker when he experienced a helmet-to-helmet collision with another child. His father recalled, "Both kids went down and didn't move. I remember someone saying, 'Those kids are really hurt.'" Brent's helmet had split in half. Yet the boy himself was not injured, according to Hannon, who added that Brent "never suffered a serious injury while playing" the sport from his youth through his college football days. In other words, a collision where two young players went down and did not move was deemed not to have resulted in a serious injury.[40]

Sports Illustrated for Kids listed three key football safety factors associated with adult supervision: proper equipment; teaching correct football techniques, specifically never leading with the helmet to make a tackle; and the small size of the young children matched against other children of a similar age and weight ("FORCE=mass x acceleration, and kids don't generate much force"). The article also quoted coaches who made familiar comparisons about the safety of football relative to other popular childhood activities. One football coach in his eleventh year of coaching Pop Warner teams stated, "Frankly, many more of our kids get hurt riding bikes, climbing trees, or in-line skating than they do playing football."[41]

Despite these reassurances, the appropriate age at which to begin participation in organized youth football, whether tackle or flag, remained a source of uncertainty. The KoP archive includes a flurry of 1996 letters between parents and league officials related to whether two flag football coaches were safely conducting games and practices. Some parents expressed concerns about inadequate practice time spread too thin among too many players, while others wrote letters of support for the coaches. Notably, parent Robert B. Leahy sent a letter to the KoP Indians Flag Football Representative to communicate his view that the coaches were not fundamentally to blame for his safety concerns and that they had performed their coaching duties well. Instead, he argued, "Five year old children are not mentally and physically prepared to play football. That is just the plain truth. State it any other way you like, they are too young. The program should start at the age of six thru eight, provided weight is a consideration. One real test for the board members will be when some five year old child is out there not paying attention and is badly hurt. God forbid."[42]

Leahy's letter suggested that children who were too young to consistently pay attention to adult coaches and follow directions were unable to sufficiently benefit from adult supervision and thus too young to play football. That the source of debate by the 1990s was whether five-year-olds should be playing organized football indicates the extent to which earlier debates about the extension of competitive sports to younger ages had moved. By this time, it was largely taken as a given that children as young as nine or ten could play football. With football framed as safe for grade-school children given the proper adult supervision, the debate had instead shifted to identifying at which age children were old enough to understand and take advantage of such supervision.

Education, Race, and Big Hits

In addition to individual character building, tackle football was presumed to enable boys to access greater social status and economic success. Race and socioeconomic status significantly influenced the value of these perceived benefits. The racial integration of school and professional football teams, the growing value of college football scholarships, and the increasing television coverage of NFL games all shaped the intersection of race, the spectator nature of football, and attitudes toward physical risk.

In the latter half of the twentieth century and into the early twenty-first century, the most dramatic racial shift in football was the increasing participation and visibility of African American players. Michael Oriard has noted that the transformation of college and professional football to "a multiracial, ultimately black-dominated sport was only beginning by the end of the 1950s."[43] The civil rights movement of the 1960s also profoundly influenced the racial demographics of youth football. To the extent that schools and communities remained segregated, their football teams remained segregated too. Furthermore, as historian Lane Demas observed of college football, the "acceptance of black athletes on the playing field did not translate into equal and adequate opportunities for African American students at integrated colleges." The same can undoubtedly be said for black athletes at the high school level. Nonetheless, these social changes, including the increasing prominence of black football stars on college teams and in the NFL, made future football success a more visible possibility for young black boys (see figure 18).[44]

Quantifying the history of racial and ethnic shifts in youth football is challenging due to the lack of systematic, comparable national data on participation in youth football and race. The NFHS, which oversees football in the majority of American high schools, has not collected historical data on race in its sports participation statistics. Neither has USA Football, the national governing body for amateur football in the United States, nor have little league organizations such as Pop Warner.[45]

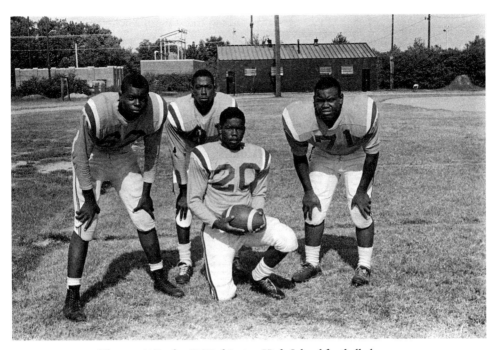

FIGURE 18 These 1968 Booker T. Washington High School football players were students from a formerly all-black high school in North Carolina. Charles S. Killebrew Photographic Collection, 1948–2001, North Carolina Collection, Louis Round Wilson Special Collections Library, University of North Carolina at Chapel Hill.

Nonetheless, some available state and local studies suggest high participation of racial minorities, particularly African Americans, in youth football after the 1960s. In 1975, two Michigan state representatives initiated a legislative inquiry into youth sports programs. The special six-member committee was tasked with examining in particular "the actual educational benefits that youth receive from these programs," as well as the medical and legal problems associated with youth sports. The first phase of the study sought to characterize the extent of sports participation by Michigan youth, including free play or recreational sports, school-sponsored sports, and agency-sponsored sports (competition between teams, clubs, or individuals not sponsored by schools). The study included eighty-nine randomly sampled Michigan school districts from across the state. A combined total of nearly 100,000 student and parent questionnaires were ultimately returned to the researchers from both private and public schools in these districts.[46]

The large sample size in conjunction with random sampling procedures meant that researchers considered the study to be representative of children from kindergarten through eleventh grade in the state of Michigan. The researchers included categories for race as well as other key variables such as age, sex, and community type. While acknowledging that the incidence of participation by race was the most difficult variable to obtain, the researchers reported finding that black participants had the highest percent participation in all agency-sponsored team sports, with the exception of soccer and ice hockey. Furthermore, the researchers found that participation in agency-sponsored sports among all youth was much higher than they had anticipated. Approximately one of every eight Michigan boys participated in agency-sponsored football. The study's findings suggested extensive youth participation in football programs outside of schools, particularly among black youth, and very little external oversight of safety. "Clearly, the extent of participation is very large with no control except that of sponsoring agencies."[47]

Football increasingly became a means by which black boys could "prove" or legitimize themselves to white-dominated communities and institutions. In 1986, Nand Hart-Nibbrig, a professor of political science and public administration, coauthored an examination of the political economy of college sports in which he recalled his own football experiences. As a black student at a Catholic high school, he felt heavy pressure from both the coaching staff and several priests to play football. When he decided to cease playing the sport at age sixteen in order to focus on his academic studies, the head football coach reportedly berated him in front of the student body, stating that "the school did not need or want" a person like him representing it. Hart-Nibbrig reflected that he was, to use Ralph Ellison's term, an "invisible man," "partly because I was black and partly because my real destiny was perceived to lie in throwing a football."[48]

Football as a means to status and success took on particular valence in racially marginalized communities. For his book *We Own This Game*, journalist Robert Andrew Powell interviewed a number of coaches, players, and former players in his examination of Pop Warner football in predominantly black, poor areas of Miami, Florida. Powell noted that although he had originally intended to spend most of his time speaking with the children who played the game, after reviewing his notes, "I realized that in talking to the people most invested in Pop Warner football, I'd spent most of my time talking to adults." The title of his book came from an interview with Miami area rapper Luther Campbell, who described the importance of football in this community: "We own this game. I mean, you can take whatever you want to take—our land, our housing, our jobs, whatever. But we got our dignity and our pride."[49]

The observations of former youth football player George Knox are particularly revealing. Born in Jacksonville, Florida, in 1943, Knox grew up in a segregated housing project where he began playing football. He recalled that "football was the most popular sport when I was growing up. When it came to following football, blacks in the community knew everything there was to know about the white high schools: who the players were, who the star was, who the mascot was, what the team colors were. We'd read the newspaper and we'd know what [all-white] Landon High School and Jackson High School were doing. On the other side of the *Florida Times-Union* newspaper was all the news 'for and about colored people.' We knew the white population wasn't reading about the activities at my high school or at any black high schools."[50]

Consequently, Knox recalled, black players yearned "to demonstrate their skills to the larger population—first to gain respect for their skills, and also to have some recognition of the very existence of the black community." He acknowledged that this desire for recognition and respect went beyond sports, but youth football became a foremost arena for these aspirations. Knox emphasized that athletic competition in many respects represented "the only direct opportunity that blacks have to demonstrate excellence, and more importantly, superiority to their white counterparts."[51] In examining the complex relationship between masculine identity and sport participation in boyhood, sociologists Kevin Young and Philip White have suggested that "to relinquish the opportunity to participate in the sporting rite of passage, or at the very least to identify with sports heroes or teams, is to risk estrangement from other boys." In racially and otherwise marginalized communities, it seems probable that participation in football not only solidified boys' relationships with one another but also with the communities they were expected to represent.[52]

The desegregation of football further fostered narratives about the sport's ability to heal across racial divides and build community among boys of differing ethnic backgrounds. For example, Bear Bryant, one of the most celebrated American college football coaches, began his twenty-five-year career with the University of Alabama in 1958 when the team—indeed, the entire Southeastern Conference (SEC)—was segregated. During the civil rights movement of the 1960s, Bryant became a "lightning rod" for criticism of segregation and racist violence. But when the league integrated, "Bryant and his biracial teams quickly became a symbol of the new paradigm of racial harmony and cooperation."[53] In fact, stories circulated that Bryant influenced notorious segregationist George Wallace by educating the governor about the benefits of racial integration. Even if these stories were overblown, they are nonetheless telling about the values fans attributed both to a popular coach and to the sport of football itself.[54]

Bryant, a teacher of a famously rough brand of football, also symbolizes another important, related later-twentieth century trend: the glorification of "big hits" and an ever more aggressive style of play. It is notable that the racial integration of college and professional football teams converged with the emergence of televised football as the most widely viewed sport on American television. In his examination of the NFL from 1920 to 1967, historian Craig Coenen observed that by 1960, televised Sunday football games were viewed by as many as 30 million to 50 million Americans, "far outpacing the weekly average for any other sport." Moreover, "Football seemed to be made for television. In the course of play all twenty-two players were compressed into a small area that could easily be captured by a single camera. In fact, the game proved easier to follow on television than at the stadium."[55]

As football became the most popular professional sport in the United States, its spectacle nature moved far beyond local communities. Television coverage heightened public fascination with brutal hits on the field. In 1960, Philadelphia Eagles player Chuck Bednarik, known as "Concrete Charlie," famously knocked opponent Frank Gifford out of play for more than eighteen months. While observers at the time debated whether the hit constituted a "cheap shot" or "a good perfect tackle," Bednarik's tackle heralded the growing celebration of big hits. Over the decades, the devastating collision would be played and replayed in highlight reels.[56] Such coverage magnified both tacit and explicit acceptance of the physical risks associated with these collisions. In 1978, after NFL safety Jack Tatum ("The Assassin") delivered a hit that paralyzed his opponent Darryl Stingley from the chest down, the chairman of the NFL Competition Committee responded that "no one liked the assassination of President Kennedy, but the world had to go on."[57]

The increasingly aggressive style of play had entertainment value; it took place as the NFL became perceived as a more viable career path and as college scholarships became more closely tied to the sport. The increasing value and attraction of a college scholarship was related to the rising cost of college, as well as the growing corporatization of college athletics. In 1957, the NCAA adopted athletic scholarships that would enable colleges to bind student athletes to one-year renewable contracts that depended upon their athletic performance. Success in football was increasingly a means by which otherwise marginalized youth might be able to access a college education. Yet while colleges depicted their athletic policies as supporting affirmative action for minority groups, the institutions benefited enormously by profiting from athletes' low-paid (or arguably unpaid) labor. Sociologist Robert Turner has observed that this feeling of exploitation on predominantly white college campuses contributed to black students leaving college early for the NFL. Moreover, "though athletes are viewed as ambassadors of the college, the demands of big-time college football rarely offer time to benefit from school resources in the same fashion as the rest of the student body." Although hopes of a future scholarship heightened the perceived value of football for boys of high school age and even younger, for many students the increased exposure to the physical risks of football did not result in full access to the benefits of higher education.[58]

Furthermore, within integrated football teams, significant racial disparities developed according to player position. The disproportionate allocation of athletes to positions according to their race or ethnicity is known as "stacking." In football, the central position of quarterback became disproportionately associated with white players, a phenomenon influenced by racist stereotypes about leadership abilities and cognitive skills.[59] Detailed college football data reveal that black athletes have become particularly overrepresented in football positions that deliver and receive the most hits (running backs, wide receivers, safeties, and cornerbacks). Stacking thus influenced not only the particular positions to which players might aspire but also the physical risks to which athletes might be exposed.[60]

College demographic data continue to suggest a racial shift in which more black boys play youth football as a means to access a college education, a football career, or both. Black college football players at top athletic programs became substantially overrepresented in relation to the racial composition of the student body as well as the overall American population. According to NCAA data from the turn of the twenty-first century, in the 1999–2000 school year, 51.3 percent of NCAA Division I college football players were white, while 39.5 percent were black. By the 2014–15 school year, a minority (40.2 percent) of Division I football players were white, while 47.1 percent were black.[61]

Football is not the only American sport that has been intimately tied to school or community identity, in which intensive feeder systems have developed, or in which racially and ethnically marginalized communities have perceived potential opportunities for social status and resources denied to them in other aspects of American life. Yet these have all been key features of youth football in the twentieth and early twenty-first centuries, and these factors are crucial to understanding the context in which doctors, educators, coaches, and parents weighed the risks and benefits of youth football.

Demographic data as well as testimony from former players and coaches suggest the extent to which the social position of children and their communities shape debates. Adult-sanctioned play carries particular resonance in a culture where children, most especially black children, can be vulnerable to violence while playing on their own. The worst-case scenario is exemplified by the 2014 death of Tamir Rice, a twelve-year-old black boy killed by a Cleveland police officer while playing in a playground with an air gun. When unsupervised children can be perceived as suspicious and dangerous, supervised play in a socially valued sport such as football affords a substantial level of social protection. Tackle football can legitimize stereotypes of male aggression and physicality as a healthy, socially sanctioned activity. This function of youth football carries particular importance for black boys and men who are especially subject to these stereotypes.

Henry Steele Commager's 1958 depiction of high school football as "burlesque performances" captured the sport's spectacle nature in conjunction with football's role as a socially sanctioned form of physical aggression. Commager's analysis highlighted the troubling implications for the teenagers expected to perform for their communities, yet largely predated the expansion of elementary and middle school football as a feeder system for future play. Commager also penned this essay before the NFL dominated American televisions and in advance of football's changing racial dynamics following school integration.

Commager's analysis does not account for the extent to which adults believed that participation in youth football conferred substantial personal and physical benefits to boys. But the expectations of adults, educators, and communities extended far beyond boys' individual development. Boys' social, economic, and educational futures were often treated as hinging on their performance on the gridiron. A 1979 examination of high school football in Texas meditated on the burden such expectations placed upon young athletes: "The prospective heroes are mostly fifteen and sixteen years old, unused to being depended upon for anything at all, justifiably haunted by the fear that they're really still just children."[62]

CHAPTER NINE

This Is Your Brain on Football

The Framing of a Concussion Crisis

I hope another player doesn't have to die before all this is taken seriously.

—James P. Kelly, 1994

In the final decades of the twentieth century, it looked like tackle football was getting safer. In 1976, the NFHS and NCAA adopted rules prohibiting "spearing," the deliberate use of the top of the helmet to strike another player.[1] Several studies attributed subsequent reductions in cervical spinal cord injuries and quadriplegia among high school and college football players to these rule changes.[2] Additionally, fatalities largely declined in the 1980s and 1990s; in fact, 1990 was the first and only year since 1931 when the AFCA's annual survey documented no direct fatalities from football.[3]

Although doctors and educators celebrated these trends, many remained concerned about the prevalence of head and neck injuries. Furthermore, the decline in severe injuries and fatalities helped bring another issue into focus: that trauma to football players' brains, even if it did not result in death or paralysis, might still constitute a serious medical problem. With new brain imaging technologies and research pointing to the risks of cumulative trauma, some doctors and scientists sounded alarm bells in scientific journals. But, for decades, their warnings did not rise above a much louder din: popular celebrations of big hits and encouragement of athletes playing through pain, from NFL broadcasts to high school football sidelines.

From Getting "Dinged" to Second-Impact Syndrome

In 1973, *Neurology*, the journal of the American Academy of Neurology (AAN), published an article describing several cases of college athletes getting "dinged" while playing football. Getting "dinged" or "getting your bell rung" were commonly used expressions to describe sustaining a hit to the head that might result in temporary confusion or even memory loss but not loss of consciousness.[4] The article's coauthors, a neurologist and an educational psychologist, cited former NFL player Dave Meggyesy's explanation of getting "dinged" as "getting hit in the head so hard that your memory is affected, although you can still walk around and sometimes even continue playing. You don't feel pain, and the only way other players or the coaches know you've been dinged is when they realize you can't remember the plays."[5]

The researchers reported on four cases of players experiencing short-term memory loss, as well as six cases of "delayed retrograde amnesia." This referred to instances where players were initially able to recall recent events immediately after their injury but permanently lost the information within minutes of being examined. This suggested that despite retaining consciousness and demonstrating immediate recall ability, a consequence of getting "dinged" might include impairment of short-term memory consolidation. Based on these findings, the *Neurology* article recommended that in order to assess "mild concussions," physicians should not ask athletes questions that evaluated their immediate memory or cognition, such as how many fingers they were holding up. Instead, they should ask questions about recent events, such as, "Where did you go after you left the playing field? What are some of your plays and assignments for this game?"[6]

Although physicians recognized that players could sustain a concussion while retaining consciousness, such concussions were considered mild. Athletes very rarely sought medical attention for getting "dinged." Consequently, studying the incidence of concussions was challenging. Simply relying on hospital data would result in a serious underestimate. Another significant problem for epidemiologists was that there was no universally agreed upon definition of concussion, let alone how to categorize different degrees or "grades" of concussion.

There had been efforts at standardization. For example, in 1966, the AMA's first standard nomenclature of athletic injuries defined an acute cerebral concussion as a clinical syndrome characterized by immediate "impairment of neural function" caused by a "direct blow to head or helmet." The AMA characterized three degrees of concussion: mild, moderate, and severe. According to this classification system, mild and moderate concussions resulted in only transient impairment, whereas a severe concussion might cause protracted impairment.[7]

Yet these definitions were repeatedly contested. In 1969, two neurosurgeons, including Richard Schneider, whose research had suggested important limitations to football helmet design (see chapter 3), noted that for years most neurosurgeons had used the term concussion to involve a state of unconsciousness. Yet, these doctors observed, loss of consciousness was not necessary for a concussion to occur, and other symptoms could be equally important. They granted that the AMA's 1966 classification system sought to enhance physicians' ability to make practical decisions about treating football injuries but stated that its categories were arbitrary. In fact, "the diagnosis of concussion has been so confusing that the British neurosurgeons recently have recommended abandoning its use." The confusion did not abate. A 2001 review article described eight different concussion grading systems that had been proposed over the previous decades. The range of definitions in use through the end of the twentieth century made comparing data across studies difficult.[8]

In 1983, public health researcher Susan Goodwin Gerberich led one of the first large-scale epidemiological studies of concussion incidence in high school football players. To address the problem that hospital records would not capture most concussion cases, her team instead mailed questionnaires to head coaches and players at more than 100 high school varsity football teams in Minnesota. The questionnaire asked players if they had lost consciousness as a result of a blow to their head or experienced other symptoms such as brief loss of awareness, headaches, dizziness, or blurred vision during the fall 1977 football season.[9]

Gerberich and her colleagues found that while only about 2 percent of players reported having diagnosed concussions in conjunction with a head injury, nearly seven times as many reported experiencing loss of consciousness or loss of awareness. Including these latter symptoms resulted in an estimated rate of about one in five players sustaining at least one probable concussion over the course of one football season. Players with a prior history of losing consciousness had a four times higher risk of losing consciousness as compared to players without such a history. While differences in players' activity levels or willingness to report symptoms may have accounted for some of this difference, Gerberich's team concluded that this result implied the need to identify previous concussions when taking players' preseason medical histories.[10]

The use of questionnaires in this study probably facilitated reporting by offering respondents confidentiality. Yet, as the researchers noted, the true incidence and severity of concussions would remain unknown without actual observation and examination of athletes by trained health professionals. Furthermore, over two-thirds of the players who had experienced loss of consciousness returned to play the same day. Many respondents reported that they had wanted to continue playing, so they did not tell anybody about their symptoms. "Better understanding of risks, by both players and coaches, is clearly in order," the researchers concluded.[11]

In addition to research suggesting that concussions were far more common than hospital diagnoses would indicate, medical reports were sounding alarms about the risks of repetitive brain trauma. A 1984 *JAMA* case report suggested that a concussion might make athletes more vulnerable to severe consequences of a second brain injury. In this article, a neurologist and a neurosurgeon reported on the death of an otherwise healthy nineteen-year-old college freshman football player. The student had collapsed "despite accounts of no unusual head trauma" after being involved as a blocker in a running play. He went into a coma and was placed on a ventilator. Despite an operation that sought to reduce the swelling in his brain, he never regained consciousness and died several days later.[12]

Disturbed by this seemingly inexplicable death, doctors made inquiries with the deceased player's family, teammates, and coaches. Four days prior to his collapse on the field, they learned, the young athlete had briefly lost consciousness following a hit to the head sustained during a fistfight. He claimed to have only a mild headache several days following the hit and had thus been given permission to return to play. The doctors suggested that this previous head trauma might have made the football player more susceptible to brain injury in the following days than he would have been otherwise. They consequently warned that even seemingly "ordinary sports violence might precipitate catastrophic brain swelling." The doctors wrote that this "second impact" phenomenon, while apparently rare, nonetheless raised serious questions about football safety. The risks warranted "a more critical view of the adequacy of clinical assessment after minor head injuries in contact sports." If some players could be identified as being at increased risk, they might need to be instructed to avoid further impact to protect them from harm.[13]

One of the readers of this article was Robert Cantu, a neurosurgeon involved in football as both a parent and a doctor. He had a young son who played in the Pop Warner league, and he also served as a sideline physician for local high school football teams. As writers Linda Carroll and David Rosner would dramatically recount in their 2010 book, *The Concussion Crisis*, reading about this second-impact syndrome greatly affected Cantu. "Cantu realized that if he missed a concussion today, some kid might get bumped next week and die." Cantu was particularly concerned about the many youth football games where neither a physician nor an athletic trainer was present to watch out for head trauma on the field. In 1986, only 5 percent of American high schools employed athletic trainers, according to the National Athletic Trainers Association. Moreover, many were uncertified. As the chairman of the New York State Athletic Trainers' Association colorfully observed, "In New

York, we're talking Joe service-station attendant who goes to games on Saturday and calls himself the trainer."[14]

To address the dangers, Cantu believed that coaches as well as medical personnel needed guidelines to determine when athletes could safely return to sports. Although there were no formal, standardized guidelines at the time, many physicians already discouraged players from continuing to play football after sustaining three concussions. Augustus Thorndike, a leader in the development of sports medicine (see chapter 4), had proposed this policy in a 1952 article describing contraindications to continued participation in sport. Thorndike had further advised that patients "with more than momentary loss of consciousness at any one time should not be exposed to further body-contact trauma." The selection of three concussions as a cutoff point was arbitrary. Nonetheless, this informal policy proved influential: it was adopted by many physicians, and was promulgated and debated in medical journals in the ensuing decades.[15]

Some specialists considered Thorndike's recommendations to be unduly conservative. For example, in a 1959 symposium issue on sports injuries, two neurosurgeons contended that multiple concussions should not necessarily represent a contraindication to further participation in contact sports, because the severity of brain trauma was a "highly individualized matter" that needed to be decided on a case-by-case basis. After careful study of an individual patient, "if no evidence of damage to the brain is found, we do not believe that they would take any greater risk in engaging in contact sports than other athletes who have not had such injuries." By contrast, other experts emphasized a more conservative approach, advising that even a single severe concussion might warrant removing an athlete from any further play.[16]

By 1980, a review of football head and neck injuries observed that while no hard-and-fast rules could be made, it was "generally agreed upon" that "three severe concussions sustained in football automatically should prohibit the player from participating in football again." Cantu agreed that ultimately a physician's clinical judgment, rather than strict adherence to any particular guideline, would need to determine concussion management. Yet he also believed that easy, practical guidelines that could be applied on the field were urgently needed. He depicted concussions as a serious medical and public health concern. Citing Gerberich and her colleagues' research, Cantu observed that one in five high school football players experienced a concussion every year, that some studies suggested that the effects of concussions might be cumulative, and that the discovery of second-impact syndrome in particular should make physicians wary.[17]

TABLE 5 Cantu 1986 guidelines for return to play after concussion

	1st concussion	2nd concussion	3rd concussion
Grade 1 (mild)	May return to play if asymptomatic* for one week.	Return to play in two weeks if asymptomatic at that time for one week.	Terminate season; may return to play next season if asymptomatic.
Grade 2 (moderate)	Return to play after asymptomatic for one week.	Minimum of one month; may return to play then if asymptomatic for one week; consider terminating season.	Terminate season; may return to play next season if asymptomatic.
Grade 3 (severe)	Minimum of one month; may then return if asymptomatic for one week.	Terminate season; may return to play next season if asymptomatic.	

*Asymptomatic was defined as "no headache, dizziness, or impaired orientation, concentration, or memory during rest or exertion." Adapted from Robert C. Cantu, "Guidelines for Return to Contact Sports after a Cerebral Concussion," *Physician and Sportsmedicine* 14 (1986): 75–83.

Thus, in 1986, Cantu published the first written guidelines on when athletes could return to play based on the degree and number of concussions they had sustained (see table 5). For example, Cantu proposed that after one mild concussion, athletes could return if they were asymptomatic after one week, but after a severe concussion, they would need to wait a minimum of one month. Cantu cited Thorndike's earlier proposal when explaining his recommendation that three mild concussions should terminate an athlete's season. Published in *The Physician and Sportsmedicine*, these guidelines were above all intended to highlight the need to take concussions seriously. Yet there were no research studies supporting any of the particular recommendations. In fact, Cantu later acknowledged that the recovery times he had proposed were "pure seat of the pants."[18]

A Silent Epidemic

Meanwhile, scientists were accumulating evidence that even minor or moderate head injuries could cause structural changes in the brain. In 1968, a British neuropathologist reported microscopic brain lesions in several patients who had sustained head trauma but died of nonneurological causes. Notably, five of these patients had sustained concussions, described as "clinically trivial" brain injuries. Yet it was impossible to examine these changes in the brains of living people, and because patients did not typically die of minor head injuries, it was not feasible to conduct routine postmortem studies of these structural changes.[19]

In the 1980s, however, studies of concussions in monkeys provided substantiating evidence that the forces associated with even mild head trauma could induce microscopic damage in primates' brains.[20] Epidemiological studies of minor head trauma in humans were also raising concerns. Notably, a 1981 study of more than 400 patients who had sustained minor head trauma (defined as a history of unconsciousness of twenty minutes or less) found a high incidence of symptoms and difficulties on follow-up three months after injury. Over three-quarters of the patients reported persistent headaches, and over half described problems with memory. Furthermore, of those who had been gainfully employed, one-third were unemployed three months later. The authors concluded that "the most striking observations of these studies are the high rates of morbidity and unemployment in patients 3 months after a seemingly insignificant head injury and the evidence that many of these patients may have, in fact, suffered organic brain damage."[21]

The *Wall Street Journal* reported on this research in a front page article dubbing head injuries a "silent epidemic." The write-up noted that new technologies such as computerized axial tomography (CAT) scanners were able to detect brain damage that had previously gone unrecognized, but that the frequent absence of obvious symptoms continued to pose a challenge. One physician was quoted as saying, "For the most part, we're dealing with people who look and act pretty much all right. This leads a lot of physicians to write off their complaints as psychosomatic, and insurance companies and government-medical bureaucrats to look askance at their requests for benefits." The article observed that most research for rehabilitation programs for patients with head injuries was of recent origin and had focused on Vietnam veterans, but that a few small, intensive, and costly programs for head-injured patients were beginning to be developed.[22]

Yet these studies and early media coverage of a "silent epidemic" did not immediately translate into changes in clinical practice. In fact, Jeffrey Barth, a neuropsychologist who coauthored the 1981 study of patients with mild head trauma, would later recall the day he presented those findings at a conference as one of his worst professional experiences. A skeptical audience peppered him with alternative explanations for his results: perhaps the patients he was testing were not very smart to begin with, or maybe they didn't return to work because they had an excuse from their doctor. Barth recalled, "I thought to myself: How can I get out of this? Maybe I can fake a seizure."[23]

As two ESPN reporters would later put it, at the time concussions were regarded "as the neurological equivalent of a stubbed toe."[24] In 2005, a clinical neuropsychologist recalled that through the 1980s, trauma physicians were still primarily focused on severe brain trauma. They typically discharged patients with minor head injuries within an hour, with no recommendation for follow-up. He dubbed the 1980s "the decade of the severe TBIs," with the 1990s as the period when less severe forms of brain injury gained greater attention from clinicians. In 1989, Barth contributed a chapter on head injuries in sports in the first published book devoted specifically to mild brain injury. He and his colleagues observed that given the relatively limited and controversial state of scientific knowledge, and the reluctance of athletes to report seemingly minor injuries, "it is not surprising that mild head injury has not been a principal concern of most athletes or their institutions and organizations."[25]

Yet emerging scientific findings, new brain imaging technology, and the introduction of Cantu's preliminary return-to-play guidelines all contributed to the beginnings of a shift in attitude regarding brain injuries that had previously been considered of little importance. An increase in the number of children playing youth sports in the 1990s may have also contributed to growing awareness. Much of the rise in youth sports participation in the final decades of the twentieth century was due to more girls playing sports following changes to school athletic programs required by Title IX. But the numbers of boys participating in high school athletics also increased, with tackle football consistently remaining one of the most popular sports for boys.[26]

Historian Howard Chudacoff has argued that the expansion of organized sports was part of a broader trend toward adult-organized activities for children, such as language programs, music lessons, and math and science after-school clubs. Sociologist Hilary Levey Friedman has described an "explosion of hypercompetitiveness" in the professionalization of youth sports beginning in the 1980s. Friedman identified three forms of professionalization: the expansion of elite programs such as travel leagues and Olympic development programs; the rise of paid youth coaches and specialized trainers; and the emergence of the year-round season with children playing the same sport throughout the year.[27]

In 1991, two sports medicine specialists reported that they were witnessing more sports injuries among children in their practice in tandem with increasing participation in adult-organized athletics. Furthermore, they had observed greater numbers of overuse injuries stemming from repetitive trauma children experienced by training in a single sport. With more participants playing in more intensely competitive programs, changes in scientific and medical understandings of brain trauma occurred in the context of broader attention to changing patterns of sports injuries among children.[28]

By the 1990s, a number of physicians and athletic trainers increasingly questioned the common practice of returning players to the field shortly after they had gotten their "bell rung." In a 1991 *JAMA* article, a team of physicians observed that repeated concussions could lead to cumulative neurological deficits and even death in rare cases. They warned against the common misconception that forces strong enough to cause loss of consciousness were necessary to produce a concussion. They described the case of a seventeen-year-old high school football player who died of brain swelling after sustaining multiple concussions, although he had not lost consciousness from his previous brain injuries. This case was consistent with previously documented reports of second-impact syndrome. The doctors thus recommended that players experiencing confusion and amnesia after a head injury, even if they did not lose consciousness, should be removed from play for at least a day. They should then be reexamined the following day and permitted to return only after one full week without symptoms.[29]

Eric Zemper, a researcher who helped design the NCAA's Injury Surveillance System in the 1980s, also urged a more cautious approach to brain injuries. In a 1994 study of college football players, he reported that athletes with any history of concussion in the previous five years were six times more likely to sustain a concussion than those without such a history. This was an even higher increased risk than Gerberich's team had found among high school students with a history of concussion, likely due to methodological differences between the studies, particularly in how they defined concussions. As a result, Zemper argued that a more conservative approach to concussion management was necessary, and that athletic trainers would likely need to bear the burden of resisting pressure to return athletes to play as quickly as possible. Zemper recalled, "For about 15 years, every paper I published ended with a statement that we really need to seriously rethink this practice of sending players back into the game as soon as they can see straight."[30]

Yet physicians' and trainers' beliefs about what constituted "serious" versus "minor" concussions, let alone how to manage them, remained in flux throughout the 1990s. A pediatric neurologist told the *New York Times* in 1997 that even just a few years earlier, "if a high school athlete had a collision and a minor concussion, he passed out for two or three minutes and was dizzy for just a few days, we'd say, 'No big deal,' and let him return to play ball. We never thought there would be a problem. But now it has come to the forefront that there is a cumulative effect from repetitive concussions, and at the same time a problem within the medical community developing a consensus on managing athletes with these injuries."[31]

These remarks indicate appreciation of the cumulative risks of repeated head injuries, yet the neurologist nonetheless continued to describe as "minor" a concussion where an athlete had lost consciousness and experienced persistent symptoms for several days. Meanwhile, that same year, the AAN issued its first guidelines for the management of concussion in sports, in which loss of consciousness was explicitly associated with the most severe form of concussion (grade three).[32]

The AAN's 1997 practice parameters categorized concussions into three grades with a number of similarities to Cantu's 1986 guidelines. Indeed, Cantu was one of the physicians who reviewed these guidelines. After a grade one concussion, where players experienced transient symptoms such as temporary confusion, athletes could be returned to play within fifteen minutes if their symptoms cleared. After a grade two concussion, where athletes did not lose consciousness but where symptoms did not resolve after fifteen minutes, they needed to be removed from play and could return only after one asymptomatic week. Players with multiple grade two concussions could return to play after two asymptomatic weeks, while players with multiple grade three concussions involving loss of consciousness would need to wait one month or longer, depending on the physician's clinical judgment.[33]

The development of the AAN guidelines was based upon a process of consensus building among experts, including physicians, research faculty, athletic trainers, and paramedics. These specialists recognized, however, that there was very little scientific evidence on which to base the guidelines. As a review of the process acknowledged, "there is still no consensus or data to guide the decision with regard to the question, 'how many concussions are too many?'" The guidelines promulgated by both Cantu and the AAN signified increased awareness that repeated head trauma might cause cumulative harm. But these recommendations were put forward with great uncertainty about how to minimize that harm on the ground.[34]

Moreover, some educators noted that enforcing the guidelines would prove far more difficult than proposing them, particularly without personnel available to ensure adherence. John Laurine, a high school athletic director, told the *New York Times* in 1997 that many high schools still lacked a medical trainer or other trained professional to evaluate students who experienced a possible concussion. Furthermore, many players and their parents prioritized keeping athletes on the field. Parents, according to Laurine, were concerned about their child losing a spot on the team or the potential for a college scholarship or financial aid. High school athletes, meanwhile, wanted to be "tough" and not admit to injury. They were thus reluctant to report concussions and were inclined to minimize them as "just another bang on the head."[35]

NFL and Youth Football

While doctors and athletic trainers increasingly worried about how to protect child athletes from head injuries, their young charges were watching their sports heroes repeatedly bang their heads on TV. By the late twentieth century, NFL games were one of the most popular sources of entertainment in the United States. The league dominated American televisions; since 1990, *Monday Night Football* games ranked among the highest-rated prime-time programs every year. By 2005, the NFL was grossing nearly $5 billion a year, with its teams' average value more than double that of clubs in other major professional sports leagues. In 2006, a sports economist would observe that "football stands like a colossus across the landscape of American sports."[36]

The NFL juggernaut strongly influenced youth football safety debates in several ways. Injuries among NFL players were frequently the most visible and dramatic examples of the dangers of football. Because NFL athletes were role models to youth, their attitude toward their injuries and decisions about when to return to play were held up as worthy of emulation. Indeed, sports media celebrated the concept of athletes playing through pain and injuries. A 1993 analysis of *Sports Illustrated* articles contended that when athletes were pressured or socialized to view injuries as an inevitable or even attractive part of the game, the players themselves could be among the strongest opponents of safety measures. "Athletes may find it difficult to escape the hold of the culture of risk and related structural influences . . . . and even take pride in their pain threshold as proof of their character as athletes, their dedication to the team, and, at least for some males, their masculinity."[37]

The NFL reinforced this culture of risk. The league's responses to injuries—from the ways it described them to the press, to the common practice of cutting away from shots of injured players during televised matches for commercial breaks, to the glorification of violent collisions with promotional videos such as *The NFL's Greatest Hits*—were seen and read by millions of Americans. In 1998, former NFL linebacker Harry Carson wrote a letter to the *New York Times* warning that "the glorification of the Big Hit by television networks and periodicals only fans the flame and encourages younger players to strive to make the hits that will be featured on 'SportsCenter.'"[38]

In addition to the collisions that were celebrated across the American media landscape, the NFL's research on brain injuries influenced understandings of the sport's risks at all levels. In the early 1990s, the NFL found itself under scrutiny after a spate of high-profile head injuries among numerous prominent stars, making concussions "the most highly publicized injury of the 1994 season." A 1994 *Time* magazine story explained: "Even in a sport long admired and abhorred for its body-crunching brutality, concern about the carnage is rising. Players, coaches and fans may never forget some of this season's scariest images: the vacant, confused stare of Dallas Cowboys quarterback Troy Aikman after he collided chin-first with a blitzing Phoenix Cardinal; the sight of Buffalo Bills receiver Don Beebe lying, out cold, on the field, with one forearm pointed stiffly into the air; the awful stillness of New York Giants quarterback Dave Brown after his head was slammed to the turf by a Houston Oilers linebacker."[39]

Perhaps most notably, in October 1994, Merril Hoge retired from the NFL at age twenty-nine after sustaining multiple concussions that left him experiencing a range of symptoms, including headaches, dizziness, numbness, and memory problems. Hoge's departure from the game focused attention not only on the risks to players' careers but also on the threat to their long-term health. *Time* magazine cited experts who warned that concussions could result in serious consequences. "The brain is shaken in the cranium much like Jell-O in a bowl," explained Cantu.[40] Other news stories that season sounded similar warnings. The director of a brain injury rehabilitation program told *Sports Illustrated* that head injuries in football needed to be taken seriously: "It isn't just cataclysmic injury or death from brain injuries that should concern people. The core of the person can change from repeated blows to the head. I get furious every time I watch a game and hear the announcers say, 'Wow, he really got his bell rung on that play.' It's almost like, 'Yuk, yuk, yuk,' as if they're joking. Concussions are no joke."[41]

In response to the flurry of concern and unflattering media attention, in 1994, the commissioner of the NFL appointed a committee to study mild traumatic brain injury (mTBI). As one essayist would later observe on the formation of this committee, "we might pause here a moment to linger upon the spooky propagandistic frisson produced by the juxtaposition of those two words: *mild, traumatic*."[42] Most of the committee was composed of NFL insiders, including team doctors, trainers, a consulting engineer, and an equipment manager. The chairman, New York Jets team doctor El-liot Pellman, was a rheumatologist with no expertise in neurology or brain trauma. In 1994, he told *Sports Illustrated* that "concussions are part of the profession, an occupational risk." Pellman further claimed that veteran play-ers could be cleared to play after a concussion more quickly than rookies. "They can unscramble their brains a little faster, maybe because they're not afraid after being dinged." Former players for the Jets would later recall how Pellman often allowed athletes back onto the field after they had sustained concussions.[43]

As extensively documented by ESPN reporters in a 2013 exposé, *League of Denial*, the NFL's mTBI committee would largely minimize the severity of concussions among professional players. But the committee would also explicitly apply its research to youth football. In 2003, when the committee first began to publish studies in peer-reviewed medical journals, NFL com-missioner Paul Tagliabue expressed confidence that NFL-supported research on concussions would "advance the cause of improving the safety of profes-sional and amateur athletes on all levels."[44]

The NFL proceeded to publish a series of articles in *Neurosurgery* claiming that NFL players did not show evidence of brain damage after multiple con-cussions. These articles even claimed that the NFL's team doctors were per-haps overly conservative in their decisions about when to allow players back on the field. Although the mTBI committee had done no research on high school and college football players, they extrapolated their findings to these age groups. "It might be safe for college/high school football players to be cleared to return to play on the same day as their injury. The authors suggest that, rather than blindly adhering to arbitrary, rigid guidelines, physicians keep an open mind to the possibility that the present analysis of professional football players may have relevance to college and high school players." Sev-eral peer reviewers, including Cantu, were so frustrated by the unsupported claims in these papers, and *Neurosurgery*'s apparent willingness to continue publishing them despite fundamental flaws, that they eventually stopped re-viewing the NFL committee's articles.[45]

While the NFL minimized the risks of concussions in respected scholarly journals, youth athletes continued to shake off symptoms of brain trauma in order to continue competing. As a sixteen-year-old high school student explained, "I've never had a concussion. I probably get my 'bell rung' or get 'dinged' once every game or every other game. I've never told a trainer because it doesn't really cause problems, it's just a short little bang. It's pounded in your head that you can play through anything. I just suck it up most of the time. You just have to suck it up if you want to play."[46]

Even news stories that expressed concern about the potential dangers indicated that child athletes were very rarely removed from play following head trauma. For example, a 1998 article told the story of a high school quarterback, Mac Mansavage, who shrugged off dizziness and a headache after a tackle, and continued to play and receive hits. Mansavage was ultimately rushed to the emergency room once his symptoms became obvious: he began slurring his speech and his teammates observed his eyes roll back in his head. Mansavage was diagnosed with a concussion. His parents insisted that he promise to report any symptoms in the future, but Mansavage admitted to a reporter that he wondered whether, when back on the field with the adrenaline flowing, he would be willing to take himself out of the game. "I probably would. But I'm not sure."[47]

Mansavage's attitude was not unusual for a high school football player at the end of the twentieth century. The description of his team's response to his concussion illustrates the extent to which the burden of addressing concussions was placed upon children themselves. Only when his symptoms became impossible to ignore might a football player be removed from the field. But in many cases, concussion symptoms such as dizziness or headaches were not obvious to parents, referees, and coaches. And given that many youth football programs did not even have trained observers such as doctors or athletic trainers on the sidelines, the chances of adult supervisors detecting the symptoms of a concussion were even smaller.

Furthermore, many adults modeled not treating concussions seriously. Boys strove to emulate their NFL heroes and to display a tough form of masculinity to their coaches and peers. They were unlikely to report symptoms that were considered minor from locker rooms to the pages of *Neurosurgery*. And after their child was rushed to the emergency room for brain trauma, parents might not require them to cease playing. The risks were perceived as small relative to the benefits of participating in youth football.

Yet this pattern—recurrent pockets of media and medical concern about the dangers of youth football that largely remained on the sidelines of a football-loving culture—began to be disrupted in the mid-2000s. Several key factors contributed to making concerns about brain injuries at all levels of football a topic of national debate. These included former athletes speaking out about their symptoms; new medical findings, including the identification of a degenerative brain disease in former football players; a series of more than 100 articles in the *New York Times* on the subject that would be nominated for a Pulitzer Prize; and an emerging framing of brain damage in football as a public health concern that had been covered up by the NFL, akin to the tobacco industry's response to the health risks of smoking.

Football and Chronic Brain Disease

The NFL had by far the largest budget available to spend on studies of football-related brain trauma. In fact, the league became the main sponsor of research on the topic.[48] Yet in the early 2000s, several studies by independent researchers challenged the NFL's narrative that football did not cause long-term harm to athletes' brains. This independent research included epidemiological studies that highlighted the cumulative impact of concussions, as well as neuropathological examinations of brain tissue that identified a disturbing disease associated with repetitive brain trauma.

The lead author of one important study on the cumulative effects of concussions among NCAA football players was motivated to conduct this research in part by the NFL injuries he had seen. Before becoming director of the University of North Carolina's education program for certified athletic trainers, Kevin Guskiewicz had worked for the Pittsburgh Steelers as an assistant trainer. There, he befriended Merril Hoge, who had retired from the NFL in 1994 due to concussion symptoms. After speaking with Hoge by phone several years later, Guskiewicz was disturbed that Hoge did not seem to sound like himself. Convinced that Hoge's symptoms were due to the brain trauma he had sustained playing football, Guskiewicz decided to set up a large-scale study of concussions at the college level.[49]

Guskiewicz assembled a team of experts, including Cantu, to follow nearly 3,000 college football players over the course of three seasons. The athletes were given neuropsychological exams at the beginning of each season to be used as a baseline. Those athletes who sustained concussions were given the exam again after their injury, and monitored until their symptoms resolved. Published in 2003, this study found that players with three or more concussions were three times more likely to sustain a new concussion. Furthermore, athletes who sustained multiple concussions experienced slower recovery times. The authors concluded that even just one previous concussion could have a cumulative effect, and that concussions caused physiological changes that left athletes vulnerable to slower recovery of neurological function following a subsequent concussion.[50]

This study's documentation of the cumulative effects of concussions would be cited by hundreds of additional articles in the medical literature. Yet when it was originally published, the research did not have a dramatic effect on football safety debates among the broader public. Although the study received brief mention in the news with its takeaway message that return-to-play policies should be stricter, at the time this research did not translate into widespread concern about the sport's risks.[51]

Another scientific finding that would influence debates over the safety of youth football—and that would ultimately form the basis of a major feature film in 2015—also did not originally make a substantial splash outside the confines of medical journals. This development was the discovery of a long-term degenerative disease among former NFL players. In 2002, Bennet Omalu, a neuropathologist based in Pittsburgh, identified clear evidence of brain damage on the autopsy of Mike Webster, a former NFL star who played for the Pittsburgh Steelers. Several years later Omalu would discover similar degenerative changes in the brain of another deceased Steelers player, Terry Long. The buildup of proteins and plaques he observed in these players resembled other brain diseases, such as Alzheimer's and dementia pugilistica, in some ways. Yet the pattern of deterioration appeared to be sufficiently different that Omalu believed he had observed a new, though related, disease resulting from repetitive head trauma.[52]

Although not the first to coin the term, Omalu referred to this degenerative disease as "chronic traumatic encephalopathy," or CTE. Omalu later explained how he chose this name for the form of brain damage he had discovered in retired football players: "Chronic means long-term, traumatic is associated with trauma, and encephalopathy refers to brain damage, disease or malfunction.... The name was sufficiently generic that if I were proven wrong and this was not a newly discovered brain disease, it still referred to a bad brain associated with trauma."[53]

Omalu first shared his finding with a mentor, neuropathologist Ronald Hamilton. Hamilton agreed with Omalu's diagnosis and realized that linking such extensive brain damage to head trauma in football was groundbreaking. "I knew this was a billion-dollar kind of finding when I saw it," Hamilton later recalled. They approached several other experts who agreed. In 2005 and 2006, Omalu, Hamilton, and their colleagues published the results of the autopsies on Webster's and Long's brains in the journal *Neurosurgery*. In the

2005 paper, they described their finding as a "sentinel case that draws attention to a possibly more prevalent yet unrecognized disease" because brain autopsies were rarely performed on former NFL players.[54]

These medical case reports received relatively limited national media attention at the time they were published. For example, in 2005 the *New York Times* published a brief note on the death of Terry Long, observing that he had died of brain inflammation according to the coroner with "chronic traumatic encephalopathy" as a contributing factor, but the article contained no mention of the possible broader implications of this finding for other players at any level of football.[55]

But the *Neurosurgery* articles on CTE did attract attention and emphatic condemnation from the NFL and its doctors. Three doctors on the NFL's mTBI committee, including committee chairman Elliot Pellman, demanded that Omalu's 2005 *Neurosurgery* paper be retracted. They wrote a lengthy and scathing letter to the journal, refuting the suggestion that the damage to Mike Webster's brain was related to his experience playing football. Without identifying their connection with the NFL, these doctors insisted that Omalu and his colleagues' claims were "based on a complete misunderstanding of the relevant medical literature." The bulk of their letter was devoted to describing CTE in boxers and suggesting that such damage was not evident in NFL players. Mike Webster had "no known history of brain trauma *inside* professional football," the NFL doctors asserted. They suggested instead that Webster's brain may have been damaged by his alcohol, steroid, or illicit drug use.[56]

The NFL similarly denied that the brain damage evident on Terry Long's autopsy resulted from football. The controversy received some coverage in the local papers in Pittsburgh, where Webster and Long had played. In 2005, the *Pittsburgh Post-Gazette* quoted the Steelers' team neurologist as saying, "Given Mr. Long's history of drug abuse and suicide attempts or whatever altercations may have contributed to his demise, I think it's just bad science to conclude that football caused his death." The debate was framed as a scientific controversy about the deaths of several individual NFL players, not as an indication of a larger health problem in football.[57]

Despite the NFL's efforts to discredit Omalu's work, the discovery of CTE moved from the sidelines to center field several years later. The reporting of *New York Times* journalist Alan Schwarz proved instrumental in communicating Omalu's findings to a broader public and in drawing sustained national attention to concussions in football at all levels. Schwarz later explained to the *Columbia Journalism Review* that he latched onto the story through a mutual friend who had put him in touch with Chris Nowinski. Nowinski was a professional wrestler who had sustained several concussions in his wrestling career as well as during his days playing college football at Harvard. Prompted by his personal experiences, Nowinski was working on a manuscript on concussions and sought the advice of a professional writer. Schwarz, impressed with what he read, introduced Nowinski to several publishers. Most, however, did not consider the topic of sufficient commercial interest.[58]

Then, "completely out of the blue," Nowinski contacted Schwarz again, this time about the 2006 suicide of former NFL player Andre Waters. Nowinski believed Waters's tragic death at the age of forty-four might have something to do with football-related brain damage. He persuaded Waters's family to donate the athlete's brain tissue. Waters's niece, Kwana Pittman, would explain that the family's decision to donate was connected to their concern about the health of other football players, particularly children. "The young kids need to understand; the parents need to be taught."[59]

Omalu agreed to examine Waters's brain, and again, he discovered signs of degeneration. Schwarz realized that the sports section of the *New York Times* would be interested in this story. In January 2007, he began his coverage of football brain injuries for the *Times* with an article announcing that Omalu had linked Waters's suicide to signs of brain damage he suspected were linked to successive concussions. He likened the damage to the characteristics of a brain of an eighty-five-year-old man in the early stages of Alzheimer's disease.[60]

Shortly after the Waters article was published, Schwarz was contacted by a former NFL player who wanted to go public with his own concussion symptoms. The *New York Times* ultimately assigned Schwarz to provide long-term, ongoing coverage of the issue, "with no responsibilities other than to broaden his new beat's focus beyond the N.F.L. to the more than four million amateur athletes who play organized football." Schwarz proceeded to write a series of more than 100 articles on sports concussions and received a Pulitzer Prize nomination for this work.[61]

Schwarz highlighted the public health implications from the first year he began reporting on concussions. For instance, a 2007 article on the reluctance of high school football players to report concussion symptoms emphasized that this was a health concern affecting more than a million teenagers. Schwarz noted that children were particularly vulnerable to the harms of head injury because their brain tissue was still developing. In a 2009 article summarizing a study that found that rates of dementia were significantly higher among retired NFL players than among the general population, Schwarz discussed the possible implications for younger athletes. "Could some players who stop playing football in high school or college face the same latent risks as professionals who lasted six more years in the N.F.L.? It is one equation that doctors of all affiliations have yet to solve."[62]

In October 2009 and January 2010, the U.S. House Judiciary Committee held a series of hearings on football head injuries. These hearings were prompted in large part by the results of a University of Michigan study of more than 1,000 retired NFL players that found the former players were much more likely to be diagnosed with dementia and Alzheimer's disease compared to men in the national population. Yet increasing media and public attention had also contributed to placing the topic on the congressional agenda. Representative Anthony Weiner (D-New York) stated that Schwarz's reporting had driven the issue. "We probably wouldn't even be here today if it were not for some of the stories that he has written."[63]

Although much of the congressional testimony came from players, doctors, and executives associated with the NFL, a recurrent theme throughout the hearings was how the NFL's handling of head injuries inevitably influenced youth football. As Representative Bob Goodlatte (R-Virginia) observed, panelists at these hearings emphasized that sports head injuries were "a problem at a very young age, in junior high school, high school, on up through college, and long before [the players] get to the NFL."[64] Representative Linda Sánchez (D-California) likened the NFL's denial of the link between football and brain damage to the behavior of tobacco companies in obfuscating the connection between smoking and health harms. Researcher Chris Nowinski and former NFL player Bernie Parrish both echoed the tobacco comparison, with Parrish testifying that "this mild traumatic brain injury committee is the sequel to the tobacco council which produced its own bogus studies, paid experts to testify that tobacco products do not cause cancer, and it exactly parallels the way that Covington & Burling partner Paul Tagliabue, who was commissioner of the NFL, set up and created the NFL's Mild Traumatic Brain Injury Committee."[65]

Such analogies between the way the NFL and tobacco companies had manufactured doubt about the health effects of their products were significant in framing debates over football safety. As legal and public health scholar Daniel Goldberg would later observe, the tobacco analogy put forward in the 2009–2010 hearings seemed to markedly influence the NFL's public behavior. Just one month after the first House judiciary hearing, the NFL announced a stricter set of guidelines for managing concussions among its players. These included requiring any player with significant concussion symptoms, such as disorientation or amnesia, to be removed from play for the game. Athletes with symptoms that were considered milder, such as headaches or dizziness, might still be returned to play at the discretion of the examining physician.[66]

As Schwarz would observe, these policy changes amounted to a silent acknowledgement that it was no longer possible for the NFL to "defend a position that conflicted with nearly all scientific understanding of head trauma." Indeed, by the end of 2009, an NFL spokesman for the first time acknowledged the long-term risks when announcing the league's decision to donate money to Boston University's Center for the Study of Traumatic Encephalopathy. "It's quite obvious from the medical research that's been done that concussions can lead to long-term problems."[67]

The NFL's shift in policy signaled the extent to which public awareness of brain trauma in football had increased. This shift was due in large part to the work of an independent researcher motivated by his personal experiences of concussions, the reporting of a career baseball journalist with relatively fewer concerns that challenging the NFL would limit his press access, and the reframing of previously overlooked research as profoundly relevant for youth football. The growing awareness of the NFL's role in downplaying such research is perhaps best encapsulated by a joke headline that the satirical newspaper *The Onion* ran in time for the 2014 Super Bowl: "Super Bowl Confetti Made Entirely from Shredded Concussion Studies."[68]

Yet the NFL's policies also indicated the league's persistent efforts to distinguish between major brain trauma and purportedly minor, insignificant bumps. As one NFL team doctor explained, "On every play there are traumatic experiences to the head. The question is one of degree." If only the biggest and most severe brain trauma was of meaningful concern, then tinkering with rule changes and helmet design might address the problem, and tackle football could persist without significant change.[69]

Framing a Concussion Crisis

By the beginning of the 2010s, public awareness of concussions in football was dramatically increasing, as were demands for reforms to address the issue. Fundamentally altering, let alone eliminating, the sport of football was largely not part of the framework advanced by those seeking policy changes to improve sports safety. Instead, advocates for reform, led by parents in response to their sons' catastrophic football injuries, asked policymakers to intervene to mandate improved coaching and medical supervision.

As sociologist Joseph R. Gusfield observed in his study of drunk driving, determining which individuals or institutions are given responsibility for addressing a problem is central to understanding how an issue is constructed as a public problem. In the case of the emergence of concussions as a public problem in the early twenty-first century, the individual adult supervisors closest to the sport on the ground—namely, parents, coaches, and trainers—were assigned primary responsibility for better identifying and managing concussions. In this context, the introduction of new laws at the state level to address the management of concussions in youth sports proved to be one of the most prominent policy responses.[70]

In 2009, Washington became the first U.S. state to legally mandate return-to-play guidelines. This law was nicknamed the "Lystedt law" in honor of Zackery Lystedt, whose injury had inspired its passage. In 2006, Lystedt sustained a concussion playing middle school football, was returned to play later in the same game, then collapsed and suffered a catastrophic brain injury. After spending a week on life support, Lystedt could not speak for nine months and required a feeding tube for two years. Years of intensive physical therapy enabled him to regain the ability to walk a few steps with a cane, but he would almost certainly require care for the rest of his life. In response to their son's devastating injury, his parents lobbied the state of Washington to pass a law requiring, among other things, that a licensed health care provider examine youth athletes who experienced a concussion and clear them before allowing them to return to play.[71]

After the successful passage of the law in Washington, the Lystedt family joined with the Sarah Jane Brain Foundation and ACSM to form the Zackery Lystedt Brain Project. Formally announced during the 2010 Super Bowl, this project's goal was the passage of similar Lystedt laws across the United States mandating how traumatic brain injuries in youth sports should be managed. "The Lystedt law became a crusade for the family of Lystedt and Dr. Stan Herring," the co-medical director of the Seattle Sports Concussion Program and a Seattle Seahawks team physician who had helped treat Lystedt.[72] With the support of advocates, medical professionals, and sports organizations, by 2014 all fifty U.S. states and Washington, D.C., had passed similar laws with return-to-play guidelines. The laws often required parents and coaches to receive educational information on how to detect and respond to brain injuries.[73]

In 2015, citing Zackery Lystedt's experience, the NFL donated $2.5 million to form the University of Washington Medicine Sports Health and Safety

Institute.[74] Herring became the institute's first director and was granted a Zackery Lystedt Sports Concussion endowed professorship. "Without the NFL, we would not have been successful in getting Lystedt Laws in all 50 states and D.C.," Herring explained.[75]

Lystedt laws primarily addressed how to manage concussions but not how to prevent them. In part, this was because there was very little research supporting methods to actually prevent brain injuries in a collision sport. As Lyle Micheli, an orthopedic surgeon and former ACSM president, observed, "There's so much work being done on how to diagnose and treat concussion, but we still are relatively not very far along as far as how to prevent concussions."[76] Meanwhile, Lystedt laws placed the responsibility for detecting and managing brain injuries with individual coaches, parents, trainers, and health professionals supervising youth sports.[77]

In addition to state-level laws intended to enhance medical supervision, parents and athletic directors sought the most advanced, state-of-the-art protective equipment to continue to allow children to play tackle football. Mike Oliver, the executive director of NOCSAE, told the *New York Times* that sales of football helmets had dramatically changed since 2011. "I see high school athletic directors submitting purchase orders for 500 five-star helmets. Parents are saying, 'I don't want a four-star helmet, I want the best for my kid.'"[78]

Much public attention on concussions focused on efforts to identify a technological solution. News teams investigated schools providing young players football helmets with outdated or poor designs.[79] Parents and players filed a class-action lawsuit against Riddell, charging that the manufacturer had put forward misleading claims that their helmets could reduce the risks of concussions.[80] Magazines highlighted helmet design research that could purportedly "save football."[81] Other companies focused on other head protection technologies, particularly headbands or helmet accessories, such as polyurethane shells to be added to helmets to add extra cushioning.[82] The technological imperative was also evident in the research and development of a "concussion collar" that would lightly constrict athletes' jugular veins. The collar would thus restrict the blood flow back to the heart, purportedly providing "cushioning" to reduce the movement of players' brains to prevent concussions.[83]

Public anxiety about concussions created an environment ripe for dubious claims about other products intended to reduce the risks. In December 2015, the University of Maryland issued a press release claiming that a study had found that high school football athletes who consumed a particular high-protein chocolate milk experienced improved cognitive and motor function, even after sustaining concussions. A critique of this release noted that the study did not appear to be peer reviewed or published, did not adequately quantify the purported benefits of the milk, and did not disclose whether the company producing the chocolate milk under study provided any funding or free product. Nonetheless, the superintendent of Washington County Public Schools in Maryland planned to purchase $25,000 worth of the chocolate milk for his district's student athletes.[84]

Meanwhile, continuing research on CTE was suggesting that even relatively young adults were vulnerable to chronic brain damage sustained in football. In 2010, researchers at Boston University diagnosed CTE in Owen Thomas, a twenty-one-year-old former football player who died by suicide. Thomas, who had started playing football at age nine and participated through several years of college, was the youngest and first amateur player to be diagnosed with a clear case of CTE. A pathologist who independently confirmed the diagnosis told the *New York Times*, "This is a call for a broader range of research into this problem that extends beyond the heavy duty N.F.L. level of athletics."[85]

In fact, emerging research evidence was suggesting that beyond the most severe and obvious cases of brain injuries, repeated "subconcussive" hits—in other words, asymptomatic head trauma that did not meet the diagnostic criteria of a concussion—might cause structural and cumulative damage to players' brains. In 2011, PBS's *Frontline* produced a documentary, *Football High*, examining the shifting debates at the high school level that highlighted research on less visible football injuries. The documentary focused on findings from studies conducted at the Purdue MRI Facility, a magnetic-resonance imaging center that was founded in 2007 at Purdue University.[86]

According to Purdue engineering professor and lead investigator Tom Talavage, the original intent for the project was to evaluate athletes who had experienced concussions. Yet for the first few weeks of their project, none of the fifty players on the high school football team the researchers were following were diagnosed with a concussion. So the researchers instead decided to bring in some players who had not experienced concussions and see if they could detect any changes resulting from the blows they were receiving to their heads.[87]

Eventually some of the athletes under study did experience concussions, so the researchers ultimately conducted computer-based neurocognitive testing and functional magnetic resonance imaging (fMRI) on both concussed and nonconcussed student athletes over the course of the fall 2009 season. These exams included preseason, in-season, and postseason tests. The researchers also installed sensors in the players' helmets to track the number of "collision events," defined as a motion or action where the helmet accelerometer registered a magnitude over 14.4 g (g forces are a standard measure of acceleration; 14.4 g is 14.4 times the force of gravity). Over the course of one season, the research team documented over 15,000 collision events among the 21 players participating in the study, meaning an average of over 700 collisions per player.[88]

Talavage's team was surprised to find that about half the players brought in ostensibly for control purposes—that is, the players who showed no clinical symptoms of concussions—exhibited significantly impaired performance on the in-season computer-based testing and/or fMRI imaging. The researchers found a strong correlation between the number of collision events detected by the helmet sensors and changes to the players' fMRI brain imaging, as well as changes to the players' performance on the computer-based tests. Initially the team thought they must have done something wrong to observe such findings. But when they reevaluated the data, they confirmed that the players whose brains looked different on fMRI were the same players who were showing a difference in neurocognitive testing. The researchers concluded that this group of high school players experiencing neurological changes after one season of subconcussive hits represented "a newly-observed category of neurological injury."[89]

Talavage and his colleagues proceeded to publish a series of studies confirming these preliminary findings. In addition to structural changes observed in the brains of high school football players, research among NFL athletes began to link multiple subconcussive hits to other potential health harms, notably hormonal dysfunction.[90] Other studies in both humans and mouse models in the 2010s also suggested that repetitive subconcussive impacts might play a larger role than individual concussions in the development of long-term brain degeneration such as CTE.[91]

The accumulating evidence that repeated, asymptomatic hits could cause neurological injury suggested a new and disturbing possibility. If subconcussive hits caused chronic brain damage, then focusing on concussions alone would not address the more fundamental problem of repetitive brain trauma inherent to the collisions involved in tackle football. As Talavage frankly observed in advance of a 2014 White House summit on concussions in youth sports, "Just increasing efforts to improve concussion diagnosis or even prevent concussions is a waste of time and taxpayer money. We need to figure out how to reduce the number of hits to these kids' heads."[92]

TABLE 6 Head impact exposure in youth football, 2014

Age Level	Median Impact	95 Percentile Impact	Impacts per Season
7–8 Years	16 g	38 g	161
High School	21 g	56 g	565
College	18 g	63 g	1,000

Adapted from Tyler J. Young, Ray W. Daniel, Steven Rowson, et al., "Head Impact Exposure in Youth Football: Elementary School Ages 7–8 Years and the Effect of Returning Players," *Clinical Journal of Sport Medicine* 24, no. 5 (2014): 416–21.

A team of Virginia Tech researchers studying head impacts in even younger football players was coming to a similar conclusion. Conducting studies where they attached sensors to the helmets of young Pop Warner players, they found that athletes as young as seven and eight years old were sustaining "head impacts similar in magnitude to severe impacts seen at the high school and collegiate level." The high-severity impacts occurred more frequently in practices than in games among the youngest players. Young players experienced fewer impacts per season overall than high school or college players, because they participated in fewer practices and games than their older counterparts. But the potential for high-magnitude impacts at even the youngest levels of the sport was troubling (see table 6). The researchers likened the need to restrict hits to children's heads to the practice of a "pitch count" in youth baseball, which limited the number of pitches a child could throw in order to prevent joint injuries. In 2015, one of the leaders of Virginia Tech's research team told *Time* magazine, "I don't see how a reasonable person would argue that we should count pitches to protect the elbow, but not count hits to protect the brain."[93]

But the idea that subconcussive hits posed a more fundamental, even existential problem for youth collision sports was largely masked by the widespread framing of a concussion crisis. According to this framing, proper diagnosis and management of concussions that caused clinical symptoms would be sufficient to alleviate the risks. Improved tackling techniques, better helmet design, and education campaigns for players and parents all similarly fit within this framework. These strategies encouraged athletes and their adult supervisors to take responsibility for preventing youth football concussions.[94]

The NFL actively participated in framing concerns about youth football head injuries as an issue to be addressed by better medical and coaching supervision. In 2010, the commissioner of the NFL sent a letter to forty-four state governors urging them to adopt Lystedt laws to regulate the management of concussions in youth sports. The NFL framed its own management of concussions as a model for youth leagues to follow: "Given our experience at the professional level, we believe a similar approach is appropriate when dealing with concussions in all youth sports. That is why the NFL and its clubs urge you to support legislation that would better protect your state's young athletes by mandating a more formal and aggressive approach to treatment of concussions."[95]

The NFL also partnered with the U.S. Centers for Disease Control and Prevention (CDC) to create a public-service announcement about concussions in youth sports. Introduced at the end of 2009, this spot aired on national media during the 2010 NFL playoffs and Super Bowl. The thirty-second voiceover emphasized the responsibility of young athletes themselves, as well as their parents and coaches, in reporting and managing concussions: "Concussions and other head injuries must be taken seriously. If you're a player, protect yourself and your teammates. If you think you're hurt, don't hide it. Report it, and take time to recover. If you're a coach or parent, know concussion symptoms and warning signs, and never let athletes return to action before a health professional says it's OK. Help take head injuries out of play."[96]

The league also provided funding to the CDC's *Heads Up* public information campaign on the risks of concussions, including videos, posters, online trainings, and fact sheets. In 2014, CDC researchers published a ten-year review of this campaign. They reported that their online training courses focused on the risks of concussions among young athletes were among their most popular materials, and that these courses had been developed through a grant from the NFL. The review did not evaluate whether the *Heads Up* program in fact reduced the incidence of concussions but instead detailed the amount of material that had been disseminated and assessed the impact of the material on recipients' attitudes. For example, among youth sports coaches who had been exposed to educational *Heads Up* print materials, 77 percent self-reported being better at identifying athletes who may have sustained a concussion, and nearly two-thirds viewed concussions as being a more serious injury.[97]

In addition, the NFL partnered with USA Football, its youth development arm, to promote "heads up" tackling. This was a purportedly safer tackling technique that taught players to keep their heads up and to lead with their shoulders while tackling. Introduced in 2012, the Heads Up football program was funded entirely by the NFL. In a 2013 open letter to NFL fans, NFL commissioner Roger Goodell promoted the program, writing that 2,800 youth leagues—including 90,000 coaches and more than 600,000 youth players—had registered for Heads Up in its first year. Several former NFL players publicly expressed their skepticism; one told ESPN in 2014 that Heads Up was intended to "create the illusion that the game is safe or can be made safe." Nonetheless, the NFL's senior vice president for health and safety insisted that "Heads Up football makes the game safer." In July 2016, a *New York Times* investigation found that the Heads Up program showed no effect in reducing concussions among youth football players.[98]

The NFL treated mothers as a primary source of opposition to the sport, consistent with a decades-long history of sports organizations and media framing "worried moms" as needing to be reassured that football was not dangerous (see chapter 2). Through USA Football, the league started conducting hundreds of "Moms Clinics" in 2013. These clinics were intended to alleviate the fears of worried moms by teaching them the principles of football safety. Commissioner Goodell even attended several of these clinics with his wife, Jane, highlighting the importance the NFL attached to them. "The biggest thing is giving people information they can understand," Goodell explained. A 2015 *New York Times* profile of these clinics quoted an NFL defensive lineman involved in teaching the mothers, "For moms, it's less X's and O's and more safety and directions." In other words, mothers were not expected to understand the most detailed football strategies and techniques. Instead, mothers simply needed to be provided enough information to be persuaded that their sons could safely play football.[99]

Major football organizations thus framed brain injuries as a problem amenable to improved supervision and information provision. Yet many youth football organizers maintained that concussion concerns did not even apply to tackle football at the pre-high school level, because the small size of prepubescent children meant that they could not hit each other as hard as the professionals. In 2010, the safety officer for the Jersey Shore Pop Warner league, a New Jersey league with about 12,000 players on 360 teams, stated, "I can probably count on one hand the number (of concussions) I've seen or that have been reported to us over the last several years." In 2014, the safety page of the Pop Warner youth football league website explained that in Pop Warner football, there was "an absence of catastrophic head and neck injuries and disruptive joint injuries found at higher levels."[100]

Supporters of youth football emphasized these claims in arguments to parents and the general public. In a 2015 op-ed in the *Star Tribune*, the largest newspaper in Minneapolis, an educator and former football player wrote that "Young kids simply do not have the combination of size and speed necessary to cause serious brain injury." He cited research from an NFL-funded study published in the *Journal of Pediatrics* stating that "youth football is a generally safe activity with regard to concussions for children aged 8–12 years."[101] The belief that football was relatively safer than driving (see chapter 5) persisted to a remarkable extent in these arguments. "I guess since football (was) so ingrained in me growing up, I think football is still safer than your teenage boy driving a car," explained one high school football coach in 2015.[102]

Other writers and even physicians also pushed back against brain injury concerns as overblown or even a form of hysteria. In 2013, Daniel J. Flynn, a conservative author and *American Spectator* columnist, penned a book characterizing football concussion concerns as a "cultural tic masquerading as a public health crusade." Flynn argued that limiting children's participation would effectively amount to a de facto ban on the sport, because the overwhelming majority of tackle football players were children. "To say you don't want kids to play football is to say you don't want football played."[103]

In 2015, Steven Rothman, a pediatric neurologist, wrote an op-ed in the *New York Times* entitled "Parents, Stop Obsessing over Youth Concussions." Rothman cited a 2014 ESPN sports poll finding that nearly 90 percent of parents were worried about the risk of injury in youth sports, with concussions representing the injury of greatest concern. Rothman argued that this was troubling given the importance of physical activity and the high rates of obesity in the United States. Data about brain damage among adults in professional football could not be applied to children, and furthermore, Rothman argued, the "crisis" could be attributed in part to the loosening of the definition of a concussion in recent decades. He cited a 1977 medical text as requiring temporary loss of consciousness as part of the definition of a concussion, whereas by the 2010s, medical definitions of mild head trauma could include a range of symptoms without loss of consciousness. Ultimately, Rothman concluded that "too many teenagers who face little chance of long-term brain injury are being kept from playing in healthy organized sports out of an excessive sense of caution."[104]

Adding to the debate, in 2015 Sony Pictures released a major film on Christmas Day, *Concussion*, which starred Will Smith as Bennet Omalu. The film told the story of Omalu's research on CTE and depicted the NFL's efforts to discredit his work. The movie also included a scene where an NFL doctor warned Omalu, "If 10 percent of mothers in this country begin to see football as a dangerous sport, that is the end of football." The movie deeply affected many former NFL players who watched it. Domonique Foxworth, an NFL veteran and former president of the NFL Players' Association, stated, "I can no longer confidently say that I would trade my quality of life for the opportunity to improve the trajectory of my family's future."[105] Pierre Woods, who played in the NFL principally with the New England Patriots, told the *Detroit Free Press* that if he had seen this movie in his freshman year of high school, "I would have never played football."[106]

The film also appeared to have an impact on younger players and their parents. For example, one eighteen-year-old high school football star in Pennsylvania had received several "full ride" football scholarships to Division I schools. He decided to turn them all down after watching *Concussion*, stating that seeing the deterioration of beloved Steelers player Mike Webster on the big screen hit him especially hard. He explained, "Yeah, it would be free college. But your whole life is in jeopardy. You're putting your body in harm's way every single week. It was definitely a tough choice, but I think I made the right choice." Similarly, in 2016, a seventeen-year-old high school junior explained his decision to quit playing despite coming from a "football family" that loved the game: "Football was such a big part of my life. But if I can find the satisfaction I got from football without taking the same risks, I'm going to do that instead."[107]

The release of the movie *Concussion* contributed to—and signaled— growing awareness of brain trauma as a major health concern in American sports. Recalling antidrug campaigns of the 1980s, the *New York Daily News* ran a cover photo of a damaged brain with the headline "This is your brain on football."[108] With football brain trauma rendered far more visible in the public eye, these debates had reached a new crossroads. The idea that the sport posed a risk to the brains of young athletes presented a seemingly new and potentially existential crisis for the sport.

Yet youth football's "concussion crisis" of the early twenty-first century was also informed by more than 100 years of debate over the harms and benefits of youth tackle football. Over the decades, there had been doctors, educators, lawyers, parents, athletes, and other observers who questioned whether tackle football was appropriate for young boys. Periodically, fatalities and catastrophic injuries received news coverage or were the subject of lawsuits that focused attention on the risks. Repeatedly, however, the sport's health risks were ultimately deemed worthwhile in comparison to the perceived physical and social benefits. It remains to be seen whether the latest round of debate will result in fundamental changes to the risks considered acceptable for adults to impose on boys in the context of youth sports. Meanwhile, young athletes continue to collide with one another on football fields across the United States.

Epilogue
No Game for Boys to Play

Football is supposed to build a sense of community, and true communities look out for everyone's kids—not out of self-interest, but because it's the right thing to do.

— Michael Baumann, 2015

Tyler Cornell played Pop Warner and high school football, mostly as an offensive lineman, every year from age eight until age seventeen. Among the sports trophies he accumulated, he kept a football with the autograph of a beloved NFL star, the San Diego Chargers' number 55, Junior Seau. Football was the love of Tyler's life. His childhood years of successful involvement in the sport seemed to have set him up for a bright future.[1]

But after graduating from high school, Tyler began suffering from severe anxiety and depression. After seven years of mental health problems and several hospitalizations, Tyler died by suicide in 2014 at age twenty-five. Although he had never been diagnosed with a concussion while playing football, his mother, Jo Cornell, had seen recent reports in the news about chronic traumatic encephalopathy (CTE). Cornell wondered after Tyler's death if the thousands of hits Tyler had taken over years of playing youth football might have contributed to the symptoms her son had experienced in young adulthood. She had his brain sent to Boston University. Several months later, the results of the autopsy confirmed her suspicions: Tyler had CTE. It was the same disease that National Institutes of Health researchers had found in the brain of Junior Seau, Tyler's football hero, after the former NFL star had killed himself in 2012.[2]

In 2016, Jo Cornell and Kimberly Archie, another mother whose son had been posthumously diagnosed with CTE, sued Pop Warner Little Scholars, Inc. U.S. district court judge Philip Gutierrez ruled that their claims could be brought to trial. Gutierrez concluded that there was sufficient evidence to support an association between brain trauma and playing youth football, and that "acts or omissions" by the Pop Warner league could potentially be linked to those injuries. The case will be the first against Pop Warner's handling of brain trauma to go to trial. Archie told the *San Diego Tribune*, "Every parent in America needs to know that they're playing Russian roulette with their kid's brain. If they're letting their kid play Pop Warner, they are knowingly taking the risk."[3]

The lawsuit, scheduled for trial in January 2020, comes amid ongoing media coverage and continuing research on brain injuries among athletes.[4] Indeed, as of 2019, concerns over the safety of youth tackle football have become focused almost exclusively on brain injuries, with relatively little discussion of bone and joint injuries, heat stroke, chronic pain, or other risks.[5] Moreover, contemporary debates over brain injuries in youth football are at a crossroads. Competing framings of the risks of traumatic brain injuries present significantly different potential responses to addressing the sport's risks.

The prevailing "concussion crisis," a framework shaped in many ways by the NFL and other sports organizations, suggests that improved adult supervision, return-to-play guidelines, better helmet design, and other similar strategies can sufficiently address the risks of youth football. An alternative interpretation of the scientific evidence indicates that the full-body collisions associated with tackling carry inherent risks of brain trauma that cannot be substantially reduced.[6]

The tension between these two framings is evident in both medical and public debates. Through Lystedt laws and programs such as "Heads Up" Football, a range of groups—state governments, youth football organizations, coaches, the CDC, professional health organizations such as the ACSM, and many parents—have all sought to reduce the risks of concussion through education, technology, and supervision. Advocates of the perspective that these strategies can make football safer frequently argue that the sport holds particular appeal for boys who, they contend, might not engage in physical activity otherwise. "Amid a crisis of youth obesity, we shouldn't take away from young men a sport that is so compelling."[7]

On the other hand, advocates who have deemed tackle football too inherently risky for children have promoted flag football as an alternative for concerned parents. A handful of schools and communities have taken this approach. For example, in December 2015, the recreation department of the city of Somerville, Massachusetts, decided to end city-sponsored tackle football for children.[8] In 2016, writer Gregg Easterbrook argued in the *New York Times* that changing science had made the risks of tackling for children unacceptable. "A generation ago, it wasn't known that sub-concussive hits to little children could have lifetime neurological consequences. Now that this is known, youth tackle football must stop."[9] In 2018, five state legislatures—California, Illinois, Maryland, New Jersey, and New York—introduced bills to ban children under age twelve or fourteen from playing tackle football.[10]

Examining the response of sports administrators and physicians to the risks of brain trauma in other contact sports in the early twenty-first century is telling. In both 2000 and 2014, the AAP's Council on Sports Medicine and Fitness recommended against body checking in ice hockey before age fifteen to cut down on concussions and other injuries. In 2015, the U.S. Soccer Federation responded to a class-action lawsuit charging the organization with negligence in managing head injuries by implementing new safety policies. The new guidelines, intended to cut down on head trauma, prohibited players age ten and younger from heading the ball and reduced the numbers of headers allowed in practice for athletes aged eleven to thirteen.[11]

But in 2015, the AAP's Council on Sports Medicine and Fitness did not recommend against tackling in youth football at any age. Although the AAP's literature review acknowledged that tackling was significantly associated with increased risk of concussions, severe injuries, catastrophic injuries, and overall injuries, the committee instead recommended enhancing supervision of the sport. The AAP committee shied away from endorsing the elimination of tackling in youth football, because doing so would fundamentally change the way the game is played. The committee instead stated that it was up to the participants themselves to determine whether the risks of the sport outweighed the benefits. Advocates for youth tackle football quickly seized upon the AAP's statement as an endorsement of the sport. In February 2016, the director of a youth tackle football program emphasized that the AAP "sets no limits as to when our children should begin playing football and realizing its rewards."[12]

Why would the preeminent professional group of American pediatricians, whose stated mission is to optimize the health and well-being of children, recommend against body-checking in youth hockey to prevent concussions but not against tackling in youth football? Understanding the history of debates over the safety of youth football and the status of football in American society is essential to answering this question.

Tackle football has nagged at American consciences for over a century. The vast amount of protective gear introduced to the sport could be considered one particularly visible indication of efforts to assuage those consciences. But ultimately, the immense popularity of the sport for children has been deeply tied to the very violence that renders the game dangerous. The collision sport was believed to have not only physical health benefits but also profound social and moral advantages in teaching boys key values of competition, toughness, leadership, discipline, teamwork, and even patriotism. The sport also fostered a form of masculinity in which physical risks were to be embraced and overcome. As football became the country's most popular enter-tainment sport, and even more deeply associated with both high school and college educational systems, football increasingly became perceived as a path to accessing higher education as well as social and economic success.

For over a century, football has been profoundly tied to what it means to be an American man and how to raise boys to meet those ideals. Conse-quently, advocates of youth football have characterized threats to the sport as existential threats to the country. In 2018, the president of the Pro Foot-ball Hall of Fame told the annual conference of USA Football that if the country lost football, "I don't know if America can survive." In this view, while football's risks could be better managed, neither football nor its risks should be eliminated. Not only the sport but also the United States is at stake.[13]

Football, of course, is far from the only risky activity in the United States where concerns about health have been overwhelmed by the strength of more powerful beliefs and framings of risk. As historian Pamela Pennock ob-served in the case of tobacco, for decades "the abstract ideology of 'public health' could not muster enough rhetorical power to serve as a rallying cry in Americans' struggle to control a profitable industry that made and sold a sub-stance that many consumers desired."[14] In their examination of lead poison-ing in the United States, Gerald Markowitz and David Rosner quoted a lead researcher as saying, "We are allowing industry to profit by using our children as uninformed research subjects of a vast experiment." A similar observation about exposing children to the uncertain harms of repetitive head trauma in tackle football can and has been made. In a 1973 textbook on football injuries, neuroscientist Richard Schneider observed, "The football fields of our nation have been a vast proving ground or laboratory for the study of the tragic neu-rologic sequelae of head and neck trauma in man."[15]

But the risks of repeated brain trauma in a competitive collision sport seemingly remained hidden for so long not only because of the corporate in-fluence of the NFL (immense as that influence was) but also because of pro-found meanings attached to football. Many American parents deeply believed that participation in tackle football enhanced their sons' lives, taught them prized and essential values, and made them into men. These beliefs were shaped by industry but also by powerful cultural and political ideologies as-sociated with competition, masculinity, and patriotism. Many athletes de-rived great meaning and pleasure from the sport, including its risks. As one commentator acknowledged in a "reluctant manifesto" against football: "You know you might get hurt playing. That's part of *why* you play, to see what you're made of, how you take a hit, to see what happens when your courage meets real hazard."[16]

In addition to these cultural values, the subtlety of symptoms associated with concussions contributed to rendering the harms of repetitive brain trauma relatively invisible. Headaches, dizziness, or nausea remain far less obvious than broken bones. Repetitive head trauma, particularly subconcussive hits with no immediate symptoms, represents a form of low-level exposure that may or may not result in symptoms or chronic disease years into the future. Again, the comparison to lead poisoning is apt. It's another instance of low-level harm that is relatively difficult for epidemiologic research to evaluate, but that in the twenty-first century cumulatively and disproportionately harms the most vulnerable children in American society. As with lead, these costs may include "silently stolen futures, lower IQs, lost productivity, narrowed life chances and well-being . . . emotional distress, and physical damage."[17]

But unlike lead poisoning, the physical experience of tackle football could include real and meaningful advantages. Athletes in many dangerous sports, including tackle football, have struggled with how to weigh the benefits they personally experience from the sport with the potential risks: "If 'doing what I loved' cost me the use of my legs and my arms, or the full use of my brain, would I say it was worth it? Could I measure the sport's rewards and stack them against the risks, and if I did, what would that balance sheet look like? What had the sport given me, and how much was I willing to pay in return?"[18]

The ethical questions about how to respond to this uncertainty are very different with child athletes as compared to adults. Children are not fully autonomous and should not be treated as having the full capacity to assess the long-term risks of repetitive brain trauma. Weighing the hazards and benefits of youth football is an adult responsibility. Tracing the history of debates over youth football safety involves examining how a wide range of adults—parents, coaches, sporting goods manufacturers, football leagues, journalists, educators, physicians, engineers, lawyers, and others—have struggled with and in many cases abdicated this responsibility. The way these debates are framed can either highlight or obscure a fundamental public health question: Are the risks of tackle football acceptable for adults to impose on children?

For over one hundred years, our society's answer for millions of boys across the United States has been yes. Throughout the late nineteenth century, twentieth century, and into the twenty-first, football withstood repeated criticisms from those doctors and educators who dubbed the sport "no game for boys to play." Instead, football became the most popular high school sport for boys and was taken up by leagues of elementary and middle school aged students. A 1964 examination of youth football, noting that the sport had undergone numerous changes over the decades, observed that "remaining unchanged is the love of contact, the desire to win, the willingness to pay the price that football has and always will demand of its practitioners. The next seventy years won't change this either."[19]

Over fifty years later, a new round of football safety debates is under way. The cumulative effects of repeated collisions on developing bodies and brains are under perhaps the harshest spotlight yet. But Americans' love affair with the sport continues. Whether parents will continue to willingly pay the price that football demands of their sons remains an open question. The answer will depend not only on the latest CTE research and brain imaging but also on how communities weigh their beliefs about boyhood and toughness with the health risks.

In the meantime, millions of boys continue to collide with one another on the gridiron. With every hit, brain cells may jiggle imperceptibly, bruises may form, and cartilage may wear down. Occasionally, bones may break or ligaments tear. But every hit also reveals social and cultural values. Each collision says something about what Americans expect of their sons, and the men they hope they will become.

Notes

Abbreviations Used in the Notes

AJPH	American Journal of Public Health
CDT	Chicago Daily Tribune
JAAHPER	Journal of the American Association for Health, Physical Education and Recreation
IJHS	International Journal of the History of Sport
JAMA	Journal of the American Medical Association
JSH	Journal of Sport History
KPHS	King of Prussia Historical Society
LAT	Los Angeles Times
NYSPHSAA	New York State Public High School Athletic Association
NYT	New York Times
SI	Sports Illustrated
WP	Washington Post

Introduction

1. "Football Reform by Abolition," *The Nation* 81 (November 30, 1905): 437–38.

2. "The Football Mortality," *JAMA* 39, no. 23 (1902): 1464–65.

3. "Annual Football Mortality," *Independent* 54 (December 11, 1902): 2977–78.

4. Guy M. Lewis, "Theodore Roosevelt's Role in the 1905 Football Controversy," *Research Quarterly* 40, no. 4 (1969): 717–24.

5. John Hammond Moore, "Football's Ugly Decades, 1893–1913," *Smithsonian Journal of History* 2 (Fall 1967): 49–68.

6. Joseph H. Burnett, "Survey of Football Injuries in the High Schools of Massachusetts," *Journal of Health and Physical Education* 2, no. 8 (October 1931): 32–33, 50.

7. Jim Murray, "Head Coach or Surgeon?" *LAT*, October 19, 1961.

8. Franklin Foer and Chris Hughes, "Barack Obama Is Not Pleased: The President on His Enemies, the Media, and the Future of Football," *New Republic*, January 27, 2013, accessed March 19, 2019, http://www.newrepublic.com/article/112190/obama-interview-2013-sit-down-president.

9. Andy Clayton, "Trump Also Slams NFL for 'Ruining the Game' with New Rules to Protect Players," *New York Daily News*, September 23, 2017, accessed March 19, 2019, http://www.nydailynews.com/sports/football/trump-slams-nfl-ruining-game-new-safety-rules-article-1.3515837.

10. Steve Fainaru and Mark Fainaru-Wada, "Why Former 49ers Chris Borland is the Most Dangerous Man in Football," *ESPN*, August 20, 2015, accessed March 19, 2019, http://www.espn.com/nfl/story/_/id/13463272/how-former-san-francisco-49ers-chris

-borland-retirement-change-nfl-forever; Chris Borland, Bill Simmons, and Kevin Clark. "The Future of Football with Chris Borland," *The Ringer NFL Show*, December 28, 2017, accessed March 19, 2019, https://www.theringer.com/2017/12/28/16803842/future-of -football-with-chris-borland.

11. Steve Almond, *Against Football: One Fan's Reluctant Manifesto* (Brooklyn, NY: Melvin House, 2014), 7–8. "Local Matters: Foot Ball," *Boston Daily Advertiser*, November 9, 1863.

12. Josh Pruce, national director of scholastics and media relations for Pop Warner, in discussion with the author, August 4, 2014.

13. Emily A. Harrison, "The First Concussion Crisis: Head Injury and Evidence in Early American Football," *AJPH* 104, no. 5 (2014): 822–33.

Chapter One

1. "From Gridiron to the Grave," *Atlanta Constitution*, October 31, 1897.

2. Christopher C. Meyers, "'Unrelenting War on Football': The Death of Richard Von Gammon and the Attempt to Ban Football in Georgia," *Georgia Historical Quarterly* 93, no. 4 (2009): 388–407.

3. Meyers, "Unrelenting War on Football"; "A Fatal Game in Atlanta," *NYT*, October 31, 1897.

4. "Football Caused His Death," *WP*, October 27, 1897.

5. "Football Kills in Stoneham," *NYT*, November 17, 1897; "A Grammar School Takes on the Appearance of a Hospital," *CDT*, November 22, 1897.

6. "No Football in Georgia: Bill Prohibiting the Game Passed by the Lower House," *NYT*, November 9, 1897; Meyers, "Unrelenting War on Football." See also Charles Martin, *Benching Jim Crow: The Rise and Fall of the Color Line in Southern College Sports, 1890–1980* (Urbana: University of Illinois Press, 2010).

7. George W. Miles, "Good Old English Game," *Baltimore Sun*, November 26, 1897.

8. "Football," *NYT*, November 10, 1897.

9. "Gov. Atkinson's Reasons for Football Bill Veto," *Atlanta Constitution*, December 8, 1897.

10. Gail Bederman, *Manliness & Civilization: A Cultural History of Gender and Race in the United States, 1880–1917* (Chicago: University of Chicago, 1995).

11. Winthrop Saltonstall Scudder, *An Historical Sketch of the Oneida Football Club of Boston, 1862–1865* (Massachusetts Historical Society, 1926).

12. Allison Danzig, *The History of American Football: Its Great Teams, Players and Coaches* (Englewood Cliffs, NJ: Prentice-Hall, 1956); Amos Alonzo Stagg and Wesley Winans Stout, *Touchdown!* (New York: Longsman, Green and Co., 1927); Emily A. Harrison, "The First Concussion Crisis: Head Injury and Evidence in Early American Football," *AJPH* 104, no. 5 (2014): 822–33. See also Douglas A. Noverr and Lawrence E Ziewacz, *The Games They Played: Sports in American History, 1865–1980* (Chicago: Nelson-Hall, 1983) for illustrations of the development of early American football.

13. Allison Danzig, *The History of American Football: Its Great Teams, Players and Coaches* (Englewood Cliffs, NJ: Prentice-Hall, 1956). See also Julie Des Jardins, *Walter Camp: Football and the Modern Man* (New York: Oxford University Press, 2015).

14. Danzig, *The History of American Football*, 88; "Football Armor: Changes in the Devices for Players this Year," *CDT*, October 3, 1897.

15. Lamont Buchanan, *The Story of Football in Text and Pictures* (New York: Stephen-Paul, 1947), 63.

16. "Football Armor."

17. Caspar Whitney, "The Athletic Development at West Point and Annapolis," *Harper's Weekly*, May 21, 1892.

18. "The Delights of Fencing as Described by Diana," *Philadelphia Inquirer*, October 23, 1898.

19. Edward H. Nichols and Homer B. Smith, "The Physical Aspect of American Football," *Boston Medical and Surgical Journal* 154, no. 1 (1906): 1–8. See also Harrison, "The First Concussion Crisis."

20. Steven W. Pope, "God, Games, and National Glory: Thanksgiving and the Ritual of Sport in American Culture, 1876–1926," *IJHS* 10, no. 2 (1993): 242–49.

21. Michael Oriard, *The Art of Football* (Lincoln: University of Nebraska Press, 2017), 8.

22. Pope, "God, Games, and National Glory."

23. "Gone Football Crazy," *WP*, October 28, 1894.

24. W. Cameron Forbes, "The Football Coach's Relation to the Players," *Outing, An Illustrated Monthly Magazine of Recreation*, December 1900, 336. On the importance of the Ivy League schools to the development of football, see Mark F. Bernstein, *Football: The Ivy League Origins of an American Obsession* (Philadelphia: University of Pennsylvania Press, 2001).

25. Mark Dyreson, "Globalizing the Nation-Making Process: Modern Sport in World History," *IJHS* 20, no. 1 (2003): 91–106.

26. Michael A. Robidoux, "Imagining a Canadian Identity Through Sport: A Historical Interpretation of Lacrosse and Hockey," *Journal of American Folklore* 115, no. 456 (2002): 209–25; Tony Collins, *The Oval World: A Global History of Rugby* (London: Bloomsbury, 2015); Inoue Shun, "The Invention of the Martial Arts," in *Mirror of Modernity: Invented Traditions of Modern Japan*, ed. Stephen Vlastos (Berkeley: University of California Press, 1998): 163–73.

27. Donald J. Mrozek, *Sport and American Mentality, 1880–1910* (Knoxville: University of Tennessee Press, 1983), 28; Varda Burstyn, *The Rites of Men: Manhood, Politics, and the Culture of Sport* (Toronto: University of Toronto Press, 1999). On U.S. nationalism and foreign policy at the turn of the twentieth century, see Paul T. McCartney, *Power and Progress: American National Identity, the War of 1898, and the Rise of American Imperialism* (Baton Rouge: Louisiana State University Press, 2006).

28. Jack W. Berryman, "Early Black Leadership in Collegiate Football: Massachusetts as a Pioneer," *Historical Journal of Massachusetts* 9 (June 1981): 17–28; Richard A. Swanson and Betty Spears, *History of Sport and Physical Education in the United States* (Dubuque, IA: WCB Brown & Benchmark, 1978), 181.

29. Sally Jenkins, *The Real All-Americans: The Team that Changed a Game, a People, a Nation* (New York: Doubleday, 2007), 122; "News," *The Indian's Friend* 10, no. 9 (June 1906): 9. See also Lori Jacobson, "'Shall We Have a Periodical?': *The Indian's Friend*," in *The Women's National Indian Association: A History* (Albuquerque: University of New Mexico Press, 2015): 46–61.

30. Arjun Appadruai, "Playing with Modernity: The Decolonization of Indian Cricket," in *Consuming Modernity: Public Culture in a South Asian World*, ed. C. A. Breckenridge (Minneapolis: University of Minnesota Press, 1995): 23–48.

31. "Lo, The Poor Indian: C.A.C. Defeats Carlisle Indian School 18 to 0," *WP*, November 25, 1894; Matthew Bentley, "Playing White Men: American Football and Manhood at the Carlisle Indian School, 1893–1904," *Journal of the History of Childhood and Youth* 3, no. 2 (Spring 2010): 187–209.

32. Mark Rubinfeld, "The Mythical Jim Thorpe: Re/presenting the Twentieth Century American Indian," *IJHS* 23, no. 2 (2006): 167–89.

33. Jim Nasium, "This Indian the Athletic Marvel of the Age," *Philadelphia Inquirer*; December 3, 1911, 12; Kate Buford, *Native American Son: The Life and Sporting Legend of Jim Thorpe* (New York: Knopf, 2010); Jennifer Guiliano, *Indian Spectacle: College Mascots and the Anxiety of Modern America* (New Brunswick: Rutgers University Press, 2015); Philip J. Deloria, *Indians In Unexpected Places* (Lawrence: University Press of Kansas, 2004), 122.

34. Jenkins, *The Real All-Americans*, 150.

35. Michael Oriard, *King Football: Sport and Spectacle in the Golden Age of Radio and Newsreels, Movies and Magazines, the Weekly and the Daily Press* (Chapel Hill: University of North Carolina Press, 2001), 226.

36. Reet A. Howell and Maxwell L. Howell, "The Myth of 'Pop Warner': Carlisle Revisited," *Quest* 30, no. 1 (1978): 19–27.

37. Carlos Montezuma, "Football as an Indian Educator," *The Red Man* (January 1900), 8.

38. "Two Curable Evils," *NYT*, November 23, 1897.

39. "The Brutal Game of Football," *CDT*, December 11, 1892.

40. "Football Apologies: The Game Is a Dangerous and Demoralizing One," *CDT*, November 30, 1894.

41. George E. Merrill, "Is Football Good Sport?" *North American Review* 177, no. 564 (November 1903): 758–65; Ira Hollis, "Intercollegiate Athletics," *Atlantic Monthly* 90 (1902): 534.

42. "Perils of the Football Field," *San Francisco Chronicle*, November 27, 1902. For further discussion of press coverage of football injuries, see Roberta J. Park, "Mended or Ended? Football Injuries and the British and American Medical Press, 1870–1910," *IJHS* 18, no. 2 (2001):110–33.

43. Nichols and Smith, "The Physical Aspect of American Football," 8.

44. Theodore Roosevelt, *The Strenuous Life: Essays and Address* (New York: The Century Co., 1900): 164.

45. See particularly the more than 100 books on prep school and sports life authored by Ralph Henry Barbour. "To Barbour, life is little more than a cosmic football game," Fred Erisman, "The Strenuous Life in Practice: The School and Sports Stories of Ralph Henry Barbour," *Rocky Mountain Social Science Journal* 7, no. 1 (April 1970): 29–37.

46. Ronald A. Smith, "Harvard and Columbia and a Reconsideration of the 1905–1906 Football Crisis," *JSH* 8, no. 3 (1981): 5–19.

47. John Corbin, "The Puritan and the Football Player," *The Independent*, December 16, 1897.

48. Stephen Hardy, *How Boston Played: Sport, Recreation, and Community 1865–1915* (Boston: Northeastern University Press, 1982); "Schoolboys Have Crack Teams: Never So Much Interest as Now Shown in Interscholastic Football," *NYT*, October 31, 1893.

49. Robert Pruter, "Chicago High School Football Struggles, the Fight for Faculty Control, and the War Against Secret Societies, 1898–1908," *JSH* 30, no. 1 (2003): 47–72;

"Brooklyn Team Beaten: Poly Prep Football Eleven Made Lamentable Showing," *NYT*, December 7, 1902; "Brooklyn vs. Hyde Park: East to Meet West for High School Football Honors," *CDT*, December 1, 1902.

50. "Football Old Game: Gridiron Sport Was Introduced Thirty Years Ago," *WP*, October 8, 1905.

51. "Fatality Dooms Football Games," *CDT*, November 5, 1905.

52. "Football Is Prohibited in New York's Public Schools," *Baltimore Sun*, December 10, 1909; "Ban on Football: Board of Education Nearly Unanimous," *New York Tribune*, December 9, 1909.

53. "Football—Why Not Make it Safe?" *Christian Science Monitor*, December 10, 1909.

54. "Lift Ban from Football: Board of Education Decides to Permit the Game Under New Rules," *NYT*, September 15, 1910. See John M. Carroll, *Red Grange and the Rise of Modern Football* (Urbana: University of Illinois Press, 1999), 30–31.

55. Jeffrey Mirel, "From Student Control to Institutional Control of High School Athletics: Three Michigan Cities, 1883–1905," *Journal of Social History* 16, no. 2 (1982): 83–100; Pruter, "Chicago High School Football Struggles."

56. Mirel, "From Student Control to Institutional Control."

57. Jane E. Good, *High School Heroes: A Century of Education & Football at Annapolis High School, 1896–2003* (Bowie, MD: Heritage Books, 2004), 43.

58. Lewis Hoch Wagenhorst, *The Administration and Cost of High School Interscholastic Athletics* (New York: Columbia University, 1926).

59. Holt-Delhi Historical Society, "History of Holt Varsity Football," March 19, 2019, http://holtdelhihistoricalsociety.webs.com/history.

60. See, for example, Deobold B. Van Dalen, Elmer D. Mitchell, and Burcle L. Bennett, *A World History of Physical Education* (Englewood Cliffs, NJ: Prentice-Hall, 1953).

61. Guy Lewis, "Adoption of the Sports Program, 1905–39: The Role of Accommodation in the Transformation of Physical Education," *Quest* 12, no. 1 (1969): 34–46.

62. S. W. Pope, *Patriotic Games: Sporting Traditions in the American Imagination, 1876–1926* (New York: Oxford University Press, 1997), 128; Brad Austin, *Democratic Sports: Men's and Women's College Athletics During the Depression* (Fayetteville: University of Arkansas, 2015), 89. See also Catherine D. Ennis, "Curriculum: Forming and Reshaping the Vision of Physical Education in a High Need, Low Demand World of Schools," *Quest* 58, no. 1 (2006): 41–59.

63. See, for example, Bruce Haley, *The Healthy Body and Victorian Culture* (Cambridge, MA: Harvard University Press, 1978).

64. A. E. Colton, "What Football Does," *Independent* 57 (September 15, 1904), 605–07. For a discussion of Colton's letter and how its litany of football-produced virtues "blurred the line between the sacred and the secular," see Mark Dyreson, "Regulating the Body and the Body Politic: American Sport, Bourgeois Culture, and the Language of Progress, 1880–1920," in *The New American Sport History: Recent Approaches and Perspectives*, ed. S. W. Pope (Urbana: University of Illinois Press, 1997), 121–44.

65. Guy Lewis, "World War I and the Emergence of Sport for the Masses," *Maryland Historian* 4, no. 2 (Fall 1973): 109–22. See also Timothy P. O'Hanlon, "School Sports as Social Training: The Case of Athletics and the Crisis of World War I," *JSH* 9, no. 1 (Spring 1982): 5–29.

66. "Wilson's Ire Roused: Rebukes Defense League's Attack on the National Guard," *WP*, January 26, 1917.

67. "Leading Educators Press for Physical Training in Public Schools," *American Physical Education Review* 22, no. 2 (1917): 113. For a discussion of the history of sports and fitness in the American military during and after World War I, see Wanda Ellen Wakefield, *Playing to Win: Sports and the American Military, 1989–1945* (Albany: State University of New York Press, 1997).

68. William J. Meadors, *The History of the National Federation of State High School Athletic Associations*, D.P.E. thesis, Springfield College, 1970, 83.

69. "Leading Educators Press for Physical Training"; H. P. Silver, "Sports for Character Building," *American Physical Education Review* 32, no. 5 (1927): 345–48.

70. Daniel Chase, "The Early Days of the NYSPHSAA, 1921–1926," *New York State Journal of Health, Physical Education and Recreation* 13, no. 2 (1960): 29–34.

71. "The Sportsmanship Brotherhood," *NYT*, November 4, 1925.

72. John M. Booth, "An Investigation in Interscholastic Athletics in Northwestern High Schools," *School Review* 36, no. 9 (1928): 696–706.

73. Mark Dyreson, *Making the American Team: Sport, Culture, and the Olympic Experience* (Urbana: University of Illinois Press, 1998), especially "The Moral Equivalent of War," 194–96.

74. "Athletics as an Inspiration for Sculpture," *Pennsylvania Gazette* 20, no. 15 (February 3, 1922): 344–45; "Moral Equivalents," *NYT*, February 5, 1922.

75. George D. Strayer and N. L. Engelhardt, "Editors' Introduction," in Frederick Rand Rogers, *The Future of Interscholastic Athletics* (New York City: Teachers College, Columbia University, 1929), vii.

76. Paul J. Zbiek, "The Importance of High School Sports in Northeastern Pennsylvania: Scholastic Football in the Wyoming Valley," in *The History of Northeastern Pennsylvania: The Last 100 Years* (Nanticoke, PA: Luzerne County Community College, 1989), 24–41.

77. Rogers, *The Future of Interscholastic Athletics*, 31n13.

78. Rogers, *The Future of Interscholastic Athletics*, 31.

79. "The Football Fatalities and Injuries of 1903," *JAMA* 42, no. 5 (1904): 316.

80. Ambrose Bierce, *The Cynic's World Book* (New York: Doubleday, Page, 1906), 9–10. Bierce's work of humorous definitions of common English words would later be published as *The Devil's Dictionary*.

Chapter Two

1. Allison Danzig, "Sweeping Changes Made in Football: Rules Committee Acts to Lessen Hazards," *NYT*, February 16, 1932; "Sheridan, Army End, Dies of Football Injury," *NYT*, October 27, 1931; "575,000 Watch Nineteen Football Games; Largest Crowd, 75,000, in Yale Bowl," *NYT*, October 25, 1931.

2. Allison Danzig, "Sweeping Changes Made in Football."

3. The *New York Herald Tribune* reprinted a significant portion of this editorial. See "Sheridan Death Called Evidence of Football Evils," *New York Herald Tribune*, October 29, 1931.

4. "Sheridan Death Called Evidence of Football Evils."

5. "Toll in Football to Date Totals 10: 9 Deaths Resulted from Play on High or Prep School Gridirons or Sandlots," *NYT*, October 25, 1932.

6. Danzig, "Sweeping Changes."

7. Robert Pruter, *The Rise of American High School Sports and the Search For Control, 1880–1930* (Syracuse, NY: Syracuse University Press, 2013), 315.

8. Jerry Shnay, "50 Years and 120,000 Fans Ago," *Chicago Tribune*, November 27, 1987. In a 1937 letter to the *New York Times*, reader Marvin Rosen explained that the large crowd at this particular game could be partially attributed to the charity nature of the event. Further, he believed that the high attendance reflected the drawing power of a star boy athlete, student Bill DeCorrevont. "Right through the season, games in which this young football hero played have drawn crowds ranging from 8,000 to 15,000 in comparatively small stadia. The average high school game in Chicago seldom attracts more than 1,500." Marvin Rosen, "Record Attendance: Explains Large Crowd at School Football Game in Chicago," letter to the sports editor, *NYT*, December 4, 1937.

9. "High School Football Nets Gratifying Financial Total," *WP*, December 1, 1938.

10. Paul J. Zbiek, "The Importance of High School Sports in Northeastern Pennsylvania: Scholastic Football in the Wyoming Valley," in *The History of Northeastern Pennsylvania: The Last 100 Years* (Nanticoke, PA: Luzerne County Community College, 1989), 24–41.

11. "False Economy of School Boards Blamed for Football Casualties," *New York Herald Tribune*, November 21, 1935.

12. Glenn S. "Pop" Warner, "Football's New Deal," *Saturday Evening Post*, October 7, 1933.

13. Warner, "Football's New Deal," 83. See also "Football as Big Business," *Kansas City Star*, October 5, 1933.

14. Glenn S. Warner, "A Football Coach Looks the Game Over," *NYT*, November 13, 1932. By "every able-bodied youngster," Warner referred, of course, only to able-bodied boys. Schools typically did not offer contact team sports for girls. For a history of women's physical education in the United States, see Martha Verbrugge, *Active Bodies: A History of Women's Physical Education in Twentieth-Century America* (Oxford: University of Oxford Press, 2012).

15. WPA: Federal Works Agency, *Final Report on the WPA Program, 1935–1943* (Washington, DC: U.S. Government Printing Office, 1946), 50. See also Steven A. Reiss, *City Games: The Evolution of American Society and the Rise of Sports* (Urbana: University of Illinois Press, 1989), 142.

16. Gavin Hadden, "Stadium Design," *American Physical Education Review* 31, no. 9 (1926): 1004–18. While a complete assessment of all WPA stadiums specifically designed for football is not available, the University of California, Berkeley's *Living New Deal*, an ongoing project to map New Deal–funded projects across the United States, provides detailed information about 126 stadiums in their database, http://livingnewdeal.org/new-deal-categories/parks-and-recreation/stadiums/, accessed March 19, 2019.

17. Valerie Brown-Kuchera, Jerrik Keller, Kyndal Maurath, and Levi Hefner, "National Register of Historical Places Registration: Oakley High School Stadium," National Park Service, May 20, 2011, accessed March 19, 2019, http://www.nps.gov/nr/feature/places/pdfs/13000150.pdf.

18. Holly Allen, *Forgotten Men and Fallen Women: The Cultural Politics of New Deal Narratives* (Ithaca, NY: Cornell University Press, 2015), 32.

19. John Wong, "FDR and the New Deal on Sport and Recreation," *Sport History Review* 29 (1998): 173–91. See also Judith Anne Davidson, "The Federal Government and the Democratization of Public Recreational Sport: New York City, 1933–1945," Ph.D. dissertation, University of Massachusetts, 1983.

20. Paul Zbiek, "Coal, Steel and Gridiron: Scholastic Football in the Pittsburgh Area," in *Pittsburgh Sports: Stories from the Steel City*, ed. Randy Roberts (Pittsburgh: University of Pittsburgh Press: 2000), 214–42. For example, see "War Depletes Coaching Staffs of 6 of 15 D.C. High Schools," *WP*, August 17, 1942.

21. Associated Press, "5% of U.S. High Schools Drop Football," *WP*, December 31, 1942.

22. "Students 'Strike' Over Ban on Football Team," *NYT*, September 18, 1943.

23. Logan Clendening, "Will Your Boy Be Injured in High School Football?" *WP*, August 27, 1942. Clendening's 1927 popular book *The Human Body* sold approximately a half million copies, and he engaged in correspondence with American author Ernest Hemingway, who called him "one hell of a fine guy." For Clendening's career, see Ralph H. Major, "Obituary: Logan Clendening, 1884–1945," *Bulletin of the Medical Library Association* 33, no. 2 (April 1945): 257–59; Paul Smith, "The Doctor and the Doctor's Friend: Logan Clendening and Ernest Hemingway," *Hemingway Review* 8, no. 1 (Fall 1988): 37–39.

24. In 1945, 78 percent of boys and girls aged 14–17 years old were enrolled in school. By 1960, the enrollment rate for this age group had reached 90 percent. The number of students aged 14–17 enrolled in school during this same period increased from 6,956,000 to 10,240,000. National Center for Education Statistics, *120 Years of American Education A Statistical Portrait*, ed. Thomas D. Snyder (Washington, DC: U.S. Department of Education, 1993), accessed March 19, 2019, http://nces.ed.gov/pubs93/93442.pdf. High school was also increasingly accessible to working class students. "In 1930, for example, about 50 percent of working-class students attend high school. By the early 1960s, this figure was estimated at over 90 percent," James Gilbert, *A Cycle of Outrage: America's Reaction to the Juvenile Delinquent in the 1950s* (Oxford: Oxford University Press, 1986), 18.

25. Roger B. Saylor, *Scholastic Football in Southwestern Pennsylvania, 1892–1982* (Enola, PA: Roger B. Saylor, 1983).

26. The number of school districts was reduced from 117,000 in 1939 to 66,452 in 1953. See Samuel Miller Brownell, "Education Is Everybody's Business," *Proceedings of the 1954 National Convention of the American Association for Health and Physical Education*, April 18–23, New York (Washington, DC: AAHPER, 1954), 22–32.

27. Zachary Johnson, *Byrnes High School Football: Rebels Gridiron History* (Charleston, SC: History Press, 2010), 25.

28. Zbiek, "Coal, Steel and Gridiron." In Spartanburg County, South Carolina, some administrators of the newly formed District 5 preferred not to spend money on a new football field for the newly created James F. Byrnes High School. Superintendent Drury M. Nixon Jr., however, felt strongly that a field should be located on the school's campus and won over enough support for the construction of Nixon Field at the high school. The football stadium came with a $75,000 price tag. Johnson, *Byrnes High School Football*, 30.

29. Michael Oriard, "Football Town under Friday Night Lights: High School Football and American Dreams," in *Rooting for the Home: Team Sport, Community, and Identity*, ed. Daniel A. Nathan (Urbana: University of Illinois Press, 2013), 68–79.

30. "Football Now Is a Major Factor in the Life of White Plains High," *NYT*, November 14, 1946.

31. "White Plains High to Curb Football," *NYT*, December 17, 1948.

32. Don Group, "I'm Through with High-School Football!" *Saturday Evening Post*, October 11, 1952, 86.

33. "Football Robbing Baseball of Material, Greenberg Says," *Baltimore Sun*, March 30, 1952.

34. Ty Cashion, *Pigskin Pulpit: A Social History of Texas High School Football Coaches* (Austin: Texas State Historical Association, 1998), 148.

35. H. V. Porter, "Symposium: 1950–1951 Athletic Picture," *JAAHPER* 21, no. 8 (1950): 32.

36. National Center for Education Statistics, *120 Years of American Education: A Statistical Portrait*, ed. Thomas D. Snyder (Washington, DC: U.S. Department of Education, 1993), accessed March 19, 2019, http://nces.ed.gov/pubs93/93442.pdf.

37. William Lewis Mather, "Athletics and National Defense," address, 35th Convention of the NCAA and the AFCA, New York, December 30, 1940, 3–4.

38. Clifford Lee Brownell, "Report to the Profession," *Proceedings of the 1954 Convention of the American Association for Health, Physical Education and Recreation*, April 18–23, New York, NY (Washington, DC: AAHPER, 1954): 13.

39. Hans Kraus and Bonnie Prudden, "Minimum Muscular Fitness Tests in School Children," *Research Quarterly* 5, no. 2 (1954): 178–98. This test of strength and flexibility of leg muscles was given to 4,264 American schoolchildren and 2,870 European children; 57.9 percent of the American children failed the test, as compared to 8.7 percent of the European children. See also Mabel Lee, *A History of Physical Education and Sports in the U.S.A.* (New York: Wiley, 1983), 231.

40. Robert H. Boyle, "The Report that Shocked the President," *SI*, August 15, 1955.

41. Jack Walsh, "Condition of Youth Alarms Eisenhower," *Washington Post and Times Herald*, July 12, 1955.

42. Boyle, "The Report that Shocked the President." For more on Bonnie Prudden's work on physical fitness, including authoring fitness columns for *Sports Illustrated* and developing fitness classes and exercise equipment, see Jonathan Black, *Making the American Body: The Remarkable Saga of the Men and Women Whose Feats, Feuds, and Passions Shaped the Fitness Industry* (Lincoln: University of Nebraska Press, 2013).

43. Leonard Buder, "Fitness Meeting Opened by Nixon," *NYT*, June 19, 1956.

44. Matthew T. Bowers and Thomas M. Hunt, "The President's Council on Physical Fitness and the Systematization of Children's Play in America," *IJHS* 28, no. 11 (2011): 1496–1511.

45. Roger Morris, *Richard Milhous Nixon: The Rise of an American Politician* (New York: Holt, 1990), 92.

46. Morris, *Richard Milhous Nixon*, 133.

47. Richard Nixon, *RN: The Memoirs of Richard Nixon* (New York: Gosset & Dunlap, 1978), 19.

48. Dwight D. Eisenhower, *At Ease: Stories I Tell to Friends* (Garden City, NY: Doubleday, 1967), 16. Eisenhower was far from the only American president to extol the unique virtues of football. In 1894, future president Woodrow Wilson asserted that football "develops more moral qualities than any other game of athletics." As discussed in chapter 1, in 1900, President Theodore Roosevelt famously used football as a metaphor in giving the following advice to American boys: "In short, in life, as in a football game, the principle to follow is: Hit the line hard; don't foul and don't shirk, but hit the line hard!" "Football or No Football," *NYT*, February 18, 1894; Theodore Roosevelt, *The Strenuous Life: Essays and Address* (New York: The Century Co., 1900), 164.

49. John F. Kennedy, "The Soft American," *SI*, December 26, 1960; John F. Kennedy, "The Vigor We Need," *SI*, July 15, 1962. For more on the council and Kennedy's appointment of Wilkinson, see Rachel Louise Moran, *Governing Bodies: American Politics and the Shaping of the Modern Physique* (Philadelphia: University of Pennsylvania Press, 2018).

50. "Registration Certificate National Pop Warner Conference," provided to Dave Vannicelli, school year 1962–1963, Dave and Mary Vannicelli Collection, KPHS, King of Prussia, PA. This certificate was signed by Joseph J. Tomlin, founder of the National Pop Warner Conference, and by Joseph A. Donoghue, secretary of the Philadelphia Eagles Football Club.

51. Dick Hyland, "Pop Warner Conference Carries on Principles of Football Coach," *LAT*, December 17, 1959.

52. Educational Policies Commission, *School Athletics: Problems and Policies* (Washington, DC: Educational Policies Commission of the NEA and the American Association of School Administrators, 1954), 3.

53. "Third-String End Honored Guest at Football Coaches' Luncheon," *NYT*, January 9, 1958. Other competitive sports were also characterized as a means to defend the American way of life. For a discussion of how Little League Baseball was promoted "as a valuable tool in the Cold War struggle against Communism" during this period, see Michael H. Carriere, "'A Diamond Is a Boy's Best Friend': The Rise of Little League Baseball, 1939–1964," *JSH* 32, no. 3 (2005): 351–78.

54. David Wallace Adams, "More than a Game: The Carlisle Indians Take to the Gridiron," *Western Historical Quarterly* 32, no. 1 (2001): 25–53.

55. Russ Crawford, *The Use of Sports to Promote the American Way of Life During the Cold War,* (Lewiston, NY: Edwin Mellen, 2008): 178–79.

56. Crawford, *The Use of Sports.*

57. Ted Key, *Saturday Evening Post*, October 19, 1946, 68. Cited in Crawford, *The Use of Sports to Promote the American Way of Life*, 49. Jeffrey Montez de Oca, *Discipline and Indulgence: College Football, Media, and the American Way of Life During the Cold War* (New Brunswick, NJ: Rutgers University Press, 2013), 20. For a discussion of juvenile fiction celebrating multi-ethnic football teams in the years after World War II, see chapter 8, "Ethnicity," in Michael Oriard, *King Football: Sport and Spectacle in the Golden Age of Radio and Newsreels, Movies and Magazines, the Weekly and the Daily Press* (Chapel Hill: University of North Carolina Press, 2001).

58. Bill McMurray, *Texas High School Football* (South Bend, IN: Icarus Press, 1985), 389; Michael Hurd, *Thursday Night Lights: The Story of Black High School Football in Texas* (Austin: University of Texas Press, 2017), 5.

59. Joel Huerta, "Red, Brown, and Blue: A History and Cultural Poetics of High School Football in Mexican America," Ph.D. dissertation, University of Texas at Austin, 2005.

60. Huerta, "Red, Brown, and Blue."

61. Dorothy Barclay, "Competitive Sports: The Pros and Cons," *NYT*, August 28, 1955.

62. "Third-String End Honored Guest at Football Coaches' Luncheon," *NYT*, January 9, 1958.

63. David Seed, "The Postwar Jeremiads of Philip Wylie," *Science Fiction Studies* 22, no. 2 (July 1995): 234–51; Rebecca Jo Plant, *Mom: The Transformation of Motherhood in America* (Chicago: University of Chicago Press, 2010), 21. See especially chapter 2, "Debunking the All-American Mom: Philip Wylie's Momism Critique."

64. Dr. Edward A. Strecker, "What's Wrong with American Mothers?" *Saturday Evening Post,* October 26, 1946, 88.

65. Mothers were blamed both for being overly emotional and protective and for not being emotional or loving enough. For instance, during this period autism was attributed to "refrigerator mothers" who were supposedly cold, emotionally distant, and insufficiently nurturing. This thesis remained popular until the 1970s. Jeffrey P. Baker, "Autism in 1959: Joey the Mechanical Boy," *Pediatrics* 125 (2010): 1101–03; Adam Feinstein, *A History of Autism: Conversations with the Pioneers* (London: Wiley-Blackwell, 2010). See also Sarah S. Richardson et al., "Don't Blame the Mothers," *Nature* 512 (2014): 131–32.

66. Steven Mintz and Susan Kellogg, *Domestic Revolutions: A Social History of American Family Life* (New York: Free Press, 1988), 190.

67. Elaine Tyler May, *Homeward Bound: American Families in the Cold War Era,* 20th anniversary edition (New York: Basic Books, 2008); Joanne Meyerowitz, *Not June Cleaver: Women and Gender in Postwar America, 1945–1960* (Philadelphia: Temple University Press, 1994).

68. Samuel Middlebrook, "The Importance of Fathers," *Parents,* December 1947, 28, 78. Cited in May, *Homeward Bound,* 140.

69. Russell Baker, "Observer: The Muscular Opiate," *NYT,* October 3, 1967.

70. Don Iddon, "American Athletes Are Sissies," *Coronet,* February 1952, 34–37.

71. William Brady, "Student Badly Hurt Averting 'Sissy' Title," *LAT,* December 11, 1952.

72. John Kord Lagemann, "How High-Pressure Sports Can Hurt Your Child," *Redbook,* July 1958, 36–39, 52. Lagemann's article both quoted health professionals and drew their attention. The *American Journal of Public Health* published a brief write-up of this article, "Credit Lines: Little League Baseball—Questions," *AJPH* 48, no. 9 (1958): 1294.

73. Lou Little, "Teach Your Boy to Play It Safe," *Baltimore Sun,* September 26, 1954.

74. Barclay, "Competitive Sports: The Pros and Cons."

75. David Reisman and Reuel Denney, "Football in America: A Study in Cultural Diffusion," *American Quarterly* 3, no. 4 (1951): 309–25.

76. Joseph Constantine Lease, "A Survey of the Attitudes and Practices of the Administrators and Coaches in the State of California Concerning Interschool Tackle Football at the Junior High School Level," M.A. thesis, California State University, Sacramento, 1962.

77. Jack W. Berryman, "From the Cradle to the Playing Field: America's Emphasis on Highly Organized Competitive Sports for Preadolescent Boys," *JSH* 2 (1976): 112–31.

78. Joint Committee on Athletic Competition for Children of Elementary and Junior High School Age, *Desirable Athletic Competition for Children: Joint Committee Report* (Washington, DC: AAHPER, 1952), 4.

79. Arthur Edson, "Educators Tee Off on Kids' Leagues," *WP,* December 19, 1952.

80. *Desirable Athletic Competition for Children,* 3.

81. Berryman, "From the Cradle to the Playing Field."

82. Joint Committee on Standards for Interscholastic Athletics, *Standards for Junior High School Athletics: Report of the Junior High School Athletics Subcommittee of the Joint Committee on Standards for Interscholastic Athletics* (Washington, DC: AAHPER, 1963), 7.

83. Lease, "Survey of the Attitudes and Practices."

84. Lease, "Survey of the Attitudes and Practices," 96.

85. Lease, "Survey of the Attitudes and Practices," 71, 76.

86. "Are Highly Competitive Sports Desirable for Juniors?" *Recreation* 46 (1952): 422–26.

87. "Are Highly Competitive Sports Desirable for Juniors?"

88. Allen Guttmann, "The Progressive Era Appropriation of Child's Play," *Journal of the History of Childhood and Youth* 3, no. 2 (2010): 147–51; Donna St. George, "Joseph J. Tomlin, 85, Pop Warner Founder," *Philadelphia Inquirer*, May 18, 1988.

89. Glenn S. Warner and Mike Bynum, *Pop Warner, Football's Greatest Teacher: The Epic Autobiography of Major College Football's Winningest Coach, Glenn S. (Pop) Warner* (Birmingham, AL: Gridiron Football Properties, 1993).

90. Joel D. Balthaser, *Pop Warner Little Scholars* (Portsmouth, NH: Arcadia, 2004): 17.

91. Francis J. Power, *Life Story of Pop Warner: Gridiron's Greatest Strategist* (St. Louis: Spink, 1947).

92. Balthaser, *Pop Warner Little Scholars*, 22.

93. Warner and Bynum, *Pop Warner, Football's Greatest Teacher*.

94. Warner and Bynum, *Pop Warner, Football's Greatest Teacher*.

95. Howard M. Tuckner, "Bowl Football Kick-Off Is Tonight," *NYT*, November 27, 1957.

96. Warner and Bynum, *Pop Warner, Football's Greatest Teacher*.

97. Charles Lowenthal, a National Pop Warner Trustee, told the *Los Angeles Times* that Pop Warner coaches must obtain copies of their players' report cards. He added, "Championships and trips to bowl games—we now have 54 of them—are awarded only to the teams with the best scholastic records among the best playing records." Dick Hyland, "Pop Warner Conference Carries on Principles of Football Coach," *LAT*, December 17, 1959.

98. Richard Edward Stuetz, *An Evaluation of the Educational Values of Pop Warner Football with Reference to the General Objectives of Secondary Education*, M.A. thesis, Chapman College, 1969.

99. "Youth Teams to Meet in Pop Warner Bowl," *LAT*, December 14, 1958.

100. "Midget Football League Starts in Newport News," *Norfolk Journal and Guide*, October 17, 1953. "CYO Football League Gets Underway Today," *WP*, September 20, 1956. The term "midget" was often used generically to refer to youth, although some leagues used the term to specifically refer to a certain age group or size category. For instance, in a 1961 YMCA Pop Warner football league, the midget league was limited to boys ages 10 to 13 years old, with a weight limit between 85 and 115 pounds. See Howard Swindell, "Midget Gridders Ready for Big Games," *CDT*, October 8, 1961. Similarly, the 1963 Bux-Mont Midget Football League in Pennsylvania include 80-, 95-, and 115-pound teams. "Bux-Mont Midget Football League 1963 Official Schedule," Dave and Mary Vannicelli collection, KPHS, King of Prussia, PA.

101. Howard M. Tuckner, "Small Fry Football League on Long Island Still Growing; Supervised Program Much Safer than Sandlot Games," *NYT*, November 18, 1956.

102. Clyde Snyder, "Hard but Safe-Hitting Midget Grid Lines Bring Cheers from Parents," *LAT*, November 17, 1957.

103. C. B. Newman and A. H. Fetherolf, "Sales of Bats, Boats and Other Gear Climb Despite the Recession," *Wall Street Journal*, June 17, 1958.

104. Bob Holbrook, "Friedman Raps Parents: Brandeis Coach Says Football Makes Men of Boys," *Daily Boston Globe*, October 28, 1958.

105. Barclay, "Competitive Sports: The Pros and Cons."

106. "Youthful Football Players Get Plenty Protection in Pop Warner Conference," *Philadelphia Tribune*, September 20, 1955.

107. Clyde Snyder, "Hard but Safe-Hitting Midget Grid Lines."

108. Carl K. Benhase, *Ohio High School Football* (West Nyack, NY: Parker, 1967), 49.

109. Barbara Fox, "Football for the Whole Family," *Christian Science Monitor*, November 24, 1959.

110. Jeane Hoffman, "Football Mom's Life Takes Crazy Bounce," *LAT*, October 26, 1960. The tropes of mothers as chauffeurs and sisters as cheerleaders featured commonly in profiles of youth football. "And when the Cleveland Park teams play other boys' outfits in Washington or tackle each other in regular games, the mothers act as chauffeurs and join the sisters in the cheering section." Hugh Morrow, "Does He Rate Some of Your Time?" *Saturday Evening Post*, January 8, 1949, 80.

111. May, *Homeward Bound*, 11. On the history of the American family, see also Steven Mintz and Susan Kellogg, *Domestic Revolutions: A Social History of American Family Life* (New York: Free Press, 1988).

112. "Who Will Wear Crown at First Indian Bowl?"; "Not a Princess but a Queen," *Montgomery Post*, November 20, 1963; "Mom's a Coach," *Valley Forge Life*, November 21, 1963, Dave and Mary Vannicelli collection, KPHS, King of Prussia, PA. For a history of cheerleading, see Mary Ellen Hanson, *Go! Fight! Win! Cheerleading in American Culture* (Bowling Green, OH: Bowling Green State University Popular Press, 1995).

113. Holbrook, "Friedman Raps Parents."

114. Gene Earl, "Laws Protect Young Gridders," *LAT*, October 8, 1961.

Chapter Three

1. "Football Old Game: Gridiron Sport Was Introduced Thirty Years Ago," *WP*, October 8, 1905.

2. Stephen Hardy, "'Adopted by All the Leading Clubs': Sporting Goods and the Shaping of Leisure, 1800–1900," in *For Fun and Profit: The Transformation of Leisure into Consumption*, ed. Richard Butsch (Philadelphia: Temple University Press, 1990), 71–101.

3. Hardy, "Adopted by All the Leading Clubs," 71–101; Rodney Freeman, Katherine C. Donahue, Eric Baxter, et al., "The Draper-Maynard Sporting Goods Company of Plymouth, New Hampshire, 1840–1937," *Journal of the Society of Industrial Archaeology* 20 (1994): 139–51.

4. SGMA, "A Commemorative Report: A Historical Reflection of the U.S. Sporting Goods Industry's Growth and Development in the 20th Century," (North Palm Beach, FL: SGMA, 2006), 6. SGMA went through several name changes, including the Athletic Goods Manufacturers Association and the Chamber of Commerce of the Athletic Goods Manufacturers of the United States of America.

5. "John Riddell, War Helmet's Inventor, Dies," *CDT*, July 3, 1945; William L. Bird and Roger R. Ebert, *Elyria: Images of America* (Charleston, SC: Arcadia, 2014); "Army Gets a 'Chute Helmet from Gridiron," *CDT*, July 6, 1941; "Riddell Sports Group, Inc." in *International Directory of Company Histories*, ed. Karen Hill, vol. 139 (Detroit: St. James Press, 2012).

6. Andrew Gaffney, "Battle Helmets," *Popular Mechanics*, October 1995: 78–81; F. Richard Ciccone, "At this Firm, 11 Heads Are Better than One," *Chicago Tribune*, October 7, 1976; "Riddell Sports Group, Inc." in *International Directory of Company Histories*. See also Mark

Fainaru-Wada and Steve Wainaru, *League of Denial: The N.F.L., Concussions, and the Battle for Truth* (New York: Random House, 2013), 135.

7. "Army Gets a 'Chute Helmet from Gridiron"; "John Riddell, War Helmet's Inventor, Dies"; F. Ciccone, "At this Firm."

8. Ciccone, "At this Firm"; "Riddell Sports Group, Inc." in *International Directory of Company Histories.*

9. Ciccone, "At this Firm."

10. Robert H. Boyle, *Sport: Mirror of American Life* (Boston: Little, Brown, 1963); C. B. Newman and A. H. Fetherolf, "Sales of Bats, Boats and Other Gear Climb Despite the Recession," *Wall Street Journal,* June 17, 1958; Richard Snyder, "The Sporting Goods Market at the Threshold of the Seventies" (Chicago: National Sporting Goods Association, 1969), 1.

11. Newman and Fetherolf, "Sales of Bats, Boats and Other Gear."

12. Newman and Fetherolf, "Sales of Bats, Boats and Other Gear"; Howard Swindell, "Midget Gridders Ready for Big Games," *CDT,* October 8, 1961.

13. "Retail Sales of Footballs Jump 60.4% Between 1960 and 1965," *American Druggist,* October 10, 1966, 77; Snyder, "The Sporting Goods Market," 1.

14. Stephen Hardy, "Entrepreneurs, Structures, and the Sportgeist: Old Tensions in a Modern Industry," in *Essays on Sport History and Sport Mythology,* ed. Donald Kyle and Gary Stark (College Station: Texas A&M Press, 1990), 45–82. For a discussion of the discrediting of the older work practices of the "high-class mechanic," as part of efforts to promote new scientific management in manufacturing, see David Montgomery, *Workers' Control in America: Studies in the History of Work, Technology and Labor Struggles* (New York: Cambridge University Press, 1978), 27.

15. Lawrence W. Fielding and Lori K. Miller, "Advertising and the Development of Consumer Purchasing Criteria: The Sporting Goods Industry, 1900–1930," *Sports Marketing Quarterly* 5, no. 4 (1996): 37–50; Theodore Levitt, "Marketing Intangible Products and Product Intangibles," *Harvard Business Review* 59, no. 3 (1981): 94–102.

16. Rawlings Advertisement, "Banish Fear of Injuries," *Athletic Journal* 15, no. 8 (1935); Wilson advertisement, "Wilson Offers You Advanced Equipment at a Price to Fit Your Budget," *Athletic Journal* 15, no. 8 (1935): 28–29; J. A. Dubow Manufacturing Company advertisement, "Dubow: What Will the Year Bring Forth????" *Athletic Journal* 16, no. 1 (1935): 45.

17. Rawlings advertisement, "Here's How to Start Playing Football Right!" *Boys' Life* (September 1959): 8.

18. MacGregor Goldsmith advertisement, "Just Like the Pros Wear!" *Boys' Life* (September 1960): 78; Wilson advertisement, "Are You Ready for Big-Time Football Equipment?" *Boys' Life* (September 1961): 42–43.

19. Institute for Motivational Research, Inc., *A Motivational Research Pilot Study of the Sales, Advertising, and Merchandising Problems of Rawlings Sporting Goods* (Croton-on-Hudson, NY: Institute for Motivational Research, Inc., 1958); Randall Rothenberg, "Advertising: Capitalist Eye on the Soviet Consumer," *NYT,* February 15, 1989. See also Barbara B. Stern, "The Importance of Being Ernest: Commemorating Dichter's Contribution to Advertising Research," *Journal of Advertising Research* 44, no. 2 (June 2004): 165–69.

20. Institute for Motivational Research, Inc., *A Motivational Research Pilot Study.*

21. Institute for Motivational Research, Inc., *A Motivational Research Pilot Study,* 24.

22. Witchell Sheill Company advertisement, "Witchell Scientific Football Shoes," *Proceedings of the Twelfth Annual Meeting of the American Football Coaches Association,* New York, December 27–28, 1932; Brooks Shoe Manufacturing Company, "Brooks Safety Football Shoes," *Scholastic Coach* 15 (June 1946): 35.

23. Spalding advertisement, "Here's the Helmet with the Big Safety Margin," *Scholastic Coach* 19 (March 1950); Rawlings advertisement, "Rawlings Triple Protection Head Cushion," *Scholastic Coach* 23 (May 1954): 3. MacGregor Goldsmith advertisement, "Game-Tested and Proven," *Scholastic Coach* 17 (September 1947): 17.

24. Martha N. Gardner and Allan M. Brandt, "'The Doctors' Choice Is America's Choice': The Physician in US Cigarette Advertisements, 1930–1953," *AJPH* 96, no. 2 (2006): 222–32; Allan M. Brandt, *The Cigarette Century: The Rise, Fall, and Deadly Persistence of the Product that Defined America* (New York: Basic Books, 2007); Nancy Tomes, "Merchants of Health: Medicine and Consumer Culture in the United States, 1900–1940," *Journal of American History* 88, no. 2 (September 2001): 519–47. On the comparative politics of alcohol and tobacco marketing, see Pamela E. Pennock, *Advertising Sin and Sickness: The Politics of Alcohol and Tobacco Marketing, 1950–1960* (DeKalb: Northern Illinois University Press, 2007).

25. Rawlings advertisement, "Defense Against Injury!" *Athletic Journal* 31, no. 1 (1951).

26. "Mar Vista Giants Kick Off First Season in Midget Football League," *LAT,* September 21, 1958.

27. Clyde Snyder, "Hard but Safe-Hitting Midget Grid Lines Bring Cheers from Parents," *LAT,* November 17, 1957.

28. Howard M. Tuckner, "Small Fry Football League on Long Island Still Growing; Supervised Program Much Safer than Sandlot Games," *NYT,* November 18, 1956.

29. "Athletic Competition for Children?" *Athletic Journal* 34, no. 5 (1954): 18, 20, 55. For an overview of Dr. Oberteuffer's career, see "In Memoriam: Delbert Oberteuffer, 1901–1981," *Journal of Physical Education and Recreation* 52, no. 7 (1981): 11–12.

30. Clifford B. Fagan, "Misconceptions about Protective Equipment and Procedures in Athletics," *Journal of School Health* 34 (1964): 168–73.

31. Fagan, "Misconceptions about Protective Equipment."

32. "Youth Will Pray, then Play Ball," *LAT,* October 26, 1958.

33. T. R. Van Dellen, "How to Keep Well: Football Mishaps," *Chicago Tribune,* September 29, 1950.

34. Randy Vanet, "Gridiron Challenge," *Dental Survey* 27 (1951): 1258–60.

35. Howard H. Dukes, "Latex Football Mouthpieces," *Journal of the American Dental Association* 49 (1954): 445–88; "The Fighting Irish Look Tough Again," *Life,* September 29, 1952. Michael Oriard has noted that Notre Dame officials were outraged by the implication of this *Life* feature that "the Irish were a bunch of roughnecks—with no mention of the fact that the featured players had insignificant roles on the team and were the only ones missing teeth. The university demanded, and received, an official apology two issues later, along with new photos of the players in coats and ties, their dental work firmly in place." Michael Oriard, *King Football: Sport and Spectacle in the Golden Age of Radio and Newsreels, Movies and Magazines, the Weekly and the Daily Press* (Chapel Hill: University of North Carolina Press, 2001), 216.

36. "Mouth Protection for Football Players," *Scholastic Coach* (January 1953): 24.

37. American Dental Association, "Evaluation of Mouth Protectors Used by High School Football Players," *Journal of the American Dental Association* 68 (1964): 430–42. For a review

of the use of mouth guards in sports, see Joseph J. Knapik et al., "Mouthguards in Sport Activities: History, Physical Properties and Injury Prevention Effectiveness," *Sports Medicine* 37, no. 2 (2007):117–44.

38. Stephen E. Reid, "Radio Telemetry in a Study of Football Helmets," in AMA Committee on the Medical Aspects of Sports, *Proceedings of the National Conference on Head Protection for Athletes* (Chicago: American Medical Association, 1962), 40–41.

39. "Parents Urged to Check Gear of Footballers," *NYT*, August 5, 1964.

40. Herbert Davis Horton, *A Survey of the Safety Features of Expensive Items of Football Equipment as Used in Texas High Schools*, M.A. thesis, Southwest Texas State University, 1955, 36.

41. Charles Trimble, "Glory Days at the Mission School," *Indian Country Today Media Network*, October 25, 2006. See also Charles Trimble, *Iyeska* (Indianapolis: Dog Ear, 2012).

42. Edward R. Dye, "Engineering Research on Protective Headgear," *American Journal of Surgery* 98, no. 3 (1959): 368–72; Allan J. Ryan, "Organized Medicine and Athletics: The Role of the American Medical Association Committee on Injury in Sports," *American Journal of Surgery* 98, no. 3 (1959): 325–27.

43. William H. White, "Armor that Does as Much Harm as Good," *SI*, October 31, 1955.

44. "Here and There Over the Nation," *Kentucky High School Athlete* (September 1948): 8–9, accessed March 19, 2019, https://encompass.eku.edu/athlete/497/.

45. Glenn Scobey Warner, "Football Rules," *Athletic Journal* 12, no. 7 (1932): 55–57; Frederick O. Mueller and Robert C. Cantu, *Football Fatalities and Catastrophic Injuries, 1931–2008* (Durham, NC: Carolina Academic Press, 2011), 59.

46. Mueller and Cantu, *Football Fatalities*, 79.

47. Mueller and Cantu, *Football Fatalities*, 98.

48. Stephen E. Reid, Joseph A. Tarkington, and Matthew Petrovick, "Radio Telemetry in a Study of Football Helmets," 83–93. Marc Michaelson, "Should Your Son Play Football?" *Popular Mechanics*, September 1962, 94.

49. Robert F. Brown, *Head Injuries in Colorado High School Football for 1957*, M.A. thesis, University of Wyoming, 1958, 42.

50. Richard C. Schneider et al., "Serious and Fatal Football Injuries Involving the Head and Spinal Cord," *JAMA* 177, no. 6 (1961): 362–67.

51. Joan Beck, "New Football Helmets Dangerous for Boys," *CDT*, November 7, 1961.

52. Jim Murray, "Head Coach or Surgeon?" *LAT*, October 19, 1961.

53. Bob Addie, "Equipment Advances: Bob Addie's Column," *WP*, November 9, 1961.

54. "Colleges Weigh Helmet Changes: Rise in Injuries Spurs Study of Current Football Gear," *NYT*, October 29, 1961.

55. "Colleges Weigh Helmet Changes."

56. "Football Armor," *San Francisco Chronicle*, October 28, 1961.

57. Mal Stevens, "It's Basically a Safe Game: Mal Stevens Sees Night Football Boosting Injuries," *Boston Globe*, September 9, 1962.

58. Fagan, "Misconceptions about Protective Equipment."

59. Murray, "Head Coach or Surgeon?"

60. "Sports Authorities Warn Against 'Spearing,'" *Journal of the Iowa Medical Society* 57, no. 9 (1967): 930–31; Ciccone, "At this Firm."

61. "Coach Group's Head Upset over Prep Grid Fatalities," *Baltimore Sun*, October 13, 1961.

62. E. S. Gurdjian, H. R. Lissner, and L. M. Patrick, "Problems in Providing Protection for the Head and Neck in Sports," AMA Committee on the Medical Aspects of Sports, *Proceedings of the National Conference on Head Protection for Athletes* (Chicago: American Medical Association, 1962), 1–14.

Chapter Four

1. Carl E. Willgoose, "Health Implications of Highly Competitive Sports at the Elementary-Junior High Level," *Journal of School Health* (1959): 224–27.

2. Willgoose, "Health Implications," 225.

3. Marcia Winn, "Fit the Exercise to the Growing Boy," *CDT*, October 20, 1955, C1.

4. Kathleen E. Bachynski, "Tolerable Risks? Physicians and Youth Tackle Football," *New England Journal of Medicine* 374 (2016): 405–7.

5. "Football Mortality Among Boys," *JAMA* 49 (1907): 2088.

6. Thomas N. Horan, "Analysis of Football Injuries," *JAMA* 103, no. 5 (1934): 325–27. On Cranbrook School and Dr. Horan's role as resident physician, see "Michigan Fosters Cranbrook Plan," *Michigan Alumnus* 38 (1932): 445–46, 450.

7. Gallagher's study included approximately 650 boarding students per year, ranging in age from 13 to 18 years old. J. Roswell Gallagher, "Athletic Injuries Among Adolescents: Their Incidence and Type in Various Sports," *Research Quarterly* 19, no. 3 (1948): 198–214.

8. Gallagher, "Athletic Injuries Among Adolescents."

9. Heather Munro Prescott, *A Doctor of Their Own: The History of Adolescent Medicine* (Cambridge: Harvard University Press, 1998). See especially chapter 2, "J. Roswell Gallagher and the Origins of Adolescent Medicine." For Gallagher's own perspective on the field, see J. Roswell Gallagher, "The Origins, Developments and Goals of Adolescent Medicine," *Journal of Adolescent Health Care* 3 (1982): 57–63. On debates in the late 1920s and early 1930s over the nature of high school interscholastic sports, see Robert Pruter, *The Rise of American High School Sports and the Search for Control, 1880–1930* (Syracuse, NY: Syracuse University Press, 2013).

10. Augustus Thorndike Jr., "Trauma Incident to Sports and Recreation," *New England Journal of Medicine* 219, no. 13 (1938): 457–65. See also Thorndike, *Athletic Injuries: Prevention, Diagnosis and Treatment* (Philadelphia: Lea & Febiger, 1938). For a brief review of Thorndike's career and his contribution to the development of sports medicine, see Bertram Zarins, "History of the Massachusetts General Hospital Sports Medicine Service," *Orthopaedic Journal at Harvard Medical School* (2007): 108–10, accessed March 19, 2019, http://www.orthojournalhms.org/volume9/manuscripts/ms13.pdf. See also his obituary, "Dr. Augustus Thorndike, 89, Sports Medicine Specialist," *NYT*, February 1, 1986.

11. "Athletes' Injuries," *Time* 36, no. 8, August 19, 1940.

12. George Maksim, "Desirable Athletics for Children," *JAMA* 168, no. 11 (1958): 1431–33. Similarly, in 1957, *Sports Illustrated* quoted Maksim as saying, "Competition is part of the growing child that should be recognized, accepted and directed." Kenneth Rudeen, "The Verdict," *SI*, August 26, 1957.

13. Diana Chapman Walsh, "Divided Loyalties in Medicine: The Ambivalence of Occupational Medical Practice," *Social Science & Medicine* 23, no. 8 (1986): 789–96.

14. John Sayle Watterson, *College Football: History, Spectacle, Controversy* (Baltimore: Johns Hopkins University Press, 2000), 155.

15. "Report of Rules Committee," *Athletic Journal* 12, no. 7 (1932): 19–24. The Heisman trophy for most outstanding college football player in the United States would later be named for John Heisman.

16. AFCA, *Proceedings of the Twelfth Annual Meeting of the American Football Coaches Association*, New York, December 27–28, 1932, 5. The AFCA's annual survey included figures for football played at the sandlot, club, high school, and college levels. Since 1931, the AFCA has tabulated the numbers of catastrophic injuries and fatalities in football occurring in children and young adults. Two doctors compiled these statistics through 2008 and have summarized some of the rules and equipment changes that were instituted during this time period. Frederick O. Mueller and Robert C. Cantu, *Football Fatalities and Catastrophic Injuries, 1931–2008* (Durham, NC: Carolina Academic Press, 2011).

17. Marvin Allen Stevens and Winthrop Morgan Phelps, *The Control of Football Injuries* (New York: A. S. Barnes, 1933), 211.

18. Stevens and Phelps, *The Control of Football Injuries,* viii.

19. H.V. Porter, "National Federation Annual Meeting," *Scholastic Coach* 18, no. 6 (1949): 44–46; 60.

20. Jess F. Kraus, "A Journey to and Through Injury Epidemiology," *Injury Epidemiology* 1, no. 3 (2014): 1–3.

21. Lucian H. Landry, "Injuries Peculiar to Modern Football," *American Journal of Surgery* 28, no. 3 (1935): 601–12.

22. John C. Burnham, "Why Did the Infants and Toddlers Die? Shift in Americans' Ideas of Responsibility for Accidents—From Blaming Mom to Engineering," *Journal of Social History* 29 (1996): 817–38.

23. William J. Haddon Jr., Edward A. Suchman, and David Klein, *Accident Research: Methods and Approaches* (New York: Harper and Row, 1964).

24. Ralph Nader, *Unsafe at Any Speed* (New York: Grossman, 1965). For a discussion of earlier conceptualizations of injuries as acts of God, see Hermann Loimer and Michael Guarnieri, "Accidents and Acts of God: A History of the Terms," *AJPH* 86, no. 1 (1996): 101–07. On developments in injury prevention as a field of public health, see Julian A. Waller, "Reflections on a Half Century of Injury Control," *AJPH* 84, no. 4 (1994): 664–70.

25. Augustus Thorndike, "Prevention of Injury in Athletics," *JAMA* 162, no. 12 (1956): 1126–32.

26. On the foundation of the National Athletic Trainers' Association and the development of athletic training education, see Gary D. Delforge and Robert S. Behnke, "The History and Evolution of Athletic Training Education in the United States," *Journal of Athletic Training* 34, no. 1 (1999): 53–61.

27. Jack W. Berryman, *Out of Many, One: A History of the American College of Sports Medicine,* (Champaign, IL: Human Kinetics, 1995).

28. Douglas W. Jackson, "The History of Sports Medicine, Part 2," *American Journal of Sports Medicine* 12, no. 4 (1984): 255–57.

29. "Round Table: Legal, Moral, and Ethical Questions in Sports Medicine," *Physician and Sportsmedicine* 3 (March 1975): 71–84. A professional athlete participant in this round-table, Keith Erickson of the Phoenix Suns, challenged the contention that physicians al-

ways put players first. He indicated that many athletes felt that team physicians were only interested in management's point of view. "If [a player] was hurt, he just had to get back and play as soon as possible."

30. Neil Amdur, "Once More, Doc, with Feeling," *NYT*, August 22, 1974.

31. Robert Markus, "Trainer Now Man of Science; Era of Aspirin Bluff Gone," *Chicago Tribune*, June 15, 1965. Dr. Ben Casey was the title character of an American TV medical drama which ran from 1961 to 1966. For a history of early athletic training written by an athletic trainer, see Matt J. Webber, *Dropping the Bucket and Sponge: A History of Early Athletic Training, 1881–1947* (Prescott, AZ: Athletic Training History Publishing, 2013).

32. Frank S. Lloyd, *Safety in Physical Education in Secondary Schools* (New York: National Bureau of Casualty and Surety Underwriters, 1933).

33. George B. Logan, "Essential Medical Supervision in Athletics for Children," *JAMA* 169, no. 8 (1959): 786–88. Logan accepted the AAP presidency in 1967. See Logan, "Acceptance of the Presidency of the American Academy of Pediatrics," *Pediatrics* 40, no. 6 (1967): 1049.

34. Richard H. Alley Jr., "Head and Neck Injuries in High School Football," *JAMA* 188, no. 5 (1964): 118–22.

35. AAP, *Report of the Committee on School Health of the American Academy of Pediatrics* (Evanston, IL: American Academy of Pediatrics, 1966), 72.

36. Jack Walsh, "Football Ban Urged for Youngsters," *WP*, May 27, 1953. The forty-four delegates who made the recommendations included representatives from twenty-nine different interested groups, including the AAP, the NEA, National Recreation Association, AMA, American School Health Association, the Pop Warner Foundation (football), Little League Baseball, and other similar medical, educational and recreational groups. For a summary of the conference, see J. Bertram Kessel, "Planning Games and Sports for Youngsters: Highlights of the National Conference on Program Planning in Games and Sports for Boys and Girls of Elementary School Age," *JAAHPER* 24 (1953): 8–9.

37. Marshall Pease, *American Academy of Pediatrics: June 1930 to June 1951* (Evanston, IL: American Academy of Pediatrics, 1952).

38. AAP Committee on School Health, "Competitive Athletics: A Statement of Policy: Report of the Committee on School Health, American Academy of Pediatrics," *Pennsylvania Medical Journal* 60, no. 5 (1957): 627–29.

39. "Doctors on Sport," *Time*, December 12, 1960.

40. "Curbs on Football for Smaller Boys Asked by Doctors," *NYT*, November 18, 1960.

41. C. L. Lowman, "The Vulnerable Age," *Journal of Health and Physical Education* 18, no. 9 (1947): 635–36, 693.

42. Lowman, "The Vulnerable Age," 636.

43. Hollis Fait, "Needed: A Policy on Junior-High Interschool Athletics," *JAAHPER* 21, no. 8 (October 1950): 20–21.

44. Paul Starr, *The Social Transformation of American Medicine* (New York: Basic Books, 1983).

45. John L. Reichert, "Competitive Athletics for Pre-Teen-Age Children," *JAMA* 166, no. 14 (1958): 1701–7. Prior to its 1958 publication in *JAMA*, Reichert had read this article before the Section on Pediatrics at the AMA's annual meeting in 1957. In 1957, he had also published a similar article to the 1958 *JAMA* piece. See John L. Reichert, "A Pediatrician's View of Competitive Sports before the Teens," *Today's Health* 35 (1957): 28–31.

46. Reichert, "Competitive Athletics for Pre-Teen-Age Children," 1703.

47. Reichert, "Competitive Athletics for Pre-Teen-Age Children," 1706. For a biography of football coach Eddie Anderson, see Kevin Carroll, *Dr. Eddie Anderson, Hall of Fame Football Coach: A Biography* (Jefferson, NC: McFarland, 2007). Anderson also spent several years coaching at the University of Iowa. Hein had served as secretary of the Joint Committee on Health Problems in Education for the NEA and the AMA from 1949 to 1957. "Fred V. Hein Receives R. Tait McKenzie Award 1973," *School Health Review* 4, no. 4 (1973): 22. The original source of the claim that tackling or being tackled was associated with 60 percent of football injuries is unclear; one possibility is a 1936 report in the Bulletin of the New York State Public School Athletic Association. See reference 15 in James T. O'Shea, "The Control of Football Injuries in High School," *Journal of School Health* 8, no. 7 (1938): 190–97.

48. Lance Van Auken and Robin Van Auken, *Play Ball! The Story of Little League Baseball* (University Park: Pennsylvania University Press, 2000), 110–111. See also Charles Euchner, *Little League, Big Dreams: The Hope, the Hype and the Glory of the Greatest World Series Ever Played* (Naperville, IL: Sourcebooks, 2006); Richard Sandomir, "Creighton Hale, 93, Inventor of Little League Helmet, Dies," *NYT*, October 20, 2017.

49. Creighton Hale, "What Research Says About Athletics for Pre-High School Age Children," *Journal of Health, Physical Education, and Recreation* 30, no. 9 (1959): 19–21, 43.

50. Hale, "What Research Says," 19.

51. Hale, "What Research Says," 19.

52. Reichert, "Competitive Athletics for Pre-Teen-Age Children," 1706.

53. Lowman, "The Vulnerable Age."

54. Lou Little, "Teach Your Boy to Play It Safe," *Baltimore Sun*, September 26, 1954.

55. Paul Costello, Massachusetts High School Football Association, email to author, June 13, 2015. See also the Gridiron Club of Greater Boston, "Dr. Joseph H. Burnett Award," accessed March 19, 2019, http://gridclubofgreaterboston.com/awards/dr-joseph-h-burnett-award.html.

56. Joseph H. Burnett, "A Review of Injuries in Boston Secondary Schools," *New England Journal of Medicine* 223, no. 13 (1940): 486–89. On the expansion of highly organized youth sports, see Jack W. Berryman, "From the Cradle to the Playing Field: America's Emphasis on Highly Organized Competitive Sports for Preadolescent Boys," *JSH* 2 (1976): 112–31.

57. Burnett, "A Review of Injuries," 489.

58. James J. Daly, "Treatment of Athletes," *California Medicine* 88, no. 6 (1958): 441–42.

59. Thorndike, "Prevention of Injury in Athletics."

60. Thorndike, "Prevention of Injury in Athletics," 1128.

61. Clark Shaughnessy, "The Football Coach and the Team Physician," *Journal of the American College Health Association* 15, no. 2 (1966): 113–20.

62. Rodney Atsatt, "The High School Football Team Physician," *California Medicine* 87, no. 4 (1957): 263–65.

63. Atsatt, "The High School Football Team Physician," 263.

64. Allan J. Ryan, "The A.M.A. and Sports Injuries," *JAMA* 162, no. 12 (1956): 1160–61.

65. Clyde Snyder, "Hard but Safe-Hitting Midget Grid Lines Bring Cheers from Parents," *LAT*, November 17, 1957.

66. Snyder, "Hard but Safe-Hitting," 18.

67. Fred V. Hein, "Educational Aspects of Athletics for Children," *JAMA* 168, no. 11 (1958): 1434–38.

68. Richard H. Alley Jr, "Analysis of Injuries to Southern California High School Football Players," in AMA Committee on the Medical Aspects of Sports, *Proceedings of the National Conference on Head Protection for Athletes* (Chicago: American Medical Association, 1962), 20–24.

69. "Third General Session: Reports from Workshop Sessions," Francis Murphy, M.D., presiding, *Proceedings of the National Conference on Head Protection for Athletes*, 59–62

70. Robert Dickerman, "Colts and Devils Practice Hard and Play Harder," *CDT*, October 15, 1961.

71. "Parents Ask for More School Football Coaches," *LAT*, October 9, 1956, 9.

72. Howard M. Tuckner, "Small Fry Football League on Long Island Still Growing; Supervised Program Much Safer than Sandlot Games," *NYT*, November 18, 1956, 222.

73. The concept of a technological imperative includes among its several definitions the notion of a strong faith in, focus on, and proliferation of technological approaches to address medical problems. See, for example, Bjørn Hoffmann, "Is There a Technological Imperative in Health Care," *International Journal of Technological Assessment in Health Care* 18, no. 3 (2002); 675–89; David J. Rothman, *Beginnings Count: The Technological Imperative in American Health Care* (New York: Oxford University Press, 1997).

74. James Michener, *Sports in America* (New York: Random House, 1976), 17.

75. Art Baker, "A Coach's Responsibility to His Players," *Journal of the South Carolina Medical Association* 63 (November 1967): 400–04.

76. "But each of us has received the same special blessing from our Creator by having the wonderful opportunity, responsibility and talent of working with and influencing the lives of these young people. I feel that we owe a debt to God for this special blessing. I believe we should use whatever influence we have on these young lives for the good of His Kingdom," Baker, "A Coach's Responsibility to His Players," 403.

77. Richard W. Godshall, "Junior League Football: Risks vs. Benefits," *Journal of Sports Medicine* 3, no. 3 (1975): 139–44.

Chapter Five

1. "Brain Injury Kills Pop Warner Gridder," *LAT*, October 4, 1964; Joseph Jares, "Pop Warner Football Stirs Enthusiasm, Controversy," *LAT*, November 29, 1964; Joseph Jares, "'Safety First' Stressed in Pop Warner Football," *LAT*, November 30, 1964.

2. AFCA Committee on Injuries and Fatalities, *The Thirty-Third Annual Survey of Football Fatalities, 1931–1964* (Chicago, IL: American Football Coaches Association, 1965), 17.

3. Jares, "'Safety First' Stressed in Pop Warner Football."

4. Jares, "Pop Warner Football Stirs Enthusiasm, Controversy."

5. Jares, "Pop Warner Football Stirs Enthusiasm, Controversy."

6. William F. Keefe, "Helping Hands for Peewee Sports," *Physicians Management* 54 (1965): 54–72.

7. Travis Vogan, *Keepers of the Flame: NFL Films and the Rise of Sports Media* (Urbana: University of Illinois Press, 2014).

8. Jares, "'Safety First' Stressed in Pop Warner Football."

9. John Hall, "Rising Rate of Football Deaths Indicates Safety Measures Needed," *LAT*, November 11, 1967.

10. Jares, "'Safety First' Stressed in Pop Warner Football."

11. Fred L. Allman Jr., "Competitive Sports for Boys Under Fifteen Beneficial or Harmful?" *J.M.A. Georgia* 55 (1966): 464–66.

12. Gerald Astor, "Block that Fracture! Midgets, Peewees, and Junior Peewees Give Their All," *NYT*, November 10, 1974.

13. Gerald Eskenazi, "Are Little League Sports Too Big For Children?" *NYT*, November 16, 1978.

14. Jody Homer, "Too Young For Sports? Marathons at Age 7, Football at 8—Doctors Debate Effect on Children," *Chicago Tribune*, June 5, 1983.

15. Chris Dufresne, "Can't Run From this Memory," *LAT*, August 6, 2001.

16. Kent Hannon, "Is Football Safe for Kids?" *Sports Illustrated for Kids* 8, no. 9 (September 1996), 22.

17. A. H. Steinhaus, "Boxer's Brains Swapped for Medals," *JAAHPER* 8 (1951): 12–14.

18. Thomas A. Gonzales, "Fatal Injuries in Competitive Sports," *JAMA* 146, no. 16 (1951): 1506–11.

19. Jeffrey Sammons argues that the enormous growth of the television industry rendered boxing a less attractive and necessary form of programming, with major networks cutting back on telecasts and NBC becoming the first to drop the sport in September 1960. "In 1952, 31 percent of the available audience watched boxing telecasts; by 1959 only 10.6 percent watched televised fights. Boxing's failure to keep pace with the expanding television audience made sponsorship of a prizefight a poor proposition for return on investment," Jeffrey T. Sammons, *Beyond the Ring: The Role of Boxing in American Society* (Urbana: University of Illinois Press, 1988), 174.

20. Herbert Davis Horton, *A Survey of the Safety Features of Expensive Items of Football Equipment as Used in Texas High Schools*, M.A. thesis, Southwest Texas State University, 1955, 8. Conversely, references to the ubiquity of football would later be employed in efforts to promote boxing. "Boxing is no more dangerous or cruel than football," one boxing trainer asserted in 1972, "Sissies Don't Make Very Good Boxers," *Sarasota Herald-Tribune*, July 16, 1972.

21. Mal Stevens, "It's Basically a Safe Game: Mal Stevens Sees Night Football Boosting Injuries," *Boston Globe*, September 9, 1962.

22. Marvin Allen Stevens and Winthrop Morgan Phelps, *The Control of Football Injuries* (New York: A. S. Barnes, 1933), ix.

23. Lou Little, "Teach Your Boy to Play It Safe," *Baltimore Sun*, September 26, 1954.

24. Charles Mather, "A Brief for Junior High School Football," *Scholastic Coach* 21, no. 2 (April 1952): 32–36.

25. Edward Mason, "A Parent Asks, a Coach Answers," *Athletic Journal* 38, no. 7 (March 1958): 8, 59–63.

26. Floyd R. Eastwood, "Athletic Injuries," *New England Journal of Medicine* 217 (1964): 411–13.

27. A. Ross Davis, "The Athletic Toll," *Texas Journal of Medicine* 60 (1964): 661–64.

28. "Helmets Tuned in to Aid Science," *NYT*, October 30, 1963.

29. It is unclear whether this *Los Angeles Times* article is referring to a hypothetical father, or quoting an actual unnamed father on the sidelines. Clyde Snyder, "Hard but Safe-Hitting Midget Grid Lines Bring Cheers from Parents," *LAT*, November 17, 1957.

30. David Condon and E. W. (Pat) Patten, "So Your Son Wants to Play Football!" *CDT*, September 16, 1962.

31. Kenneth S. Clarke, "Calculated Risk of Sports Fatalities," *JAMA* 197, no. 11 (1966): 172–74.

32. Metropolitan Life Insurance Company, "Competitive Sports and Their Hazards," *Statistical Bulletin of the Metropolitan Life Insurance Company* 46 (1965): 1–3. The *Statistical Bulletin* circulated Metropolitan Life Insurance Company data and health findings among policyholders and health activists. For a history of how American life insurance companies quantified risk, see Dan Bouk, *How Our Days Became Numbered: Risk and the Rise of the Statistical Individual* (Chicago: University of Chicago Press, 2015). The *Boston Globe* reported that auto racing and football had been shown to cause the largest number of deaths in competitive sports. Nonetheless, the reporter cautioned that while the statistical survey provided interesting information, "it is not possible to measure accurately the relative hazards because adequate data on the number of participants and the frequency and duration of participation is lacking." George Vass, "Auto Racing, Football Account for Most Deaths in in Sports," *Boston Globe*, January 2, 1966.

33. Jaime W. Schultz, Larry Kenney, and Andrew D. Linden, "Heat-Related Deaths in American Football: An Interdisciplinary Approach," *Sport History Review* 45, no. 2 (2014): 123–44; Milton Gross, "School Ignored Board Warning on Illegal Drills," *Boston Globe*, September 2, 1962.

34. Clarke, "Calculated Risk of Sports Fatalities," 173. To collect data on football fatalities, the AFCA relied on "the assistance of coaches, athletes, trainers, athletic directors, executive officers of state and national athletic organizations, a national newspaper clipping service, and professional associates of the researchers." Frederick O. Mueller, "Catastrophic Head Injuries in High School and Collegiate Sports," *Journal of Athletic Training* 36, no. 3 (2001): 312–15.

35. Clarke, "Calculated Risk of Sports Fatalities," 173.

36. Clarke, "Calculated Risk of Sports Fatalities," 174.

37. Tabrah writes that he computed injury frequency and severity rates for hazardous occupations according to the American Standard Method of Recording and Measuring Work Injury Experience, Code Z 16.1-1954. Frank L. Tabrah, "High School Football: Valuable Sport or Sado-Masochistic Excess?" *Hawaii Medical Journal* 3, no. 2 (1963): 106–8. See also page 23 of Blyth and Mueller's epidemiological study of high school football injuries for a discussion of Tabrah's analysis. Carl S. Blyth and Frederick O. Mueller, *An Epidemiologic Study of High School Football Injuries in North Carolina, 1968–1972* (Washington, DC: U.S. Government Printing Office, 1974), 23.

38. Tabrah, "High School Football."

39. Mather, "A Brief for Junior High School Football," 34.

40. Joseph H. Burnett, "Survey of Football Injuries in the High Schools of Massachusetts," *Journal of Health and Physical Education* 2, no. 8 (October 1931): 32–33, 50.

41. George W. Haniford, "New Body-Contact Game Offers Fewer Hazards," *Recreation* 46, no. 5 (October 1952): 303–4. American ball did not widely catch on.

42. William C. Menninger, "Recreation and Mental Health," *Recreation* 42, no. 6 (November 1948): 340–46.

43. Paul Weiss, *Sport: A Philosophic Inquiry* (Carbondale: Southern Illinois University Press, 1969), 220. While Weiss's examination of sports undoubtedly reflected numerous popular assumptions about sports and gender, academic philosophers were not impressed

by his analysis. One reviewer concluded, "He who is fond of either sport or philosophy can save himself from a thoroughly distasteful experience by avoiding Weiss's book." Joseph S. Ullian, "Sport: A Philosophic Inquiry" (review) *Journal of Philosophy* 70, no. 10 (1973): 299–301. On how beliefs about sex differences influenced the separate development of physical education programs for boys and girls in the late nineteenth and early twentieth century, see Martha Verbrugge, *Active Bodies: A History of Women's Physical Education in Twentieth-Century America* (Oxford: University of Oxford Press, 2012).

44. Mason, "A Parent Asks, A Coach Answers."

45. Joan Bescos, "Junior Grid Loop Gives Boys Boost," *LAT*, November 6, 1957. For an examination of beliefs about juvenile delinquency in the United States in the 1950s, see James Gilbert, *A Cycle of Outrage: America's Reaction to the Juvenile Delinquent in the 1950s* (Oxford: Oxford University Press, 1986).

46. James Nolan, "Athletics and Juvenile Delinquency," *Journal of Educational Sociology* 28, no. 6 (1955): 263–65.

47. Snyder, "Hard but Safe-Hitting Midget Grid Lines."

48. A. Ross Davis, "The Athletic Toll," *Texas Journal of Medicine* 60 (1964): 661–64.

49. Fred L. Allman Jr., "Competitive Sports for Boys Under Fifteen Beneficial or Harmful?" *J.M.A. Georgia* 55 (1966): 464–66. Allman likely derived the Herbert Hoover quote from a 1960 speech where Hoover accepted a gold medal award from the National Football Foundation. Hoover described sportsmanship as "the greatest teacher of morals except religion.... From true sportsmanship radiates moral inspiration to our whole nation." "Hoover Praises Sports as Teacher of Morals," *Christian Science Monitor*, December 7, 1960.

50. Condon and Patten, "So Your Son Wants to Play Football!"

51. Condon and Patten, "So Your Son Wants to Play Football!"

52. Little, "Teach Your Boy to Play It Safe."

53. Snyder, "Hard but Safe-Hitting."

54. Condon and Patten, "So Your Son Wants to Play Football!"

55. Donald B. Slocum, "The Mechanics of Football Injuries," *JAMA* 170 (1959): 1640–46.

56. Slocum, "The Mechanics of Football Injuries." In 1975, Dr. Slocum would be named "Mr. Sports Medicine" by the American Orthopedic Society for Sports Medicine. Clinton L. Compere, "Donald B. Slocum, MD: Mr. Sports Medicine of the Year," *Journal of Sports Medicine* 3, no. 5 (1975): 260.

57. Stephen E. Reid, Edward J. Helbing, Jr. and Thomas E. Helion, "Knee and Ankle Injuries in Football," *Quarterly Bulletin of the Northwestern University Medical School* 33 (1959): 250–53.

58. Slocum, "The Mechanics of Football Injuries," 1959; "Football Injuries—A Symposium," *United States Navy Medical Newsletter* 40, no. 6 (September 21, 1962): 3–10.

59. Frederick O. Mueller and Robert C. Cantu, *Football Fatalities and Catastrophic Injuries, 1931–2008* (Durham, NC: Carolina Academic Press, 2011), 12.

60. Larry Cappiello, "New Football Seasoning," *Scholastic Coach* 19, no. 9 (1950): 7, 57–59. Whether or how much players ought to be allowed to scrimmage during practice was an ongoing debate. See, for example, Bob Priestly, "Scrimmage: Yes or No," *Scholastic Coach* 22, no. 1 (1952): 16, 71.

61. Richard C. Schneider, "Serious and Fatal Neurosurgical Football Injuries," *Clinical Neurosurgery* 12 (1964): 2226–36.

62. Joseph M. Sheehan, "Football Warned of Curb on Head Blocking if Heavy Injury Toll Continues," *NYT*, October 24, 1962.

63. Richard H. Alley, "Head and Neck Injuries in High School Football," *JAMA* 188 (1964): 418–22.

64. "National Federation Meeting," *Kentucky High School Athlete* (February 1963): 1, 9 accessed March 19, 2019, https://encompass.eku.edu/athlete/86/.

65. "Sports Authorities Warn Against 'Spearing,'" *Journal of the Iowa Medical Society* 57, no. 9 (1967): 930–31.

Chapter Six

1. John Barry, "Insured Squad for Nashua High," *Daily Boston Globe*, September 16, 1931.

2. Barry, "Insured Squad for Nashua High."

3. Willard Walter Patty and Paris John Van Horn, "Athletic Insurance," *Athletic Journal* 16, no. 6 (February 1936): 38–41.

4. Fred Wittner, "Wisconsin Insures 22,560 Boys Against School Sport Injuries," *New York Herald Tribune*, March 20, 1932. See also C. Frazier Damron, *Accident Surveillance Systems for Sports* (Washington, DC: American Alliance for Health, Physical Education, and Recreation, 1977) for a discussion of how such insurance plans as Wisconsin's provided data on injuries sustained by student athletes.

5. Wittner, "Wisconsin Insures 22,560 Boys." See also Michael Loren McCormick, "An Analysis of the Arizona High School Athletic Insurance Program," Ph.D. thesis, Montana State University–Bozeman, 1970.

6. Robert Lynn Cox, *The New York State Public High School Athletic Association in Historical Perspective, 1922 to 1972*, D.P.E. thesis, Springfield College, 1973.

7. Paul W. Kearney, "What Price Football?" *The Rotarian* (October 1946): 37–38.

8. Donald R. MacArthur, "Accident Insurance in Sports," *Scholastic Coach* 20, no. 6 (February 1951): 34–36.

9. R. J. Kidd, "Athletic Benefit Plan is Adopted," *Interscholastic Leaguer* 24, no. 1 (September 1940): 1, 4.

10. For example, statistician Frederick L. Hoffman of the Prudential Life Insurance Company used the company's large data sets to conduct wide-ranging research on a variety of health and safety issues, including workplace hazards, cancer, and suicide. See Megan Wolff, "The Money Value of Risk: Life Insurance and the Transformation of American Public Health, 1896–1930," Ph.D. dissertation, Columbia University, 2011.

11. For example, as described in chapter 4, in 1948 the NFHS published simple injury counts derived from an insurance company to inform its membership of the percentage of football injuries sustained according to age. See also Damron, "Accident Surveillance Systems for Sports."

12. New York State Bureau of Physical Education, *Safety in Physical Education for Junior and Senior High School Boys* (Albany, NY: State Education Department, 1963), 1.

13. New York State Bureau of Physical Education, *Safety in Physical Education*, 22.

14. Subcommittee on Classification of Sports Injuries, Committee on the Medical Aspects of Sports, *Standard Nomenclature of Athletic Injuries* (Chicago: American Medical Association, 1966), vii.

15. Marvin McClelland, "High School Football Injuries," *JAMA* 193, no. 7 (1965): 158; William F. Garrahan, "The Incidence of High School Football Injuries," *Rhode Island Medical Journal* 50, no. 12 (1967): 833–35.

16. Garrahan, "The Incidence of High School Football Injuries." The rate of injury found in the Ohio study was 19.5 percent (550 injuries among 2,826 players) as compared to 19.9 percent in the Rhode Island study (2,191 injuries among 11,020 players).

17. Cox, *The New York State Public Health School Athletic Association in Historical Perspective.*

18. Cox, *The New York State Public High School Athletic Association in Historical Perspective*; William T. Callahan, Francis J. Crowley, J. Kenneth Hafner, *A Statewide Study Designed to Determine Methods of Reducing Injury in Interscholastic Football Competition by Equipment Modification* (Albany: New York State Public High School Athletic Association, 1969).

19. Cox, *The New York State Public High School Athletic Association*; Callahan et al., *A Statewide Study*; M. Laurens Rowe, "1968 Varsity Football Knee and Ankle Study," in *Second Annual Symposium on the Medical Aspects of Sports*, New York, February 8, 1969, 57–63; Murle Laurens Rowe, "Varsity Football Knee and Ankle Injury," *New York State Journal of Medicine* 69, no. 23 (1969): 3000–3003.

20. Callahan et al., *A Statewide Study*, 1.

21. Callahan et al., *A Statewide Study*, 43.

22. Callahan et al., *A Statewide Study*, 43.

23. M. Laurens Rowe, "The Cleatless Heel," in *Medical Aspects of Sports: A Symposium Sponsored by the Medical Society of the State of New York on the Medical Aspects of Sports*, New York, February 10, 1968, 4–6.

24. Anthony J. Pisani, "Anatomy with Reference to the Mechanics of Injury," in *Medical Aspects of Sports: A Symposium*, 1–3. After ten years with the New York Giants, Pisani would retire from working for the NFL team one month before being named in a 40-count indictment issued against two bookmakers involved in a $26 million/year gambling operation. While Pisani would never be charged, his involvement led a *New York Times* writer to reflect that team physicians, "like players and fans, are only human." Neil Amdur, "Once More, Doc, with Feeling," *NYT*, August 22, 1974; "Giants' Ex-Doctor Tied to Bookies in a Conspiracy," *NYT*, August 21, 1974.

25. Arturo Gonzalez, "The Pain Behind the Paycheck in Pro Football," *Chicago Tribune*, June 9, 1968.

26. "Use of Helmets Rapped by Doctor," *LAT*, January 9, 1969.

27. Edward B. Becker, "Helmet Development and Standards," in *Frontiers in Head and Neck Trauma: Clinical and Biomedical*, ed. Narayan Yoganandan et al. (Amsterdam: IOS Press, 1998), 113–30; Edward B. Becker, "The Snell Memorial Foundation, Past and Present," *Motorcycle Safety Foundation*, February 7, 2001, accessed March 19, 2019, http://www.msf-usa.org/downloads/imsc2001/Becker.pdf.

28. George G. Snively, Charles Kovacic, and C. O. Chichester, "Design of Football Helmets," *Research Quarterly* 32, no. 2 (1961): 221–28; Edward B. Becker, "Helmet Development and Standards," in *Frontiers in Head and Neck Trauma: Clinical and Biomedical*, ed. Narayan Yoganandan et al. (Amsterdam: IOS Press, 1998): 113–30, Becker, "The Snell Memorial Foundation, Past and Present." See also George G. Snively, "Skull Busting for Safety," *Sports Car Illustrated* (July 1957): 22.

29. Harold A. Fenner Jr., "Football Injuries and Helmet Design," *General Practice* 30, no. 4 (1964): 106–13; "Fenner: Doctor Helped Develop Safer Football Helmets," *Albuquerque Journal*, May 4, 2011, accessed March 19, 2019, http://www.abqjournal.com/obits/profiles /042133249981obitsprofiles05-04-11.htm.

30. Fenner, "Football Injuries and Helmet Design," 112.

31. Richard C. Schneider and Bartley E. Antine, "Visual-Field Impairment Related to Football Headgear and Face Guards," *JAMA* 17, no. 192 (1965): 616–18.

32. "Conference Planning Committee," *National Conference on Protective Equipment in Sports*, University of Wisconsin, Madison, June 14–16, 1968, ii.

33. "Introduction," *National Conference on Protective Equipment in Sports*, 1.

34. Allan J. Ryan, "What Injuries in Sports Can Be Prevented by the Use of Protective Equipment," *National Conference on Protective Equipment in Sports*, 4–16.

35. "Recommendations of the Conference," *National Conference on Protective Equipment in Sports*, 75–85.

36. James M. Robey, Carl S. Blythe, and Frederick O. Mueller, "Athletic Injuries: Application of Epidemiologic Methods," *JAMA* 217, no. 2 (1971): 184–85.

37. James M. Robey, "Contribution of Design and Construction of Football Helmets to the Occurrence of Injuries," *Medicine and Science in Sports* 4, no. 3 (1972): 170–74.

38. Kyle Graham, "Strict Products Liability at 50: Four Histories," *Marquette Law Review* 98, no. 2 (2014): 555–24.

39. William L. Prosser, "The Fall of the Citadel (Strict Liability to the Consumer)," *Minnesota Law Review* 50 (1966): 791–848; Aaron Gershonowitz, "The Strict Liability Duty to Warn," *Washington and Lee Law Review* 44, no. 1 (1987): 71–107; Kenneth S. Abraham, *The Liability Century: Insurance and Tort Law from the Progressive Era to 9/11* (Cambridge, MA: Harvard University Press, 2008).

40. Prosser, "The Fall of the Citadel," 793–94; Abraham, *The Liability Century*, 146. On the limits of such legal changes and regulatory reform to address the fundamental reality that the physical risks of defective products first materialize "on the bodies and lives of individuals," see Barbara Young Welke, "The Cowboy Suit Tragedy: Spreading Risk, Owning Hazard in the Modern America Consumer Economy," *Journal of American History* 101 (2014): 97–121.

41. Amy Beth Gangloff, "Medicalizing the Automobile: Public Health, Safety, and American Culture, 1920–1967," Ph.D. dissertation, State University of New York at Stony Brook, 2006; Julian A. Waller, "Reflections on a Half Century of Injury Control," *AJPH* 84, no. 4 (2004): 664–70; Jerry L. Mashaw and David L. Harfst, "Regulation and Legal Culture: The Case of Motor Vehicle Safety," *Yale Journal on Regulation* 4 (1987): 257–316.

42. "It was our expectation, of course, that the commission's deliberations would lead inexorably to a legislative proposal for the creation of a permanent consumer product safety commission, with full authority to set product safety standards and to order recalls. . . . Since Morton Mintz sought, and was assigned by the *Washington Post*, to follow the commission from city to city, the hearings and revelations were assured not only of intense regional coverage and interest, but of a national (i.e., Washington, D.C.) audience as well." Michael Pertschuk, *Revolt Against Regulation: The Rise and Pause of the Consumer Movement* (Berkeley: University of California Press, 1982), 41–43. Senator Magnuson, himself a cigar smoker, was also notably involved in efforts to stop tobacco companies from

marketing their products to children. See Shelby Scates, *Warren G. Magnuson and the Shaping of Twentieth-Century America* (Seattle: University of Washington Press, 1997).

43. "Statement of Larry Csonka," *National Commission on Product Safety Hearings, Washington, Jan-Feb 1969* (New York: Law-Arts Publishers, 1970), 391–94.

44. "Statement of Thomas R. McClelland" and "Statement of Mrs. Dorothy McClelland," *National Commission on Product Safety Hearings*, 394–96.

45. "Statement of Mr. Harry M. Philo," *National Commission on Product Safety Hearings, Washington*, 396–401; American Association for Justice, "Remembering Harry M. Philo, 1924–2012," American Association for Justice, accessed March 19, 2019, https://www.justice.org/membership/memoriam/remembering-harry-m-philo-1924-2012.

46. "Statement of Mr. Harry M. Philo," *National Commission on Product Safety Hearings*, 413; Morton Mintz, "Hill Witnesses Rap Helmet Makers for Huge Injury Toll," *WP*, February 19, 1969; Arthur L. Dickinson, "The Incidence of Graded Cerebral Concussions Sustained by Athletes Participating in Intercollegiate Football," *Journal of the National Athletic Trainers Association* 2, no. 2 (Summer 1967): 14–15.

47. "Statement of David Rust," *National Commission on Product Safety Hearings*, 430.

48. "Statement of David Rust." See also Morton Mintz, "Hill Witnesses Rap Helmet Makers."

49. Joshua Eilberg, "Statement of Hon. Joshua Eilberg, a Representative in Congress from the State of Pennsylvania," National Commission on Product Safety Extension and Child Protection Act: Hearings Before the Subcommittee on Commerce and Finance of the Committee on Interstate and Foreign Commerce, House of Representatives, Ninety-First Congress, first session, May 20 and 22, 1969, 93.

50. The sixteen categories of products highlighted in the final report as including unreasonably hazardous models or types were "architectural glass, color television sets, fireworks, floor furnaces, glass bottles, high-rise bicycles, hot-water vaporizers, household chemicals, infant furniture, ladders, power tools, protective headgear, rotary lawnmowers, toys, unvented gas heaters, and wringer washers." *National Commission on Product Safety: Final Report Presented to the President and Congress, June 1970* (Washington, DC: U.S. Government Printing Office, 1970), 1; Jules Witcover, "Panel Details Perils of 16 Home Products," *LAT*, June 29, 1970.

51. *National Commission on Product Safety: Final Report*, 28.

52. Jules Witcover, "Commission Warns of Product Hazards," *LAT*, June 24, 1970; "Excerpts from Product Safety Report," *WP*, June 24, 1970; Witcover, "Panel Details Perils."

53. Pub. Law No. 92-573 (October 28, 1972); Antonin Scalia and Frank Goodman, "Procedural Aspects of the Consumer Product Safety Act," *UCLA Law Review* 20 (1973): 899–953; Carl Tobias, "Revitalizing the Consumer Product Safety Commission," *Montana Law Review* 50, no. 2 (1989): 237–41; Robert S. Adler, "From 'Model Agency' to Basket Case—Can the Consumer Product Safety Commission be Redeemed?" *Administrative Law Review* 41, no. 1 (1989): 61–129.

54. Susan P. Baker and William Haddon Jr., "Reducing Injuries and Their Results: The Scientific Approach," *Milbank Memorial Fund Quarterly, Health and Society* 52, no. 4 (1974): 377–89; Division of Hazard and Injury Systems, "NEISS: The National Electronic Surveillance System: A Tool for Researchers," U.S. CPSC (March 2000), accessed March 19, 2019, https://www.cpsc.gov//PageFiles/106626/2000d015.pdf; U.S. CPSC, *Together We Can Reduce Injury* (Washington, DC: U.S. CPSC, 1975).

55. U.S. CPSC, *Hazard Analysis: Football: Activity and Related Equipment* [NIIC 1211-74 H010] (Washington, DC: Bureau of Epidemiology, 1974), 6.

56. U.S. CPSC, *Hazard Analysis: Football*, 20.

57. U.S. CPSC, *Hazard Analysis: Football*, 16.

Chapter Seven

1. Condolences guest book, "Ernest Wayne 'Ernie' Pelton," *Sacramento Bee* obituary, September 20, 2017, accessed March 11, 2019, http://www.legacy.com/guestbooks/sacbee/ernest-wayne-pelton-ernie-condolences/94511474.

2. Melody Guttierez, "Football Horror from 1967 Still Haunts Family," *Sacramento Bee*, November 28, 2007.

3. Guttierez, "Football Horror"; Melody Guttierez, "A Tragic Injury Brings Change: Family Lost Suit but Spurred Era of Safer Football Gear," *Sacramento Bee*, November 29, 2007; "Victory, but Equipment Improvement Still Sought," *NCAA News* 7, no. 10 (November 1970): 3; Morton Mintz, "Hill Witnesses Rap Helmet Makers for Huge Injury Toll," *WP*, February 19, 1969; "Jury Clears Company in Head Injury Case," *Interscholastic Leaguer*, November 1970, accessed March 19, 2019, http://www.uiltexas.org/files/leaguer/leaguer-archives/LE-1970-11.pdf.

4. "Statement of Dr. George G. Snively, M.D.," *National Commission on Product Safety Hearings, Washington, Jan-Feb 1969* (New York: Law-Arts Publishers: 1970), 438–42; Edward B. Becker, "Helmet Development and Standards," in *Frontiers in Head and Neck Trauma: Clinical and Biomedical*, ed. Narayan Yoganandan et al. (Amsterdam: IOS Press, 1998): 113–30.; American National Standards Institute, "1918–2008: ANSI: An Historical Overview," *ANSI Public Document Library*, accessed March 19, 2019, http://publicaa.ansi.org/sites/apdl/Documents/News%20and%20Publications/Links%20Within%20Stories/ANSI%20-%20A%20Historical%20Overview.pdf; Edward B. Becker, "The Snell Memorial Foundation, Past and Present," *Motorcycle Safety Foundation*, February 7, 2001, accessed March 19, 2019, http://www.msf-usa.org/downloads/imsc2001/Becker.pdf.

5. "Statement of Dr. George G. Snively, M.D.," 441.

6. ASTM, "Football Injury Conference Called for November," *Materials Research and Standards* 8, no. 10 (October 1968): 26–27; Becker, "Helmet Development and Standards."

7. ASTM, "Football Injury Conference Called for November," 26–27.

8. ASTM, "New Technical Committees: What They Are and What They Do," *Materials Research and Standards* 9, no. 10 (October 1969): n.p., center insert; ASTM, "Dr. Creighton J. Hale Named Chairman of Protective Sports Equipment Committee," *Materials Research and Standards* 9, no. 12 (December 1969): 40; William F. Hulse, "Sports Equipment Standards," in *Sports Injuries: The Unthwarted Epidemic*, ed. Paul F. Vinger and Earl F. Hoerner (Littleton, MA: PSG, 1981): 378–82. Committee F-8 held its first meeting on September 15–16, 1969, at ASTM headquarters in Philadelphia.

9. ASTM, "ASTM Newsfront," *Materials Research and Standards* 9, no. 9 (September 1969): 5; Hulse, "Sports Equipment Standards."

10. Creighton J. Hale, "Significant Trends and Complex Barriers in the Engineering of Protective Sports Equipment," *Materials Research and Standards* 11; 10 (October 1971): 8–12.

11. "Doctors Plan Defense to Stop Injuries," *The Journal* [Ogdensburg, NY], September 9, 1971; Hale, "Significant Trends and Complex Barriers."

12. "Activities subcommittees focus on individual sports—namely, football, gymnastics, wrestling, fencing, skiing, and hockey. Resource subcommittees address medical aspects and biomechanics, playing surfaces and facilities, headgear, footwear, padding, and apparel." "Female Athletes Seek Equal Time on Committee F-8," *ASTM Standardization News* 4, no. 9 (September 1976): 29. See also Hulse, "Sports Equipment Standards."

13. J. Nadine Gelberg, "The Lethal Weapon: How the Plastic Football Helmet Transformed the Game of Football, 1939–1994," *Bulletin of Science, Technology & Society* 15, no. 5–6 (1995): 302–9.

14. "Round Table Discussion: Standards for Sports Equipment and Facilities," *Proceedings of the Second National Sports Safety Conference, Chicago, IL, October 15–17, 1976* (Washington, DC: American Alliance for Health, Physical Education, and Recreation: 1977), 105–7; William F. Hulse, "ASTM—F-8 Committee on Sports Equipment and Facilities," *Proceedings of the Second National Sports Safety Conference*, 97–101.

15. Hulse, "ASTM—F-8 Committee," 99.

16. "Kenneth S. Clarke, "Epidemiology of Athletic Head Injury," *Clinics in Sports Medicine* 17, no. 1 (1998): 1–12.

17. "Victory, But Equipment Improvement Still Sought," 3.

18. "Victory, But Equipment Improvement Still Sought," 3.

19. "Victory, But Equipment Improvement Still Sought," 3.

20. "Committee to Set Equipment Standards Is Created," *NCAA News* 7, no. 6 (June 1970): 5.

21. Elmer A. Blasco, "What Every Football Coach Should Know About NOCSAE and Football Helmets," *Athletic Journal* 61, no. 10 (1981): 63. Blasco had worked for Rawlings in the 1950s, and later served as publisher of several sports-related magazines, including *Athletic Journal*. Graydon Megan, "Inventor of Gold Glove Award Dies," *Chicago Tribune*, August 11, 2008, accessed March 19, 2019, http://articles.chicagotribune.com/2008-08-11 /news/0808100291_1_gold-glove-award-first-award-major-league-baseball.

22. Frederick O. Mueller and Robert C. Cantu, *Football Fatalities and Catastrophic Injuries, 1931–2008* (Durham, NC: Carolina Academic Press, 2011).

23. Gary Delforge, "The Professional Services Division: What Is It Doing for You?" *Journal of the National Athletic Trainers Association* 6, no. 4 (1971): 176–78; Voigt R. Hodgson, "National Operating Committee on Standards for Athletic Equipment Football Helmet Certification Program," *Medicine and Science in Sports* 7, no. 3 (1975): 225–32; Charles Gadd, "Tolerable Severity Index in Whole-Head, Nonmechanical Impact," in *15th Stapp Car Crash Conference Proceedings*, Coronado, CA, November 17–19, 1971, 809–16.

24. On the critiques of using head impact criteria based on translational motion, as well as a review of biomechanical research on skull/brain injury tolerance from 1960–1980, and how these research findings were used in the context of motor vehicle safety, see Robert L. Hess, Kathleen Weber, and John W. Melvin, "Review of Literature and Regulation Relating to Head Impact Tolerance and Injury Criteria" (Ann Arbor: University of Michigan Highway Safety Research Institute, 1980). See also Arthur E. Hirsch and Ayub K. Ommaya, "Protection from Brain Injury: The Relative Significance of Translational and Rotational Motions of the Head after Impact," (SAE Technical Paper 700899)

in *14th Stapp Car Crash Conference Proceedings*, Ann Arbor, MI, November 17–18, 1970, 144–51.

25. Hodgson, "National Operating Committee on Standards for Athletic Equipment."

26. "Question and Answer Period," *Proceedings of the Second National Sports Safety Conference*, 101–4.

27. NFHS, "NOCSAE Questions and Answers: Certification, Recertification and Reconditioning," *Kentucky High School Athlete* (November 1979): 6, accessed March 19, 2019, https://encompass.eku.edu/athlete/249/.

28. "Question and Answer Period," *Proceedings of the Second National Sports Safety Conference*: 102.

29. Voigt R. Hodgson, "Here Is What NOCSAE is Doing in Its Helmet Standards Program," *Athletic Purchasing & Facilities* 1 (August 1977): 27–28.

30. G. Rex Bryce and Ruel M. Barker, "Variability and Sampling Inspection in the NOCSAE Standards for Football Helmets," *Research Quarterly for Exercise and Sport* 55, no. 2 (1984): 103–8.

31. James Brady, "Gleisner Was a True Icon," *Morning Journal*, February 11, 2012, accessed March 19, 2019, http://www.morningjournal.com/general-news/20120211/gleisner-was-a-true-icon; Grant Segall, "Don Gleisner Starred in Football and Championed Safer Helmets: News Obituary," *Cleveland Plain Dealer*, February 6, 2012, accessed March 19, 2019, http://www.cleveland.com/obituaries/index.ssf/2012/02/post_52.html.

32. Bryce and Barker, "Variability and Sampling Inspection," 107.

33. Harry M. Philo and Gregory Stine, "The Liability Path to Safer Helmets," *Trial* 13 (1977): 38–40.

34. John Friend, "Sport Opinion: Prep Football Surviving," *Chicago Tribune*, August 5, 1979; Marvin's Sport City advertisement, "Special Football Sale," *WP*, August 16, 1979; Michael Sperling, "Uniforming a Football Team is Complex, Costly Procedure," *WP*, August 16, 1984.

35. Joe Gieck and Frank C. McCue III, "Fitting of Protective Football Equipment," *American Journal of Sports Medicine* 8, no. 3 (1980): 192–96.

36. Blasco, "What Every Football Coach Should Know," 63.

37. A. Ross Davis, "The Athletic Toll," *Texas Journal of Medicine* 60 (1964): 661–64.

38. On the assumption of risk, see the *Restatement of Torts (Second)* section 496A cmt. c (1977).; Alexander J. Drago, "Assumption of Risk: An Age-Old Defense Still Viable in Sports and Recreation," *Fordham Intellectual Property, Media and Entertainment Law Journal* 12, no. 2 (2002): 583–608.

39. Patrick K. Thornton, Walter T. Champion Jr., and Lawrence S. Ruddell, *Sports Ethics for Sports Management Professionals* (Sudbury, MA: Jones & Bartlett Learning, 2012): 136.

40. *Vendrell v. School District No. 26C, Malheur County*, 376 P.2d 406, 412–13 (Or. 1962). See also Eric F. Quandt, Matthew J. Mitten, and John S. Black, "Legal Liability in Covering Athletic Events," *Sports Health* 1, no. 1 (2009): 84–90.

41. *Vendrell v. School District No. 26C*.

42. *Whipple v. Salvation Army*, 495 P.2d 739 (Oregon 1972). For a brief discussion of this case, see Herbert Thomas Appenzeller, *An Analysis of Court Decisions Involving Injuries to Participants and Spectators in Youth Sport Activities* (Greensboro: University of North Carolina, 1988): 37–38.

43. Samuel Langerman, "Contact Sports Injury Cases," *American Jurisprudence Trials* 7 (1964): 213–78. For more on the relevance of charitable immunity and sovereign immunity to American sports law, see Chapter 4, "Application of Tort Law to Sports," in Glenn M. Wong, *Essentials of Sports Law*, 4th ed. (Santa Barbara, CA: ABC-CLIO, 2010), 105–55.

44. Samuel Langerman and Noel Fidel, "Responsibility Is Also Part of the Game," *Trial* 13, no. 1 (1977): 22–25.

45. Langerman and Fidel, "Responsibility Is Also Part of the Game," 25.

46. David Rosner and Gerald Markowitz, "'Educate the Individual . . . to a Sane Appreciation of the Risk': A History of Industry's Responsibility to Warn of Job Dangers Before the Occupational Safety and Health Administration," *AJPH* 106, no. 1 (2016): 28–35. On how new financial practices in the nineteenth and twentieth century United States converted various hazards into "risk-taking" as an economic phenomenon, see Jonathan Levy, *Freaks of Fortune: The Emerging World of Capitalism and Risk in America* (Cambridge, MA: Harvard University Press, 2012).

47. The Athletic Institute, *Coaching Pop Warner: A Reference Manual to the Basics of the Game of Football for Pop Warner Coaches* (Chicago: Athletic Institute, 1974), 12. On the distinction between the duty to warn and the duty to design a safe product, see Aaron Gershonowitz, "The Strict Liability Duty to Warn," *Washington and Lee Law Review* 44, no. 1 (1987): 71–107.

48. Samuel H. Adams and Mary Ann Bayless, "Helping Your Coaches Understand Their Role in Preventing Injuries," *Athletic Purchasing & Facilities* (January 1983): 18–22; "Football Player Wins $6 Million Suit," *Chicago Tribune*, February 13, 1982; Byron Rosen, "Jury in Seattle Trims Award to $6,316,000," *WP*, February 13, 1982; Sharon Huddleston, "The Coach's Legal Duty to Properly Instruct and to Warn Athletes of the Inherent Dangers in Sport," in *Sports and the Law: Major Legal Cases*, ed. Charles E. Quirk (New York: Garland, 1996), 14–17.

49. Adams and Bayless, "Helping Your Coaches Understand Their Role," 18–19; Appenzeller, *An Analysis of Court Decisions*.

50. "Protect the Children, Protect Your Program," *Athletic Business* (March 1986): 12–18.

51. Tracy Dodds, "Helmet Makers Look for Some Protection," *LAT*, June 13, 1982; Adams and Bayless, "Helping Your Coaches Understand Their Role."

52. "Football Rule Changes Announced for '86 Season," *Kentucky High School Athlete* (February 1986): 4, accessed March 19, 2019, https://encompass.eku.edu/athlete/315/. See also NFHS, "NFHS Rules Changes Affecting Risk (1982–2011)," available at http://www.nfhs.org, accessed March 19, 2019.

53. Thomas Appenzeller, interviewed by author, December 14, 2014.

54. *Rawlings Sporting Goods Co., Inc. v. Daniels*, 619 S.W.2d 435 (Tex.Civ.App.1981); William L. Siler, "In Jeopardy: Football Helmet Manufacturers and Wearers," in *Sports and the Law: Major Legal Cases*, 8–10.

55. "Helmet Maker Must Pay $5.3m to Injured Player," *Boston Globe*, December 12, 1975; David Dupree, "Sports Equipment on Trial," *WP*, December 31, 1977.

56. "Sports People; Damaging Lawsuits," *NYT*, December 9, 1984, accessed March 19, 2019, http://www.nytimes.com/1984/12/09/sports/sports-people-damaging-lawsuits.html. For more on the trend in products liability cases beginning in the mid-1970s toward imposing liability for harm on manufacturers, see James A. Henderson Jr. and Theodore Eisenberg,

"The Quiet Revolution in Products Liability: An Empirical Study of Legal Change," *UCLA Law Review* 37 (1990): 479–553.

57. *Proceedings of the MAAC Liability Reform Conference*, Washington, D.C., September 7–8, 1976. Sponsored by SGMA; publisher not identified. MAAC was later renamed Product Liability Sports (PLS). See SGMA, *A Commemorative Report: A Historical Reflection of the U.S. Sporting Goods Industry's Growth and Development in the 20ᵗʰ Century* (North Palm Beach, FL: SGMA, 2006), 11.

58. Howard J. Bruns, "Statement on Product Liability," *Proceedings of the MAAC Liability Reform Conference*, 95–97.

59. Howard J. Bruns, "Testimony for Select Committee on Small Business, U.S. Senate," *Proceedings of the MAAC Liability Reform Conference*, 20–23; John Husar, "Liability Suits Threaten Helmet Makers," *Chicago Tribune*, June 5, 1977. Bruns would repeatedly return to the claim that football and competitive sports generally were under threat of extinction. In 1982, he told the *Journal of Commerce*, "If we don't get tort reform, we are going to see the elimination of football and other sports activities." Susan Fass, "Helmet Liability Costs Threaten Football's Future," *Journal of Commerce*, November 3, 1982.

60. Husar, "Liability Suits Threaten Helmet Makers"; Jean Tally, "Reward for Increasing Football Helmet Safety? Legal Hassles," *Physician and Sportsmedicine* 13, no. 2 (1985): 161–68; Adele Lubell, "Insurance, Liability, and the American Way of Sport," *Physician and Sportsmedicine* 15, no. 9 (1987): 192–200.

61. Terry Morehead Dworkin, "Product Liability Reform and the Model Uniform Product Liability Act," *Nebraska Law Review* 60, no. 1 (1981): 50–80; Victor E. Schwartz and Mark A. Behrens, "The Road to Federal Product Liability Reform," *Maryland Law Review* 55, no. 4 (1996): 1363–83.

62. "The New Insurance Crisis," *WP*, February 24, 1977.

63. Letter from William C. Merritt to Mr. Cameron, "Re: *Stead v. Riddell, Inc.*, Claim No.: 010787 267 71 55, D/A: September 30, 1971, our file No.: 75-252 WCM," in *Product Liability Insurance Hearings Before the Subcommittee for Consumers of the Committee on Commerce, Science, and Transportation*, United States Senate, Ninety-Fifth Congress, first session, on S. 403, April 27, 28, and 29, 1977, 406–13.

64. Letter from William C. Merritt to Mr. Cameron, "Re: *Stead v. Riddell, Inc.*"; Patricia Elich, "Butting Heads: Miami Lawyer Carl Rentz Tackles the Country's Biggest Helmet Manufacturer," *South Florida Sun-Sentinel*, February 16, 1987, accessed March 19, 2019, http://articles.sun-sentinel.com/1987-02-16/news/8701100894_1_riddell-helmet-miami-lawyer.

65. John Husar, "Liability Suits Threaten Helmet Makers"; Shea Sullivan, "Football Helmet Product Liability: A Survey of Cases and Call for Reform," *Sports Lawyers Journal* 3 (1996): 233–60; John Underwood, "An Unfolding Tragedy," *SI*, August 14, 1978, https://www.si.com/vault/1978/08/14/822885/an-unfolding-tragedy-as-football-injuries-mount-lawsuits-increase-and-insurance-rates-soar-the-game-is-headed-toward-a-crisis-one-that-is-epitomized-by-the-helmet-which-is-both-a-barbarous-weapon-and-inadequate-protection; Bill Sing, "Helmet Making Perilous as Football," *LAT*, October 8, 1979; Mark Potts, "Helmet Makers Clipped by Insurance Costs," *WP*, March 10, 1987.

66. Tamar Lewin, "The Liability Insurance Spiral," *NYT*, March 8, 1986.

67. Sing, "Helmet Making Perilous as Football."

68. Theodore Eisenberg and James A. Henderson Jr., "Inside the Quiet Revolution in Products Liability," *UCLA Law Review* 37 (1992): 731–810. See table A-10 for changes in plaintiff success rate in published opinions by product category.

69. John H. Knowles, "The Responsibility of the Individual," *Daedalus* 106, no. 1 (1977): 57–80.

70. Richard Feldman, *Ricochet: Confessions of a Gun Lobbyist* (Hoboken, NJ: Wiley, 2007), 136; "Statement of the Sporting Goods Manufacturers Association," *Product Liability Reform Act: Hearings Before the Subcommittee on the Consumer of the Committee on Commerce, Science, and Transportation*, United States Senate, One Hundred and First Congress, second session, on S. 1400, February 22, April 5, and May 10, 1990, 595–97.

71. Sharon M. Lincoln, "Sports Injury Risk Management & the Keys to Safety," *Journal of Physical Education, Recreation & Dance* 63, no. 7 (1992): 40–42, 63.

72. Lincoln, "Sports Injury Risk Management."

73. Some industry front groups promoting personal responsibility are associated with both the tobacco and fast-food industries. For example, the tobacco industry originally funded the Center for Consumer Freedom to lobby against public smoking restrictions, but this D.C.-based lobbying group evolved to advocate for food and sugar-sweetened beverage manufacturers. See Lissy C. Friedman, Andrew Cheyne, Daniel Givelber, Mark A. Gottlieb, and Richard A. Daynard, "Tobacco Industry Use of Personal Responsibility Rhetoric in Public Relations and Litigation: Disguising Freedom to Blame as Freedom of Choice," *AJPH* 105, no. 2 (2015): 250–60.

74. Mike Reilley, "Players' Safety Costly Aspect for Programs," *LAT*, September 19, 1990.

Chapter Eight

1. Henry Steele Commager, "A Historian Looks at the American High School," *School Review* 66 (Spring 1958): 1–18.

2. Commager, "A Historian Looks at the American High School," 10–11.

3. Paul J. Zbiek, "The Importance of High School Sports in Northeastern Pennsylvania: Scholastic Football in the Wyoming Valley," in *The History of Northeastern Pennsylvania: The Last 100 Years* (Nanticoke, PA: Luzerne County Community College, 1989), 24–41; Gerhard Falk, *Football and American Identity* (New York: Haworth, 2005), 31.

4. The tradition of presenting male newborn babies in Massillon with footballs persisted and is featured in the 2001 documentary *Go Tigers!* that examines both the town and its football team. See Michael Oriard, "Go Tigers!" [review] *JSH* 30, no. 1 (2003): 139–43.

5. Walter Bingham, "Football from the Cradle," *SI*, November 13, 1961.

6. Bingham, "Football from the Cradle."

7. Carl K. Benhase, *Ohio High School Football* (West Nyack, NY: Parker, 1967), 185.

8. Geoff Winningham and Al Reinert, *Rites of Fall: High School Football in Texas* (Austin: University of Texas Press, 1979), 8.

9. Benhase, *Ohio High School Football*, 82.

10. Benhase, *Ohio High School Football*.

11. Mark Kauffman (photographer), "Rocky Cradle of Football," *Life*, November 2, 1962; John R. McDermott, "Rule One: Win or Else," *Life*, November 2, 1962.

12. Robert "Bubba" Kapral, "LIFE in the Mill Towns: Magazine Paints Eastern Ohio in Negative Light," *Martins Ferry Times Leader*, November 2, 2012. Accessed December 31, 2015 at http://www.timesleaderonline.com/news/local-news/2012/11/life-in-the-mill-towns/.

13. John Laslo, "Re: Rocky Cradle of Football," letter to the editor, *Life*, November 23, 1962; John C. Vargo, "Re: Rocky Cradle of Football," letter to the editor, *Life*, November 23, 1962.

14. Taylor H. A. Bell, *Dusty, Deek, and Mr. Do-Right: High School Football in Illinois* (Urbana: University of Illinois Press, 2010), 176.

15. Bell, *Dusty, Deek, and Mr. Do-Right*, 179.

16. H. G. Bissinger, *Friday Night Lights: A Town, a Team, and a Dream* (New York: HarperPerennial, 1991), 20.

17. Benhase, *Ohio High School Football*, 191.

18. Benhase, *Ohio High School Football*, 49. Ron Jones served as the head football, basketball, baseball, and track coach at Piketon High School until 1969 and was inducted into the Ohio Interscholastic Athletic Administrators Association Hall of Fame in 1990. "Hall of Fame," Otterbein University Athletics, accessed March 19, 2019, http://otterbeincardinals.com/hof.aspx?hof=28. Coach Tony Mason arrived in Niles, Ohio, in 1958 and remained there as head coach for six years. He would later serve as head coach at the University of Cincinnati and the University of Arizona. Corky Simpson, "Mason Never Quite the Same After His Tucson Experience," *Tucson Citizen*, July 25, 1994; Steve Ruman, "Mason, Staff Kept Red Dragons Going Despite Graduation Losses," *The Vindicator* [Youngstown, Ohio], August 25, 2013, accessed March 19, 2019, http://www.vindy.com/news/2013/aug/25/mason-staff-kept-red-dragons-going-despi/.

19. Ellsworth Tompkins and Virginia Roe, *A Survey of Interscholastic Athletic Programs in Separately Organized Junior High Schools; A Project of the NASSP Committee on Junior High-School Education* (Washington, DC: National Association of Secondary-School Principals, 1958).

20. Tompkins and Roe, *A Survey of Interscholastic Athletic Programs*, 34.

21. Joint Committee on Standards for Interscholastic Athletics, *Standards for Junior High School Athletics; Report of the Junior High School Athletics Subcommittee of the Joint Committee on Standards for Interscholastic Athletics* (Washington: AAHPER, 1963), 18.

22. Bell, *Dusty, Deek, and Mr. Do-Right*, 178.

23. Bob Reade, *Coaching Football Successfully* (Champaign, IL: Human Kinetics, 1994), 37. In 2011, Penn State dismissed Joe Paterno following the arrest of Jerry Sandusky, a former assistant football coach who was accused and subsequently convicted of sexually abusing multiple children. Mark Viera, "Paterno Is Finished at Penn State, and President Is Out," *NYT*, November 9, 2011, accessed March 19, 2019, http://www.nytimes.com/2011/11/10/sports/ncaafootball/-joe-paterno-and-graham-spanier-out-at-penn-state.html. See also Ronald A. Smith, *Wounded Lions: Joe Paterno, Jerry Sandusky, and the Crises in Penn State Athletics* (Urbana: University of Illinois Press, 2016).

24. Interview with Robert Carr by Alan P. Peppard, May 19, 1967, in Alan P. Peppard, *The Status of Programs for the Care and Prevention of Athletic Injuries in Schools Within a Geographic Region of the New York State Public Health School Athletic Association*, M.S. thesis, University of Massachusetts, 1969, 81–102.

25. Richard Edward Stuetz, *An Evaluation of the Educational Values of Pop Warner Football with Reference to the General Objectives of Secondary Education*, M.A. thesis, Chapman College, 1969, 11.

26. Stuetz, *An Evaluation of the Educational Values*, 36.

27. Stuetz, *An Evaluation of the Educational Values*, 34, 48.

28. "Indians Celebrate 40th Year," *The Reporter* [Upper Merion Area School District] (March 1995): 15; "30 Years on the Reservation" (n.d., estimated 1986), Dave and Mary Vannicelli Collection, KPHS, King of Prussia, PA; Sandy Vannicelli, interviewed by author, February 15, 2015.

29. Sandy Vannicelli, interviewed by author, February 15, 2015.

30. "30 Years on the Reservation"; Francis J. Rubert, Ann R. Shronk, and Mary P. Vannicelli, "Articles of Incorporation: King of Prussia Football Association," November 19, 1963, Dave and Mary Vannicelli Collection. The Dave and Mary Vannicelli Collection is full of newspaper clippings dating as early as the 1960s; see, for instance, "Indian 85s Win by 13–7 Against Warrington Club," *Philadelphia Evening Bulletin*, October 3, 1963.

31. Letter, David E. Vannicelli to Mr. John D. Scott, National Pop Warner Office, Philadelphia Athletic Club, August 23, 1964, Dave and Mary Vannicelli Collection.

32. "Constitution of the King of Prussia Football Association, Inc.," May 4, 1976, page 1, Dave and Mary Vannicelli Collection.

33. "History," n.d., Dave and Mary Vannicelli Collection. I estimate the date of this "History" Q&A document to be from the late 1980s or early 1990s based on the statement it contains that since 1963, "approximately 2,700 boys have participated in the Indians program." An average of 100 boys participating per year would lead to an estimate of 2,700 boys over twenty-seven years, leading to an estimate of 1990 as the date of creation of this document (twenty-seven years after 1963). The KFPA's 1986 Constitution and By-Laws noted that the KFPA previously had up to six or seven weight teams and had recently transitioned to four weight teams. Additionally, the paper and typeset of the document is similar to that of other documents in the archive dated from the late 1980s.

34. "1999 King of Prussia Indians Football" (1999), p. 4, Dave and Mary Vannicelli Collection. "History," Dave and Mary Vannicelli Collection.

35. "History," Dave and Mary Vannicelli Collection.

36. Letter, Fran Littlewood to Mike Adelsberger, President, King of Prussia Indians Football Association, November 12, 1996, Dave and Mary Vannicelli Collection.

37. "KPFA Board Meeting of 10-8-1997" and "KPFA Board Meeting of 11-12-97," Dave and Mary Vannicelli Collection.

38. Bob Gray, "Helmets—Purchases, Inventory, Notes, and Comments," March 19, 2000, Dave and Mary Vannicelli Collection.

39. Kent Hannon, "Is Football Safe for Kids?" 20–22. For an example of certifying that all football helmets in use each season had been approved by NOCSAE, see untitled letter from Michael Adelsberger, KPFA president, to the Keystone State League Commissioner, August 1, 1994, in Dave and Mary Vannicelli Collection.

40. Hannon, "Is Football Safe for Kids?" 20.

41. Hannon, "Is Football Safe for Kids?" 22.

42. Letter, Robert B. Leahy to Fran Littlewood, King of Prussia Indians Flag Football Representative, n.d. (c. November 1996), Dave and Mary Vannicelli Collection. While the letter is undated, Leahy indicates that he is replying to a communication from Fran Littlewood that was written on November 4, 1996, making it likely this letter in response was also written in November 1996.

43. Michael Oriard, *King Football: Sport and Spectacle in the Golden Age of Radio and Newsreels, Movies and Magazines, the Weekly and the Daily Press* (Chapel Hill: University of North Carolina Press, 2001), 284.

44. Lane Demas, *Integrating the Gridiron: Black Civil Rights and American College Football* (New Brunswick, NJ: Rutgers University Press, 2010), 137.

45. NFHS, "Participation Survey History Book," accessed March 19, 2019, http://www .nfhs.org/ParticipationStatics/PDF/Participation%20Survey%20History%20Book.pdf. Data available include U.S. state, year, number of participants, number of schools, type of sport played, and gender.

46. Youth Sports Study Committee, *Joint Legislative Study on Youth Sports Programs* (Lansing: State of Michigan, November 18, 1976).

47. "The lower return of questionnaires from the Detroit Public School System was the only noteable [*sic*] bias that may have been introduced into the analysis of participation in specific sports, by race," Youth Sports Study Committee, *Joint Legislative Study*, 111, 124.

48. Nand Hart-Nibbrig and Clement Cottingham, *The Political Economy of College Sports* (Lexington, MA: D. C. Heath, 1986), x.

49. Robert Andrew Powell, *We Own This Game: A Season in the Adult World of Youth Football* (New York: Atlantic Monthly Press, 2003), xvi, 19.

50. Powell, *We Own This Game*.

51. Powell, *We Own This Game*, 114, 118. Football, of course, has not been the only risky activity or occupation in American life through which African American men have striven to assert their manhood and equality. Understanding the ways in which African American men sought to prove themselves through other lauded forms of male accomplishment, and the ways that American attitudes toward these activities have been reconfigured by their changing racial demographics, could prove fruitful in understanding the racial and gender dynamics of youth football.

52. Kevin Young and Philip White, "Researching Sports Injury: Reconstructing Dangerous Masculinities," in *Masculinities, Gender Relations, and Sport*, ed. Jim McKay, Michael A. Messner, and Don Sabo (Thousand Oaks: Sage Publications, 2000): 108–27.

53. Andrew Doyle, "Bear Bryant: Symbol for an Embattled South," *Colby Quarterly* 32, no. 1 (1996): 72–86.

54. Demas, *Integrating the Gridiron*, 76.

55. Craig R. Coenen, *From Sandlots to the Super Bowl: The National Football League, 1920–1967* (Knoxville: University of Tennessee Press, 2005): 161–62. See also "The Creation of the Modern NFL in the 1960s," in Michael Oriard, *Brand NFL* (Chapel Hill: University of North Carolina Press, 2007), ch. 1.

56. "Bednarik Disbelieves 'Cheap Shot' Charges of Gifford Tackle," *Chicago Daily Defender*, November 23, 1960.

57. Jack Craig, "Football Violence: It's Profits vs. Safety," *Boston Globe*, August 18, 1978.

58. John Sayle Watterson, *College Football: History, Spectacle, Controversy* (Baltimore: Johns Hopkins University Press, 2000); Robert Winston Turner II, *NFL Means Not For Long: The Life and Career of the NFL Athlete*, Ph.D. dissertation, City University of New York, 2010, 58. On the changes in the structure of American college athletics and efforts at reform, see Allen L. Sack, *Counterfeit Amateurs: An Athlete's Journey through the Sixties to the Age of Academic Capitalism* (University Park: Penn State University Press, 2012); Ronald A.

Smith, *Pay for Play: A History of Big-Time College Athletic Reform* (Urbana and Chicago: University of Illinois Press, 2011).

59. Gregg A. Jones, Wilbert M. Leonard, Raymond L. Schmitt, et al., "Racial Discrimination in College Football," *Social Science Quarterly* 68, no. 1 (1987): 70–83.

60. Lori Latrice Martin, *White Sports/Black Sports: Racial Disparities in Athletic Programs* (Santa Barbara, CA: ABC-CLIO, 2015).

61. By contrast, college coaches and administrators remain predominantly white; in the 2014–2015 academic year, over 80 percent of Division I head coaches and coordinators were white. See Michael Baumann, "The Bleak Future of College Football," *The Atlantic*, November 29, 2015, accessed March 19, 2019, http://www.theatlantic.com/entertainment/archive/2015/11/football-risks/416862/

62. Geoff Winningham and Al Reinert, *Rites of Fall: High School Football in Texas* (Austin: University of Texas Press, 1979), 10.

Chapter Nine

1. Lawrence K. Altman, "Increase Is Reported in Paralyzing Football Injuries," *NYT*, April 8, 1979. On the complexity of the history of NCAA spearing rules, including changing definitions of spearing, see Appendix 2 of David M. Nelson, *The Anatomy of a Game: Football, the Rules, and the Men Who Made the Game* (Newark: University of Delaware Press, 1994). Thanks to Steve Hardy for drawing my attention to this source.

2. Joseph S. Torg, Joseph J. Vesgo, Brian Sennett, and Marianne Das, "The National Football Head and Neck Injury Registry: 14-Year Report on Cervical Quadriplegia, 1971 through 1984," *JAMA* 254, no. 24 (1985): 3439–4; Centers for Disease Control and Prevention, "Football-Related Spinal Cord Injuries Among High School Players-Louisiana, 1989," *MMWR* 39 (1990): 586–87. Yet other research indicated that despite the rule change, the actual incidence of spearing did not decrease, and thus could not account for the decline of catastrophic, paralyzing high school football injuries. See Jonathan F. Heck, "The Incidence of Spearing During a High School's 1975 and 1990 Football Seasons," *Journal of Athletic Trainers* 31, no. 1 (1996): 31–37. Despite declining numbers, the tragedy of such cases nonetheless continued to receive significant media attention. See, for example, Frank Hughes, "Few Neck Injuries Still Leave Many Questions for Players, Coaches," *WP*, November 19, 1993.

3. Frederick O. Mueller and Robert C. Cantu, *Football Fatalities and Catastrophic Injuries, 1931–2008* (Durham, NC: Carolina Academic Press, 2011).

4. As an example of the colloquial use of the phrase "getting your bell rung" to distinguish a hit to the head from medical harm, a character in one 1992 novel states, "Brain damage? Hell no. He just got his bell rung, as they say in football." Sheila Bosworth, *Slow Poison: A Novel* (New York: Knopf, 1992), 297.

5. Philip R. Yarnell and Steve Lynch, "The 'Ding': Amnestic States in Football Trauma," *Neurology* 23, no. 2 (1973): 196–97; Dave Meggyesy, *Out of Their League* (Berkeley, CA: Ramparts, 1970), 125.

6. Yarnell and Steve Lynch, "The 'Ding,'" 197. See also Steve Lynch and Philip R. Yarnell, "Retrograde Amnesia: Delayed Forgetting After Concussion," *American Journal of Psychology* 86, no. 3 (September 1973): 643–45.

7. Subcommittee on Classification of Sports Injuries, Committee on the Medical Aspects of Sports, *Standard Nomenclature of Athletic Injuries* (Chicago: American Medical Association, 1966), 20.

8. Richard C. Schneider and Frederick C. Kriss, "Decisions Concerning Cerebral Concussions in Football Players," *Medicine and Science in Sports* 1, no. 2 (June 1969): 112–15; Robert C. Cantu, "Posttraumatic Retrograde and Anterograde Amnesia: Pathophysiology and Implications in Grading and Safe Return to Play," *Journal of Athletic Training* 36, no. 3 (2001): 244–48.

9. Susan Goodwin Gerberich et al., "Concussion Incidences and Severity in Secondary School Varsity Football Players," *AJPH* 73, no. 12 (1983): 1370–75.

10. Gerberich et al., "Concussion Incidences and Severity."

11. Gerberich et al., "Concussion Incidences and Severity."

12. Robert L. Saunders and Robert E. Harbaugh, "The Second Impact in Catastrophic Contact-Sports Head Trauma," *JAMA* 252, no. 4 (1984): 538–39.

13. Saunders and Harbaugh, "The Second Impact," 539. See also Linda Carroll and David Rosner, *The Concussion Crisis: Anatomy of a Silent Epidemic* (New York: Simon & Schuster, 2011).

14. Carroll and Rosner, *The Concussion Crisis*, 14; Rich Cimini, "Having HS Trainers: What Price for Safety?" *Newsday*, November 23, 1986.

15. Augustus Thorndike, "Serious Recurrent Injuries of Athletes: Contraindications to Further Competitive Participation," *New England Journal of Medicine* 247, no. 15 (1952): 554–56.

16. Francis Murphey and James C. H. Simmons, "Initial Management of Athletic Injuries to the Head and Neck," *American Journal of Surgery* 98, no. 3 (1959): 379–83; Schneider and Kriss, "Decisions Concerning Cerebral Concussions." Schneider and Kriss cited a personal communication from Thomas Quigley, another sports medicine specialist, as also supporting the policy of removing players for a season after three concussions.

17. Joseph C. Maroon, Paul B. Steele, and Ralph Berlin, "Football Head and Neck Injuries—An Update," *Clinical Neurosurgery* 27 (1980): 414–29; Robert C. Cantu, "Guidelines for Return to Contact Sports after a Cerebral Concussion," *Physician and Sportsmedicine* 14 (1986): 75–83.

18. Cantu, "Guidelines for Return to Contact Sports"; Carroll and Rosner, *The Concussion Crisis*, 15.

19. David R. Oppenheimer, "Microscopic Lesions in the Brain Following Head Injury," *Journal of Neurology, Neurosurgery & Psychiatry* 31 (1968): 299–306.

20. Thomas A. Gennarelli, Lawrence E. Thibault, J. Hume Adams, et al., "Diffuse Axonal Injury and Traumatic Coma in the Primate," *Annals of Neurology* 12 (1982): 564–74.

21. Rebecca W. Rimel, Bruno Giordani, Jeffrey T. Barth, et al., "Disability Caused by Minor Head Injury," *Neurosurgery* 9, no. 3 (1981): 221–28. See also John T. Povlishock and Thomas H. Coburn, "Morphological Changes Associated with Mild Head Injury," in *Mild Head Injury*, ed. Harvey S. Levin, Howard M. Eisenberg, and Arthur L. Benton (New York: Oxford University Press, 1989), 37–53.

22. Frederick C. Klein, "Silent Epidemic: Head Injuries, Often Difficult to Diagnose, Are Getting Attention," *Wall Street Journal*, November 24, 1982.

23. Mark Fainaru-Wada and Steve Fainaru, *League of Denial: The N.F.L., Concussions, and the Battle for Truth* (New York: Random House, 2013).

24. Fainaru-Wada and Fainaru, *League of Denial*, 32.

25. Jeffrey T. Barth, Wayne M. Alves, Thomas V. Ryan, et al., "Mild Head Injury in Sports: Neuropsychological Sequelae and Recovery of Function," in *Mild Head Injury*, 257–75; Ronald Ruff, "Two Decades of Advances in Understanding of Mild Traumatic Brain Injury," *Journal of Head Trauma Rehabilitation* 20, no. 1 (2005): 5–18.

26. According to the NFHS, from the 1990–1991 school year to the 2000–2001 school year, the total number of participants in high school athletics per school year increased by about 1.4 million; nearly 900,000 of these additional participants were girls. "Sports Participation Survey," accessed March 19, 2019, http://www.nfhs.org/ParticipationStatics /PDF/Participation%20Survey%20History%20Book.pdf. On the influence of Title IX on high school sports, see Betsy Stevenson, "Title IX and the Evolution of High School Sports," *Contemporary Economic Policy* 25, no. 4 (2007): 486–505. See also Donald Huff, "Athletic Participation on Increase after Years' Long Decline," *WP*, October 1, 1991; Hal Bock, "Prep Athletes Still at Risk," *Seattle Times*, October 6, 1991, accessed March 19, 2019, http://community.seattletimes.nwsource.com/archive/?date=19911006&slug=1309237.

27. Howard Chudacoff, *Children at Play: An American History* (New York: New York University Press, 2007); Hilary Levey Friedman, *Playing to Win: Raising Children in a Competitive Culture* (Berkeley: University of California Press, 2013). See also Jay Coakley, "The 'Logic' of Specialization: Using Children for Adult Purposes," *Journal of Physical Education, Recreation & Dance* 81, no. 8 (2010): 16–25.

28. Lyle J. Micheli and J. D. Klein, "Sports Injuries in Children and Adolescents," *British Journal of Sports Medicine* 25, no. 1 (1991): 6–9.

29. James P. Kelly, John S. Nichols, Christopher M. Filley, et al., "Concussion in Sports: Guidelines for the Prevention of Catastrophic Outcome," *JAMA* 266, no. 20 (1991): 2867–69.

30. Eric D. Zemper, "Analysis of Cerebral Concussion Frequency with the Most Commonly Used Models of Football Helmets," *Journal of Athletic Training* 29 (1994): 44–50; Austin Meek, "No Denying His Work on Concussions," *Register-Guard* [Eugene, OR], December 25, 2015, accessed March 19, 2019, http://registerguard.com/rg/sports/33890906-81 /no-denying-his-work-on-concussions.html.csp. Meek's article also includes an overview of Zemper's background and career.

31. Linda Saslow, "Head Injuries Force Schools to Ponder Policy," *NYT*, May 11, 1997.

32. AAN, "Practice Parameter: The Management of Concussion in Sports (Summary Statement). Report of the Quality Standards Subcommittee," *Neurology* 48 (1997): 581–85.

33. AAN, "Practice Parameter." See also James P. Kelly and Jay H. Rosenberg, "Diagnosis and Management of Concussion in Sports," *Neurology* 48 (1997): 575–80.

34. James P. Kelly and Jay H. Rosenberg, "The Development of Guidelines for the Management of Concussion in Sports," *Journal of Head Trauma Rehabilitation* 13, no. 2 (1998): 53–65.

35. Saslow, "Head Injuries."

36. Craig R. Coenen, *From Sandlots to the Super Bowl: The National Football League, 1920–1967* (Knoxville: University of Tennessee Press, 2005): 232; Michael Leeds, "American Football," in *Handbook on the Economics of Sport*, ed. Wladimir Andreff and Stefan Szymanski (Northampton, MA: Elgar: 2006): 514–22.

37. Howard L. Nixon, "Accepting the Risks of Pain and Injury in Sport: Mediated Cultural Influences on Playing Hurt," *Sociology of Sport Journal* 10 (1993): 183–96.

38. Gerald Eskenazi, "Pro Football: Experts Disagree on Football Injury Prevention," *NYT*, December 2, 1992; Harry Carson, "Concussions: The Hidden Injury," [letter] *NYT*, April 19, 1998.

39. David E. Thigpen and Julie Grace, "Chin Music: Doctors Warn that Relentless Blows to the Head May Be Giving Football Players Lasting Brain Damage," *Time*, December 12, 1994, 71–72.

40. Thigpen and Grace, "Chin Music," 71–72; Jerry Crasnick, "Dazed and Confused: Merril Hoge and Other Veterans Are Finding Out Why Concussions Have Become Serious Head Games," *Denver Post*, November 20, 1994; Laura Vecsey, "Post-Concussion Syndrome Turns Heads in NFL," *Seattle Post-Intelligencer*, October 28, 1994; Alexander N. Hecht, "Legal and Ethical Aspects of Sports-Related Concussions: The Merril Hoge Story," *Seton Hall Journal of Sport Law* 12 (2002): 17–64.

41. James P. Kelly, quoted in Michael Farber, "The Worst Case," *SI*, December 19, 1994. Kelly also told *Sports Illustrated* that concussions definitely had a cumulative effect, while NFL team doctor Joe Torg asserted, "I know of no football player who has had residual neurological impairment from repeated insults to the head." Torg claimed that "punch-drunk" syndrome in boxers did not apply to football, because football players were rarely knocked out cold.

42. Steve Almond, *Against Football: One Fan's Reluctant Manifesto* (Brooklyn, NY: Melvin House, 2014), 44.

43. There is no evidence that professional football experience enables players to acquire the nonexistent skill of "unscrambling" their own brains. Paul Tagliabue, "Tackling Concussions in Sports," *Neurosurgery* 53, no. 4 (October 2003): 796; Fainaru-Wada and Fainaru, *League of Denial*; Michael Farber, "The Worst Case." In the same *Sports Illustrated* article, Joseph Maroon, a neurosurgeon who consulted with the Pittsburgh Steelers, likened a concussion to lights going out. He stated that sometimes concussions were akin to a light bulb dimming for an instant. "Does a very mild concussion need to be reported? Probably not."

44. Tagliabue, "Tackling Concussions in Sports," 796.

45. Elliot J. Pellman, David C. Viano, Ira R. Casson, et al., "Concussion in Professional Football: Players Returning to the Same Game: Part 7," *Neurosurgery* 56, no. 1 (2005): 79–92; Fainaru-Wada and Fainaru, *League of Denial*.

46. Chris Nowinski, *Head Games: Football's Concussion Crisis From the NFL to Youth Leagues* (East Bridgewater, MA: Drummond, 2007), 49.

47. Julie Deardorff, "Concussions Make Players Think Twice," *Chicago Tribune*, October 7, 1998, accessed March 19, 2019, http://articles.chicagotribune.com/1998-10-07/news /9810070149_1_concussions-second-impact-syndrome-athletes.

48. See Fainaru-Wada and Fainaru, *League of Denial*, 346.

49. Carroll and Rosner, *The Concussion Crisis*, 25–26.

50. Kevin M. Guskiewicz, Michael McCrea, Stephen W. Marshall, et al., "Cumulative Effects Associated with Recurrent Concussions in Collegiate Football Players: The NCAA Concussion Study," *JAMA* 290, no. 19 (2003): 2549–55. See also Carroll and Rosner, *The Concussion Crisis*, 25–26.

51. John O'Neil, "Sports Medicine: For Concussions, Bench Remedy," *NYT*, November 25, 2003, accessed March 19, 2019, http://www.nytimes.com/2003/11/25/health/vital -signs-sports-medicine-for-concussions-bench-remedy.html. In 2011, Guskiewicz would be

awarded a MacArthur Foundation "genius" grant for his work studying sports-related head injuries. "MacArthur Fellows/Meet the Class of 2011," *MacArthur Foundation*, September 20, 2011, accessed March 19, 2019, https://www.macfound.org/fellows/7/.

52. Carroll and Rosner, *The Concussion Crisis*; Fainaru-Wada and Fainaru, *League of Denial*.

53. Bennet Omalu, "Concussions and NFL: How the Name Came About," *CNN*, December 21, 2015, accessed March 19, 2019, http://edition.cnn.com/2015/12/21/opinions/omalu-discovery-of-cte-football-concussions/.

54. Fainaru-Wada and Fainaru, *League of Denial*, 161; Bennet I. Omalu, Steven T. DeKosky, Ryan L. Minster, et al., "Chronic Traumatic Encephalopathy in a National Football League Player," *Neurosurgery* 57, no. 1 (2005): 128–34; Bennet I. Omalu, Steven T. DeKosky, Ronald L. Hamilton, et al., "Chronic Traumatic Encephalopathy in a National Football League Player: Part II," *Neurosurgery* 59, no. 5 (2006): 1086–93.

55. "Pro Football; Brain Trauma Cited," *NYT*, September 14, 2005, accessed March 19, 2019, https://www.nytimes.com/2005/09/14/sports/pro-football-brain-trauma-cited.html.

56. Ira R. Casson, Elliot J. Pellman, and David C. Viano, "Chronic Traumatic Encephalopathy in a National Football League Player," *Neurosurgery* 58, no. 5 (2006): E1003. See also Fainaru-Wada and Fainaru, *League of Denial*.

57. Robert Dvorchak, "Cause of Death Sparks Debate: Steelers Doctor Says Concluding Football Led to Long's Demise is Bad Science," *Pittsburgh Post-Gazette*, September 16, 2005.

58. Brent Cunningham, "Head Cases," *Columbia Journalism Review*, January 5, 2010, accessed March 19, 2019, http://www.cjr.org/behind_the_news/head_cases.php.

59. Alan Schwarz, "Expert Ties Ex-Player's Suicide to Brain Damage," *NYT*, January 18, 2007, accessed March 19, 2019, http://www.nytimes.com/2007/01/18/sports/football/18waters.html; Greg Marx, "Power of Dispassion: Alan Schwarz Changed Football," *Columbia Journalism Review*, November/December 2011, accessed April 18, 2019, https://archives.cjr.org/feature/power_of_dispassion.php.

60. Schwarz, "Expert Ties Ex-Player's Suicide to Brain Damage."

61. Ben McGrath, "Does Football Have a Future?" *New Yorker*, January 31, 2011, accessed March 19, 2019, http://www.newyorker.com/magazine/2011/01/31/does-football-have-a-future.

62. Alan Schwarz, "Silence on Concussions Raises Risk of Injury," *NYT*, September 15, 2007, accessed March 19, 2019, http://www.nytimes.com/2007/09/15/sports/football/15concussions.html; Alan Schwarz, "Players Face Head-Injury Risk Before the N.F.L.," *NYT*, October 1, 2009, accessed March 19, 2019, http://www.nytimes.com/2009/10/02/sports/football/02dementia.html.

63. *Legal Issues Relating to Football Head Injuries (Part I & II): Hearings Before the Committee on the Judiciary House of Representatives*, 111th Congress, first and second sessions (Washington, DC: US Government Printing Office, 2010).; David R. Weir, James S. Jackson, and Amanda Sonnega, *National Football League Player Care Foundation Study of Retired NFL Players* (Ann Arbor: University of Michigan Institute for Social Research, 2009); Tom Goldman, "House Hears Testimony on Football, Head Injuries," NPR, October 28, 2009, accessed March 19, 2019, http://www.npr.org/templates/story/story.php?storyId=114253880.

64. *Legal Issues Relating to Football Head Injuries (Part I & II): Hearings Before the Committee on the Judiciary House of Representatives*, 111th Congress. See above. See also Alan Schwarz,

"N.F.L.'s Influence on Safety at Youth Levels Is Cited," *NYT*, October 29, 2009, accessed March 19, 2019, http://www.nytimes.com/2009/10/30/sports/football/30concussion.html.

65. *Legal Issues Relating to Football Head Injuries (Part I & II): Hearings Before the Committee on the Judiciary House of Representatives,* 111th Congress. See above.

66. Alan Schwarz, "N.F.L. Issues New Guidelines on Concussions," *NYT*, December 9, 2009, accessed March 19, 2019, http://www.nytimes.com/2009/12/03/sports/football/03concussion.html; Daniel S. Goldberg, "Mild Traumatic Brain Injury, the National Football League, and the Manufacture of Doubt: An Ethical, Legal, and Social Analysis," *Journal of Legal Medicine* 34, no. 2 (2013): 157–91.

67. Alan Schwarz, "N.F.L. Acknowledges Long-Term Concussion Effects," *NYT*, December 20, 2009, accessed March 19, 2019, http://www.nytimes.com/2009/12/21/sports/football/21concussions.html.

68. "Super Bowl Confetti Made Entirely from Shredded Concussion Studies," *The Onion*, February 2, 2014, accessed March 19, 2019, http://www.theonion.com/graphic/super-bowl-confetti-made-entirely-from-shredded-co-35146.

69. Schwarz, "N.F.L. Issues New Guidelines on Concussions."

70. Joseph R. Gusfield, *The Culture of Public Problems: Drinking-Driving and the Symbolic Order* (Chicago: University of Chicago Press, 1987).

71. Wash. Rev. Code Ann. § 28A.600.190 (2009); Sheila Mickool, "The Story Behind the Zachary Lystedt Law," *Seattle Magazine*, April 9, 2013, accessed March 19, 2019, http://www.seattlemag.com/article/story-behind-zackery-lystedt-law.

72. Tim Booth, "Using Head on Concussions," *Boston Globe*, September 20, 2009.

73. The Sarah Jane Brain Foundation is a national advocacy organization focused on pediatric brain injury. It was founded in 2007 by a father whose four-year-old daughter suffered a brain injury after being shaken by a nurse. Alan Schwarz, "States Taking the Lead Addressing Concussions," *NYT*, January 30, 2010, accessed March 19, 2019, http://www.nytimes.com/2010/01/31/sports/31concussions.html; Carol Kreck, "States Address Concerns About Concussions in Youth Sports," *Education Commission of the States*, March 2014, accessed March 19, 2019, http://files.eric.ed.gov/fulltext/ED561938.pdf; Hosea H. Harvey, "Reducing Traumatic Brain Injuries in Youth Sports: Youth Sports Traumatic Brain Injury State Laws, January 2009–December 2012," *AJPH* 103, no. 7 (July 2013): 1249–54.

74. JoNel Aleccia, "NFL Gives $2.5M to Launch UW Center to Study Concussions," *Seattle Times*, August 12, 2015, accessed March 19, 2019, https://www.seattletimes.com/seattle-news/health/nfl-gives-25m-to-launch-uw-center-to-study-concussions/.

75. "Sports as Medicine," *UW Medicine*, Fall 2015, accessed March 19, 2019, https://uwmedmagazine.org/fall-2015/sports-as-medicine/.

76. Lyle Micheli, interviewed by author, March 17, 2015.

77. Kathleen E. Bachynski and Daniel S. Goldberg, "Youth Sports & Public Health: Framing Risks of Mild Traumatic Brain Injury in American Football and Ice Hockey," *Journal of Law, Medicine & Ethics* 42, no. 3 (2014): 323–33.

78. Jeff Z. Klein, "Spartan Hockey Helmets Going Under Microscope," *NYT*, July 22, 2014, accessed March 19, 2019, http://www.nytimes.com/2014/07/23/sports/hockey/for-safety-hockey-helmets-going-under-microscope.html.

79. Dave Savini, "2 Investigators: Schools Using Football Helmets with Low Safety Ratings," *CBS Chicago*, November 3, 2014, accessed March 19, 2019, http://chicago.cbslocal

.com/2014/11/03/2-investigators-schools-using-football-helmets-with-low-safety-ratings
/; Michaelle Bond, "Firms Proliferate to Prevent Concussions but Evidence Lags," *Philadelphia Inquirer*, January 22, 2016. Accessed April 17, 2019 at https://www.philly.com/philly
/business/20160121_Firms_proliferate_to_prevent_concussions_but_evidence_lags
.html; Matthew Futterman, "Rethinking the Next-Generation Helmet," *Wall Street Journal*,
December 24, 2015, accessed March 19, 2019, http://www.wsj.com/articles/rethinking-the
-next-generation-helmet-1450998090.

80. Thomas Zambito, "Judge's Ruling Puts Football Helmet Lawsuit Back in Play," *NJ
.com*, August 4, 2015, accessed March 19, 2019, http://www.nj.com/news/index.ssf/2015/08
/judge_rules_football_helmet_lawsuit_back_in_play.html.

81. Tom Foster, "The Helmet that Can Save Football," *Popular Science*, December 18,
2012, accessed March 19, 2019, http://www.popsci.com/science/article/2013-08/helmet
-wars-and-new-helmet-could-protect-us-all.

82. Gary Mihoces, "More Padding the Issue of Concussions and Better Helmets," *USA
Today*, August 23, 2013, accessed March 19, 2019, http://www.usatoday.com/story/sports
/ncaaf/2013/07/30/concussions-college-football-nfl-guardian-caps/2601063/.

83. Mike Orcutt, "New Collar Promises to Keep Athletes' Brains from 'Sloshing' During
Impact," *MIT Technology Review*, February 3, 2016, accessed March 19, 2019, https://www
.technologyreview.com/s/600691/new-collar-promises-to-keep-athletes-brains-from
-sloshing-during-impact/.

84. University of Maryland press release, "Concussion-Related Measures Improved in
High School Football Players Who Drank New Chocolate Milk, UMD Study Shows," December 22, 2015. Accessed April 17, 2019 at: https://web.archive.org/web/20160115010727
/http://www.mtech.umd.edu/news/press_releases/releases/5QF/concussions/; Andrew
Holtz, Yoni Freedhoff, and Kathlyn Stone, "Release Claiming Chocolate Milk Improves
Concussion Symptoms in Student Athletes Is Out-of-Bounds," *Health News Review*, January 5, 2016, accessed March 19, 2019, http://www.healthnewsreview.org/news-release
-review/concussion-related-measures-improved-high-school-football-players-drank
-new-chocolate-milk-umd-study-shows/; Ike Swetliz, "Can Chocolate Milk Speed Concussion Recovery? Experts Cringe," *Stat News*, January 11, 2016, accessed March 19, 2019, http:
//www.statnews.com/2016/01/11/chocolate-milk-concussion/.

85. Alan Schwarz, "Suicide Reveals Signs of a Disease Seen in N.F.L.," *NYT*, September 13, 2010, accessed March 19, 2019, http://www.nytimes.com/2010/09/14/sports
/14football.html. CTE would later be diagnosed in other young football players. See, for
example, Nadia Kounang, "Football's Dangers, Illustrated by One Young Man's Brain,"
CNN, January 11, 2016, accessed March 19, 2019, http://www.cnn.com/2016/01/11/health
/football-brain-damage-cte/.

86. Cynthia Sequin, "Purdue, Community Officials Celebrate Opening of New MRI
Center to Focus on Patient Care, Research," Purdue University press release, November 2,
2007, accessed March 19, 2019, http://www.purdue.edu/uns/x/2007b/071102OlsenMRI
.html.

87. "Interview: Tom Talavage," *PBS Frontline*, April 12, 2011, accessed March 19, 2019,
http://www.pbs.org/wgbh/pages/frontline/football-high/interviews/tom-talavage.html.

88. "Interview: Tom Talavage," *PBS Frontline*; Thomas M. Talavage, Eric A. Nauman,
Evan L. Breedlove, et al., "Functionally-Detected Cognitive Impairment in High School

Football Players Without Clinically-Diagnosed Concussion," *Journal of Neurotrauma* 31 (2014): 327–38.

89. Talavage et al., "Functionally-Detected Cognitive Impairment."

90. Daniel F. Kelly, Charlene Chaloner, Diana Evans, et al., "Prevalence of Pituitary Hormone Dysfunction, Metabolic Syndrome, and Impaired Quality of Life in Retired Professional Football Players: A Prospective Study," *Journal of Neurotrauma* 31 (2014): 1161–71.

91. Kausar Abbas, Trey E. Shenk, Victoria N. Poole, et al., "Effects of Repetitive Sub-Concussive Brain Injury on the Functional Connectivity of Default Mode Network in High School Football Athletes," *Developmental Neuropsychology* 40, no. 1 (2015): 51–56; Chad A. Tagge, Andrew M. Fisher, Olga V. Minaeva, et al., "Concussion, Microvascular Injury, and Early Tauopathy in Young Athletes After Impact Head Injury and an Impact Concussion Mouse Model," *Brain* 141, no. 2 (2018): 422–58.

92. "Purdue Expert at White House Sports Summit: Subconcussive Blows Damage Kids' Brains," *Purdue University News*, May 29, 2014, accessed March 19, 2019, http://www.purdue.edu/newsroom/releases/2014/Q2/purdue-expert-at-white-house-sports-summit-subconcussive-blows-damage-kids-brains.html.

93. Tyler J. Young, Ray W. Daniel, Steven Rowson, et al., "Head Impact Exposure in Youth Football: Elementary School Ages 7–8 Years and the Effect of Returning Players," *Clinical Journal of Sport Medicine* 24, no. 5 (2014): 416–21; Sean Gregory, "Why We Need Hit Counts in Football," *Time*, October 12, 2015, accessed March 19, 2019, http://time.com/4069037/football-brain-injury-hit-counts-cte/. For research supporting pitch counts in Little League baseball, see, for example, Stephen Lyman, Glenn S. Fleisig, James R. Andrews, et al., "Effect of Pitch Type, Pitch Count, and Pitching Mechanics on Risk of Elbow and Shoulder Pain in Youth Baseball Pitchers," *American Journal of Sports Medicine* 30, no. 4 (2002): 463–68.

94. Bachynski and Goldberg, "Youth Sports & Public Health."

95. Jason La Canfora, "NFL Urges States to Adopt Legislation to Protect Young Athletes," *NFL.com*, May 23, 2010, accessed March 19, 2019, http://www.nfl.com/news/story/09000d5d81847223/printable/nfl-urges-states-to-adopt-legislation-to-protect-youth-athletes.

96. Carroll and Rosner, *The Concussion Crisis*, 255–56; "Prepared Statement of Stanley Herring," in *H.R. 6172, Protecting Student Athletes from Concussions: Hearings Before the Committee on Education and Labor, House of Representatives*, 111th Congress, second session (September 23, 2010), accessed March 19, 2019, https://www.gpo.gov/fdsys/pkg/CHRG-111hhrg58256/pdf/CHRG-111hhrg58256.pdf. The public-service announcement the NFL introduced on concussions in 2009 was also shared on YouTube. "CDC NFL Head Injuries PSA," *YouTube*, December 29, 2009, accessed March 19, 2019, https://www.youtube.com/watch?v=NhgIfWl4om4.

97. Kelly Sarmiento, Rosanne Hoffman, Zoe Dmitrovsky, et al., "A 10-Year Review of the Centers for Disease Control and Prevention's *Heads Up* Initiatives: Bringing Concussion Awareness to the Forefront," *Journal of Safety Research* 50 (2014): 143–47; Testimony of Vikas Kapil, "Protecting School-Age Athletes from Sports-Related Concussion Injury," Centers for Disease Control and Prevention, September 8, 2010, accessed March 19, 2019, http://www.cdc.gov/washington/testimony/2010/t20100908.htm. On the conflict of interest involved in the NFL funding CDC programs to address sports-related brain

trauma, see Kathleen E. Bachynski and Daniel S. Goldberg, "Time Out: NFL Conflicts of Interest with Public Health Efforts to Prevent TBI," *Injury Prevention* 24, no. 3 (2018): 180–84.

98. Steve Fainaru and Mark Fainaru-Wada, "Questions About Heads-Up Tackling," *ESPN*, January 13, 2014, accessed March 19, 2019, http://espn.go.com/espn/otl/story/_/id /10276129/popular-nfl-backed-heads-tackling-method-questioned-former-players; Alan Schwarz, "N.F.L.-Backed Youth Program Says It Reduced Concussions. The Data Disagrees," *NYT*, July 27, 2016, accessed March 19, 2019, https://www.nytimes.com/2016/07 /28/sports/football/nfl-concussions-youth-program-heads-up-football.html.

99. Mike Reiss, "Goodell Joins Pats for 'Moms Safety Clinic,'" *ESPN*, May 29, 2014, accessed March 19, 2019, http://espn.go.com/blog/boston/new-england-patriots/post/_/id /4763492/goodell-joins-pats-for-moms-safety-clinic; Ken Belson, "To Allay Fears, N.F.L. Huddles with Mothers," *NYT*, January 28, 2015, accessed March 19, 2019, http://www .nytimes.com/2015/01/29/sports/football/nfl-tries-to-reassure-mothers-as-polls-and -studies-rattle-them.html.

100. Jaime Aron, "Concussions: Youth Football Begins Prevention Work," *WP*, September 30, 2010, accessed March 19, 2019, http://www.washingtonpost.com/wp-dyn/content /article/2010/09/30/AR2010093000815.html; Pop Warner Little Scholars, Inc., "Football Safety," accessed April 18, 2019 at https://web.archive.org/web/20140331064509/http: //www.popwarner.com/football/footballsafety.htm. Pop Warner removed the claim that there was an "absence of catastrophic head and neck injuries" in youth football from its website sometime after April 2014.

101. Gary Lussier Jr., "Parents Are Overreacting to Football Risks," *Star Tribune*, August 24, 2015, accessed March 19, 2019, http://www.startribune.com/parents-are-overreacting -to-football-risks/322746741/; Anthony P. Kontos, R. J. Elbin, and Vanessa C. Fazio-Sumrock, "Incidence of Sports-Related Concussions Among Youth Football Players Aged 8–12 Years," *Journal of Pediatrics* 163, no. 3 (2013): 717–20.

102. Matt Riedel and Joanna Chadwick, "Luke Schemm's Death Puts Spotlight on High School Football Safety," *Wichita Eagle*, November 7, 2015, accessed March 19, 2019, http://www.kansas.com/sports/high-school/article43613757.html.

103. Daniel J. Flynn, *The War on Football: Saving America's Game* (Washington, DC: Regnery, 2013), 2, 14.

104. Steven M. Rothman, "Parents, Stop Obsessing over Youth Concussions," *NYT*, December 22, 2015, accessed March 19, 2019, http://www.nytimes.com/2015/12/22/opinion /parents-stop-obsessing-over-concussions.html; Tom Farrey, "ESPN Poll: Most Parents Have Concerns About State of Youth Sports," *ESPN*, October 13, 2014, accessed March 19, 2019, http://espn.go.com/espnw/w-in-action/article/11675649/parents-concern-grows -kids-participation-sports.

105. Domonique Foxworth, "7-Year NFL Veteran Domonique Foxworth Saw 'Concussion' and It Made Him Question Everything," *USA Today Sports*, January 5, 2016, accessed March 19, 2019, http://ftw.usatoday.com/2016/01/domonique-foxworth-concussion.

106. Mark Synder, "Movie Makes Ex-Wolverine Consider Cost of Football," *Detroit Free Press*, December 20, 2015, accessed March 19, 2019, http://www.freep.com/story/sports /college/university-michigan/wolverines/2015/12/20/concussion-movie-michigan -wolverines-pierre-woods/77657692/.

107. Mike White, "With Concussions on the Brain, Mars Standout Castello Shuns Football for Basketball," *Pittsburgh Post-Gazette*, February 2, 2016, accessed March 19, 2019, http://www.post-gazette.com/sports/highschool/2016/02/02/With-concussions-on-the-brain-Mars-standout-Castello-shuns-football-for-basketball/stories/201602020018; Julia Jacobo, "'Concussion' Film Inspires High School Football Star to Reject Scholarship," *ABC News*, February 3, 2016, accessed March 19, 2019, http://abcnews.go.com/US/high-school-football-star-rejects-full-scholarships-amid/story?id=36692778; Garrison Pennington, "Quitting the Gridiron When Football Runs Through the Family," *NPR*, February 4, 2016, accessed March 19, 2019, http://www.npr.org/2016/02/04/465421757/quitting-the-gridiron-when-football-runs-through-the-family.

108. *New York Daily News*, January 30, 2016; Nathaniel Vinton, "Concussions Are on the Rise in the NFL," *New York Daily News*, January 30, 2016, accessed March 19, 2019, http://www.nydailynews.com/sports/football/concussions-rise-nfl-league-data-reveals-article-1.2513828.

Epilogue

1. Tod Leonard, "Mothers Take on Football, Suing Pop Warner for Sons' Head Trauma, Deaths," *San Diego Union-Tribune*, January 28, 2018, accessed March 19, 2019, http://www.sandiegouniontribune.com/sports/sd-sp-moms-sue-pop-warner-for-cte-damage-20180128-story.html.

2. Leonard, "Mothers Take on Football,"

3. Leonard, "Mothers Take on Football,"

4. Ryan Kartje. "Pop Warner Facing 2020 Trial in Lawsuit Alleging Negligence, Wrongful Death," *Orange County Register*, July 26, 2018, accessed April 13, 2019. https://www.ocregister.com/2018/07/26/pop-warner-facing-2020-trial-in-lawsuit-alleging-negligence-wrongful-death/.

5. Kathleen Bachynski, Lisa Kearns, and Art Caplan. "Football-Related Injuries Extend Far Beyond Concussions," *Stat News*, November 22, 2017, accessed March 19, 2019, https://www.statnews.com/2017/11/22/concussions-football-injuries.

6. Kathleen E. Bachynski and Daniel S. Goldberg, "Youth Sports & Public Health: Framing Risks of Mild Traumatic Brain Injury in American Football and Ice Hockey," *The Journal of Law, Medicine & Ethics* 42, no. 3 (2014): 323–33.

7. Francis Shen, "You Can Love the Brain and Football Too," *Star Tribune*, January 31, 2018, accessed March 19, 2019, http://www.startribune.com/youth-football-and-concussions-i-love-the-brain-but-think-you-can-like-football-too/472033803/.

8. Rachel Bachman, "Flag Football: The Alternative for Concerned Parents," *Wall Street Journal*, November 9, 2015, accessed March 19, 2019, https://www.wsj.com/articles/flag-football-the-alternative-for-concerned-parents-1447093342; Joe Lipovich, "Concussion Dangers: City Eliminates Tackle Football for Kids," *Somerville Patch*, December 30, 2015, accessed March 19, 2019, http://patch.com/massachusetts/somerville/concussion-dangers-prompt-city-eliminate-youth-contact-football-0.

9. Gregg Easterbrook, "Take the Tackle Out of Youth Football," *NYT*, February 9, 2016, accessed March 19, 2019, http://www.nytimes.com/2016/02/10/upshot/take-the-tackle-out-of-youth-tackle-football.html.

10. Jason Hopkins, "4 State Legislatures Look to Ban Tackle Football," *Western Journal*, February 12, 2018, accessed March 19, 2019, https://www.westernjournal.com/4-state -legislatures-look-ban-tackle-football/; "N.J. Assemblywoman Proposes Tackle Football Ban for Kids Under 12," *CBS New York*, April 4, 2018, accessed March 19, 2019, https://newyork .cbslocal.com/2018/04/04/nj-proposed-tackle-football-ban/.

11. AAP Committee on Sports Medicine and Fitness, "Safety in Youth Ice Hockey: The Effects of Body Checking," *Pediatrics* 105, no. 3 (2000): 657–58; AAP Committee on Sports Medicine and Fitness, "Reducing Injury Risk from Body Checking in Boys' Youth Ice Hockey," *Pediatrics* 133, no. 6 (2014): 1151–57. Ben Strauss, "U.S. Soccer, Resolving Lawsuit, Will Limit Headers for Youth Players," *NYT*, November 9, 2015, accessed March 19, 2019, http://www.nytimes.com/2015/11/10/sports/soccer/us-soccer-resolving-lawsuit-will -limit-headers-for-youth-players.html.

12. AAP Committee on Sports Medicine and Fitness, "Tackling in Youth Football," *Pediatrics* 136, no. 5 (2015): e1419–e1430; Kathleen E. Bachynski, "Tolerable Risks? Physicians and Youth Tackle Football," *New England Journal of Medicine* 374 (2016): 405–7; Ron White, "Ban Youth Tackle Football in Kern County? Not So Fast," *Bakersfield Californian*, February 15, 2016, accessed March 19, 2019, http://www.bakersfield.com/news/opinion/2016/02 /15/ban-youth-tackle-football-in-kern-county-not-so-fast-1.html. White was responding to an op-ed by a former football player arguing that children should not begin tackling until age thirteen due to the risks of long-term brain disease. Clay Farr, "Ban Youth Tackle Football and Keep Our Kids CTE-Free," *Bakersfield Californian*, February 10, 2016, accessed March 19, 2019, http://www.bakersfield.com/news/opinion/2016/02/10/ban-youth-tackle -football-and-keep-our-kids-cte-free.html.

13. Ken Belson, "Football's True Believers Circle the Wagons and Insist the Sport Is Just Fine," *NYT*, January 30, 2018, accessed March 19, 2019, https://www.nytimes.com/2018/01 /30/sports/football/nfl.html.

14. Pamela E. Pennock, *Advertising Sin and Sickness: The Politics of Alcohol and Tobacco Marketing, 1950–1960* (DeKalb: Northern Illinois University Press, 2007).

15. Gerald Markowitz and David Rosner, *Lead Wars: The Politics of Science and the Fate of America's Children* (Berkeley: University of California/Milbank Fund, 2013), 228; Richard C. Schneider, *Head and Neck Injuries in Football: Mechanisms, Treatment and Prevention* (Baltimore: Williams & Wilkins, 1973), vii.

16. Steve Almond, *Against Football: One Fan's Reluctant Manifesto* (Brooklyn, NY: Melvin House Publishing, 2014), 31.

17. Markowitz and Rosner, *Lead Wars*, 216.

18. Eva Holland, "Why We Play: Doing What We Love, Despite the Risks," *SB Nation*, June 25, 2014, accessed March 19, 2019, http://www.sbnation.com/longform/2014/6/25 /5838366/why-we-play-doing-what-we-love-despite-the-risks.

19. Kern Tips, *Football Texas Style: An Illustrated History of the Southwest Conference* (New York: Doubleday, 1954): 267.

Index

Note: Figures and tables are indicated by page numbers in *italics*.

Studies in Social Medicine

Nancy M. P. King, Gail E. Henderson, and Jane Stein, eds., *Beyond Regulations: Ethics in Human Subjects Research* (1999).

Laurie Zoloth, *Health Care and the Ethics of Encounter: A Jewish Discussion of Social Justice* (1999).

Susan M. Reverby, ed., *Tuskegee's Truths: Rethinking the Tuskegee Syphilis Study* (2000).

Beatrix Hoffman, *The Wages of Sickness: The Politics of Health Insurance in Progressive America* (2000).

Margarete Sandelowski, *Devices and Desires: Gender, Technology, and American Nursing* (2000).

Keith Wailoo, *Dying in the City of the Blues: Sickle Cell Anemia and the Politics of Race and Health* (2001).

Judith Andre, *Bioethics as Practice* (2002).

Chris Feudtner, *Bittersweet: Diabetes, Insulin, and the Transformation of Illness* (2003).

Ann Folwell Stanford, *Bodies in a Broken World: Women Novelists of Color and the Politics of Medicine* (2003).

Lawrence O. Gostin, *The AIDS Pandemic: Complacency, Injustice, and Unfulfilled Expectations* (2004).

Arthur A. Daemmrich, *Pharmacopolitics: Drug Regulation in the United States and Germany* (2004).

Carl Elliott and Tod Chambers, eds., *Prozac as a Way of Life* (2004).

Steven M. Stowe, *Doctoring the South: Southern Physicians and Everyday Medicine in the Mid-Nineteenth Century* (2004).

Arleen Marcia Tuchman, *Science Has No Sex: The Life of Marie Zakrzewska, M.D.* (2006).

Michael H. Cohen, *Healing at the Borderland of Medicine and Religion* (2006).

Keith Wailoo, Julie Livingston, and Peter Guarnaccia, eds., *A Death Retold: Jesica Santillan, the Bungled Transplant, and Paradoxes of Medical Citizenship* (2006).

Michelle T. Moran, *Colonizing Leprosy: Imperialism and the Politics of Public Health in the United States* (2007).

Karey Harwood, *The Infertility Treadmill: Feminist Ethics, Personal Choice, and the Use of Reproductive Technologies* (2007).

Carla Bittel, *Mary Putnam Jacobi and the Politics of Medicine in Nineteenth-Century America* (2009).

Samuel Kelton Roberts Jr., *Infectious Fear: Politics, Disease, and the Health Effects of Segregation* (2009).

Lois Shepherd, *If That Ever Happens to Me: Making Life and Death Decisions after Terri Schiavo* (2009).

Mical Raz, *What's Wrong with the Poor? Psychiatry, Race, and the War on Poverty* (2013).

Johanna Schoen, *Abortion after Roe* (2015).

Nancy Tomes, *Remaking the American Patient: How Madison Avenue and Modern Medicine Turned Patients into Consumers* (2016).

Mara Buchbinder, Michele Rivkin-Fish, and Rebecca L. Walker, eds., *Understanding Health Inequalities and Justice: New Conversations across the Disciplines* (2016).

Muriel R. Gillick, *Old and Sick in America: The Journey through the Health Care System* (2017).

Michael E. Staub, *The Mismeasure of Minds: Debating Race and Intelligence between* Brown *and "The Bell Curve"* (2018).

Mari Armstrong-Hough, *Biomedicalization and the Practice of Culture: Globalization and Type 2 Diabetes in the United States and Japan* (2018).

Kathleen Bachynski, *No Game for Boys to Play: The History of Youth Football and the Origins of a Public Health Crisis* (2019).